Biological and Clinical Aspects of
THE FETUS

Edited by

YUKIO NOTAKE, M. D.

Former Professor and Chairman, Department of Obstetrics
and Gynecology, School of Medicine, Keio University, Tokyo;
Visiting Director, The Kitasato Institute, Tokyo

and

SHUETU SUZUKI, M. D.

Associate Professor, Department of Obstetrics
and Gynecology, School of Medicine,
Keio University, Tokyo

UNIVERSITY PARK PRESS
BALTIMORE   AND   LONDON
IGAKU SHOIN LTD. TOKYO

Library of Congress Cataloging in Publication Data

Main entry under title:
Biological and clinical aspects of the fetus.

    Includes index.
    1. Fetus—Growth.   2. Maternal-fetal exchange.
    3. Prenatal diagnosis.   I. Notake, Yukio, 1908–
    II. Suzuki, Shuetu. [DNLM: 1. Embryo. 2. Fetus.
    3. Growth.   4. Maternal-fetal exchange.   5. Placental
    function texts. 6. Prenatal diagnosis. WQ205 B616]
    RG600. B48   1976   612.6'47   76-57177
    ISBN 0–8391–0986–5

PUBLISHERS
© First Edition, 1977 by IGAKU SHOIN LTD., 5-24-3 Hongo, Bunkyo-ku, Tokyo.
    Sole distribution rights in the United States of America, the Dominion of Canada and Latin
America granted to
UNIVERSITY PARK PRESS: Chamber of Commerce Building Baltimore, Maryland 21202.

Printed in Japan. Composed and printed by Gakujutsu Tosho Printing Co., Ltd., Tokyo and bound by Kojima Binding Co., Ltd., Tokyo. The photographic engravings for the illustrations were made by Gakujutsu Photoengraving Co., Ltd., Tokyo.

Preface

During the past decade there have been tremendous progresses in the field of human reproduction and a rapid expansion of our knowledge relevelant to such important areas as fertilization, implantation, fetal development, materno-fetal interrelationship and placentation has been obtained. However, most of accumulating informations in these basic concepts have been come from anatomists, biologists and other basic scientists and it is quite recent that the data have become possible to apply to clinical medicine for preventive and therapeutic purposes. Therefore, it is still needed newer approaches to clarify the process leading to embryonal, fetal and neonatal medicine.

Contributors in this monograph have engaged in both basic and clinical research and are experts in the practical application of basic knowledge to clinical problems—vice versa—through their daily clinical working they have a lot of chances to spread ideas beyond the clinical level.

In the first paper, the morphology and physiology of the early mammalian embryos were reported and in the second article fetal growth in relation to the intrauterine environment, primarily, placental transfer was discussed. The following three papers dealt with the dynamic relationship of the morphological and biochemical changes between the feto-maternal functions. In two articles on diagnostic procedures, sonar method and amniocentesis were introduced and as another interesting paper, normal and abnormal human developments in the early prenatal stage were described with excellent survey on fascinating materials.

Although we would not say this book could cover all the boundaries of fetal medicine, but we believe this small monograph will give extensive contributions for clinicians and researchers at this moment.

Yukio NOTAKE, M.D.

Contributors

Erika M. BÜHLER, M.D.
Department of Genetics, Basle University Children's Hospital, Basle

Yasuo HAMADA, M.D.
Department of Obstetrics and Gynecology, School of Medicine, Keio University, Tokyo

Masato INOUE, M.D.
Department of Obstetrics and Gynecology, School of Medicine, Tokai University, Isehara, Kanagawa

Koichi ITAKURA, M.D.
Department of Obstetrics and Gynecology, School of Medicine, Keio University, Tokyo

Mitsunao KOBAYASHI, M.D.
Associate Professor, Department of Obstetrics and Gynecology, National Defense Medical College, Tokorozawa, Saitama

Tetsuya NAKAYAMA, M.D.
Professor, Department of Obstetrics and Gynecology, School of Medicine, Showa University, Tokyo

Yukio NOTAKE, M.D.
Former Professor, Department of Obstetrics and Gynecology, School of Medicine, Keio University, Tokyo; Visiting Director, The Kitasato Institute, Tokyo

Kenichi SEKI, M.D.
Department of Obstetrics and Gynecology School of Medicine, Keio University, Tokyo

Hiroaki SOMA, M.D.
Professor, Department of Obstetrics and Gynecology, Tokyo Medical College, Tokyo

Kotaro SUZUKI, M.D., Ph. D.
Assistant Professor, Department of Obstetrics and Gynecology, Harvard Medical School, Beth Israel Hospital, Boston, Massachusetts
Present Address: Chief, Department of Obstetrics and Gynecology, Boston City Hospital, Boston, Massachusetts

Shuetu SUZUKI, M.D.
Associate Professor, Department of Obstetrics and Gynecology, School of Medicine, Keio University, Tokyo

Shigeo TAKAGI, M.D.
Professor, Department of Obstetrics and Gynecology, School of Medicine, Nihon University, Tokyo

Takashi TANIMURA, M.D.
Associate Professor, Department of Anatomy, Faculty of Medicine, Kyoto University, Kyoto

Ryutaro TOJO, M.D.
Department of Obstetrics and Gynecology, School of Medicine, Keio University, Tokyo

Katsuo TSUBATA, M.D.

Assistant Professor, Department of Obstetrics and Gynecology, School of Medicine, Nihon University, Tokyo

Taiso TSUCHIMOTO, M.D.

Department of Genetics, Basle University Children's Hospital, Basle
Present Address: Sandoz LTD, Medical and Biological Research Division, 4002 Basle

Takao YOSHIDA, M.D.

Associate Professor, Department of Obstetrics and Gynecology, School of Medicine, Nihon University, Tokyo

Contents

Biology of the mammalian embryos in the pre-implantation stages

SHUETU SUZUKI, M.D., MASATO INOUE, M.D.,
KOICHI ITAKURA, M.D., YASUO HAMADA, M.D., KENICHI SEKI, M.D.
and RYUTARO TOJO, M.D.

Department of Obstetrics and Gynecology, School of Medicine, Keio University, Tokyo

INTRODUCTION

During the past several years, considerable attempts have been made to investigate the biology and physiology of the early mammalian embryos. Especially, the maturation process and subsequent development of oocytes have been carefully reported in several mammalian species, and the temporal relationship between maturation, ovulation and fertilization has been clarified. However, our understanding of the events which occur in the pre-implantation stages is still rather fragmentary and most of informations have been come from only several experimental animals.

We have studied on the morphological characteristics of the early mammalian embryo including the human ova by light and electron microscopies and have published several reports on the new findings in this field [1–18, 75].

In the present paper we would like to summarize the literatures mainly concerning the morphology and physiology of the early mammalian embryos introducing our recent investigations.

A BRIEF OUTLINE OF THE PROCESS OF OOGENESIS, OVULATION, FERTILIZATION AND IMPLANTATION

In the majority of mammalian species, the germ cells undergo several mitotic division during the fetal life. Consequently the female germ cells are already in the first meiotic prophase at the time of birth with the exception of the rabbit and to lesser extent the human. Immediately post partum, the oocyte nucleus passes into a resting state in late prophase. This stage is characterized by the possession of a large nucleus which appears as an empty vesicular structure being called germinal vesicle and within the nucleus the large nucleolus is floating. This stage is named dictye, dictyotene, or dictyate. Most investigators have pointed out this stage as a sequence to diplotene, but in the mouse, it is known it follows the pachytene stage. However, in the case of human, it has been clarified that the oocyte nucleus does not pass through a dictyate period and seems to be replaced by a prolongation of the deplotene stage.

The dictyate stage lasts until several hours prior to ovulation. During this nuclear resting stage, there is an increase in the follicular fluid and it is generally believed that the ovum attains its mature size at the time of antrum formation in the follicle.

Preparatory to ovulation, the follicular oocyte undergoes maturation. This involves a reduction of the chromosomal number to haploid. The nucleolus undergoes to be faded and gradually vanished, and the chromosomes condense into small, rounded bodies scattered through the nucleus. Then the nuclear membrane disappears in the cytoplasma. Diakinesis is named for the latter half of the prophase of which ending is marked by the disappearance of the nuclear membrane. The second meiotic division is arrested at metaphase and proceeds to completion only after ovulation and penetration by the spermatozoon. When the ova are shed from the ovarian follicles, they are ordinarily surrounded by a variable number of layers of granulosa cells consisting of two parts: the cumulus oophorus and the corona radiata. With time, both the corona and the cumulus become removed from the ova, which is then said to be denuded. Although the barriers interposed by the cumulus and corona are formidable, they do not prevent the entrance of sperm into the ova. The passage of sperm through the zona pellucida is less well understood in mammals.

Approximately two hours after sperm penetration, the primary nucleoli make their appearance within the enlarged sperm nucleus. The male pronucleus grows at a more rapid rate than that of the female, and this differentiation is maintained even until karyogamy. It is rather difficult to differenciate between the male and female pronuclei. The zygotes of the mammals are remarkably similar in their appearance and rate of development through the various stages of cleavage and formation of the blastocyst. Cleavage consists of a succession of mitotic divisions of the zygote at specific time intervals after karyogamy.

In mammalian species the fertilized ovum is normally retained in the fallopian tube for approximately three days. Therefore it is very important to analyze the intristic factors for the early embryonic development in the fallopian tubes. The fertilized ova pass over the utero-tubal junction at the morula stage and they start to implant in the uterine endometrium. The inter-relationship between the blastocyst and the endometrium at the time of attachment and implantation is exceedingly complex and highly variable in different species (Fig. 1).

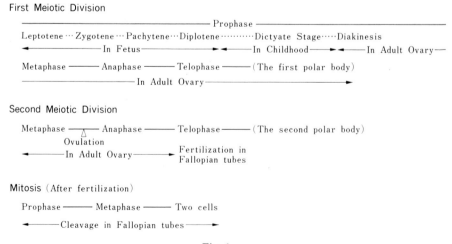

Fig. 1

THE FINE STRUCTURE OF THE HUMAN OOCYTE CULTURED IN VITRO

It is well known that mammalian oocytes reach to the prophase of the first meiotic division during embryonal life and the maturation process remain at this stage for a long period until resuming meiosis in the growing follicles prior to ovulation. On the other hand, mammalian oocytes cultured in vitro after liberation from the follicles have been reported to mature at a rate similar to that observed in the ovary after stimulation by gonadotropin. In the study of monkey follicular oocytes, although the time required for maturation through polar body extrusion was variable, after 46–48 hours in culture, postdictyate stages of meiosis were observed in 79.7 per cent and 26 of 47 ova revealed a polar body, suggesting that nuclear stages preparatory to fertilization were completed in vitro [1]. The fertilizability of such oocytes was assessed by transferring them into the fallopian tubes of inseminated recipients [3]. However, since the early studies of Rock and Menkin [19], relatively few reports on human follicular oocytes have been appeared. Edwards [20] reported that the germinal vesicle began to break down at 25 hours in culture and the great majority of human oocytes were proceeded through the first metaphase within 35 hours. Suzuki [6] cultured 84 ovarian follicular oocytes recovered from 18 patients in the medium TC 199 supplimented with 10 per cent fetal calf serum and obtained matured oocytes in the first of second metaphase after 46–48 hours in culture.

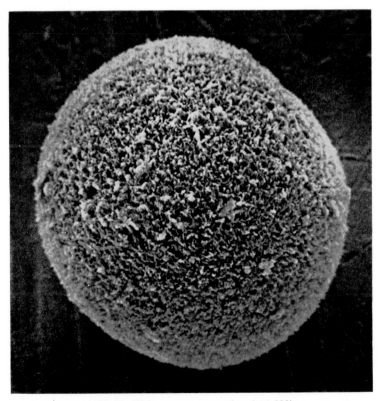

Fig. 2 Human oocyte-zona-free (×1,600).

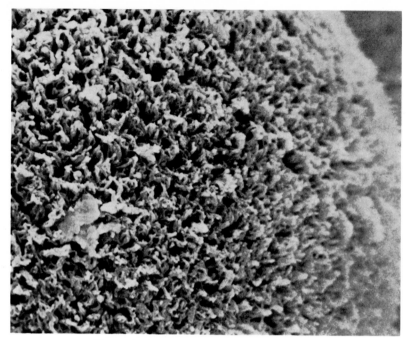

Fig. 3 High magnification of Fig. 2 (×4,200).

Although several electron microscopic studies on the human oocyte have been reported, there have been few reports on the cultured human oocytes observed by both scanning and transmission electron microscopies [14, 15, 18].

The whole ovary or a wedge of ovarian tissue was excised from the patients who were laparotomized for elective gynecological surgery. Immediately after excision, the ovarian tissue was washed in warmed tissue culture medium and placed in a sterile watch glass containing medium. The comparatively large follicles were dissected out intact and punctured to liberate the oocytes under dissecting microscope (10–30×). Oocytes which were devoid of granulosa cells believed to be recovered from atretic follicles, were discarded. Representative oocytes from each ovarian tissue were examined at the time of recovery as whole mounts under the phase contrast microscope and stained for detailed examination after fixation. The remainders, in cumulus, were transferred to depression slides containing medium Ham F-12 supplemented with 3mg/ml bovine serum albumin. After collection the depression slides were gently agitated and the medium was changed 3 times because of removal of debris in medium. By gently moving the slide, the ova were brought together and 2 or 3 oocytes were transferred in small drops of culture medium under light weight paraffin oil in a plastic culture dish (Falcon Plastics; 35×10 mm). The oil was first mixed with sterile culture medium in a ratio of 20 to 1, and the mixture was equilibrated with 5 per cent carbon dioxide in air before use. The dish was gassed with 5 per cent carbon dioxide in air in an incubator at 37°C. Randomly selected groups of oocytes were placed in the center of 4 petroleum jelly spots on a slide, and the coverslip placed over each oocyte, gently depressed until the structure within the oocyte were clearly visible under the phase contrast microscope. Throughout these experiments aseptic procedures were followed at all times, and all glassware was sterilized and warmed before and during use.

For transmission electron microscopy, oocytes were fixed at a temperature of 4°C for two hours in fresh phosphate buffered 2.5 per cent glutaraldehyde, then placed overnight

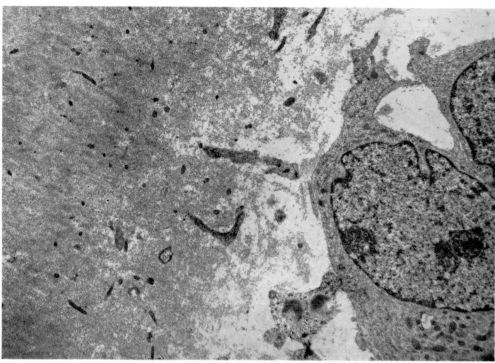

Fig. 4 A human oocyte recovered from the follicle. Granulosa cells are sticking around the zona pellucida (× 7,500).

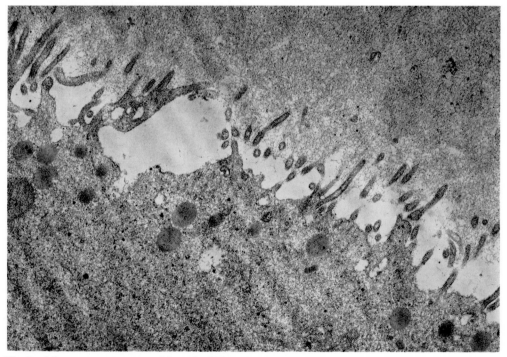

Fig. 5 A human oocyte recovered from the follicle. Cortical granules can be seen under beneath the vitelline membrane (× 8,400).

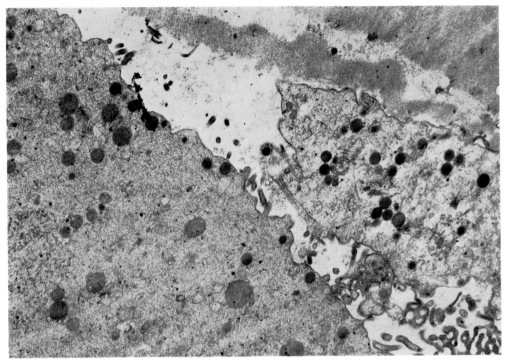

Fig. 6 A human oocyte cultured in vitro for 48 hours. The first polar body can be seen in the peri-vitelline space ($\times$ 8,400).

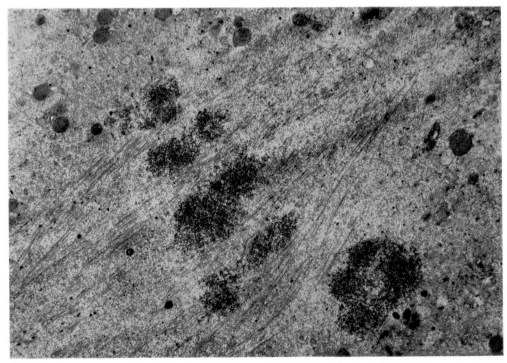

Fig. 7 A human oocyte cultured in vitro for 48 hours. Spindle formation and chromosomes can be seen in the cytoplasm ($\times$ 8,400).

in the buffer and postfixed at 4°C for one hour in 1 per cent osmium tetroxide. After fixation, oocytes were embedded in 5 per cent solid agar that was previously fixed in 2.5 per cent glutaraldehyde and trimmed about 3mm cube in order to handle easily. Then the specimens were rapidly dehydrated in graded series of ethanol, and 100 per cent aceton, infiltrated with a 4 : 6 mixture of Epon 812. The samples were trimmed, sectioned and then stained with methylene blue for the purpose of orientation. The thin section for electron microscopy were doubly stained with uranyl acetate and lead citrate. The observation was performed by HU-11-B with an accelerating voltage of 50 and 75KV.

For scanning electron microscopy, before or after fixation in glutaraldehyde, surrounding cumulus masses and zona pellucida were removed enzymatically with pronase or manually. Fixation was performed as same method as transmission electron microscopy, dehydrated in graded series of ethanol and replaced into 100 per cent amyl acetate. After mounting the samples on about 0.5 mm square slide glass from amyl acetate, critical point drying was performed. Specimen was placed on the supporter and coated with carbon and gold in the thickness of about 400Å. Observation and photography were made with JSM S-1 with an accelerating voltage of 10KV.

At the time of recovery, the follicular oocyte is normally surrounded by granulosa cells in thick layers. However, after culture in vitro for several hours, most of granulosa cells are dispersed in the culture medium. The processes of granulosa cell traverse the zona pellucida and reach until the vitelline membrane. As numerous microvilli exist at the termination, functional relationship between oocyte and granulosa cell during the maturation process could be imagined. In the postovulatory or fertilized oocyte the processes might be retracted from the zona pellucida.

The oocyte is completely enveloped by the zona pellucida which is a elastic membrane consisting of mucoprotein.

The nucleus of oocyte is relatively large and the nuclear membrane consists of two leaflets. The process of germinal vesicle breakdown in the cultured oocyte is seen to occur through fragmentation of both inner and outer leaflets and form numerous irregular gaps all over the nucleal surface. In the mouse, a sequence of germinal vesicle breakdown has been reported to take approximately 3.5 hours in vitro and in the human oocyte, within 25 hours.

In the matured oocyte, the polar body is expelled into the peri-vitelline space and the second meiotic spindle and chromosomes could be visible in the ooplasm.

The cytoplasmic organizations in the polar body are found to be similar to the oocyte matured in vivo. Numerous electron dense cortical granules are contained in the first polar body.

According to INGRAM [21], the oocyte which undergo atretic changes would go through the normal maturation stages including germinal vesicle breakdown and polar body formation before disintegrating. Therefore, the existing of the first polar body could not be proved to be a sign of normal maturation.

On the surface of the follicular oocyte microvilli distribute regularly but on the cultured oocyte they distribute unevenly. In the matured human oocyte, they become scarse in distribution and short in length. They vary in arrangements, but have always constant diameter. In the present study, clearly arbolizating microvilli were observed by both transmission and scanning electron microscopies.

BACA and ZAMBONI [22] reported that the mitochondria in the follicular oocyte had low electron opaque matrix and a few cristae which were oriented in an arch-like pattern were existed. They distributed all through the ooplasm and remarkably increased in the matured oocyte. In our study, the same observation was obtained and a lot of dumb-bell shaped mitochondria were seen in the matured oocyte. It might be suspected that in order to maintain a constant number of mitochondria in the ooplasm, their duplications has to precede the polar body extrusion. ZAMBONI and MASTROIANNI [23] found that the endoplasmic reticulum was closely associated with the mitochondria in the rabbit oocytes. This relationship had been observed also in the human oocyte [24]. Many investigators reported that the golgi complex of the quiescent oocyte were located closely to the nucleus and migrated to the cortex in the later stage. In the cultured human oocyte they could not be found so prominent as the follicular oocyte [25]. In our study, these structures were observed throughout the ooplasm. Cortical granules have been observed in various mammalian oocyte. It is said to be produced by golgi complex and migrate to beneath the plasma membrane. In the dictyate stage, they are rare but increase in numbers when the oocytes grow to mature. Sometimes, they make arrangement in multiple layers. The role of cortical granules has been suggested to be a block for polyspermy. MERCHANT and CHANG [26] observed these granules in the aged mouse tubal ova recovered 26 hours after HCG administration. On the basis of these observations it can easily be understood that the oocyte continue to produce cortical granules. ZAMBONI et al. [25] reported that prominent tubular aggregates surrounded by a peripheral corona of mitochondria occupied large parts of ooplasm irrespective of their stage of maturation. The role of these structures is not yet elucidated but they probably show some contribution for the maturation process. Annulate lamellae could not be found in the present study. ZAMBONI et al. [25] reported they presented in the meiotically inactive oocyte or in the degenerating oocyte. They stated that probably they might be a sign of atretic degeneration.

The cytoplasmic changes reported by ITAKURA [10] in the rabbit tubal aged ova were vesicular elements in the perivitelline space, vacuolae inter-mitochondriales, the disappearance of the regular microvilli and the decrease of cortical granules.

Recently, several trials have been reported on the in vitro fertilization of the human follicular ova cultured in vitro and claimed to be successful in fertilization and normal cleavage. These kinds of experiments are very important for clarifying the mechanism of the human reproduction, but still many problems should be resolved prior to the clinical application. Furthermore, the aging process of the human oocyte in the fallopian tube has not been clearly understood.

THE FINE STRUCTURE OF THE MAMMALIAN
BLASTOCYST IN THE PRE-IMPLANTATION STAGES

On the biology of the early mammalian embryos in the pre-implantation stages, numerous studies have been reported in the past decade. Electron microscopic observations on the pre-implantation embryos have been made in the rabbit [27–29], deer mouse, hamster, guinea pig and mink [30], armadillo [31, 32] and rat [36]. However, it has not been fully made to clarify the morphology of the blastocyst prior to or after implantation.

In recent years, the scanning electron microscopes have been widely applied in the biomedical fields and this new technique has deeply contributed for the understanding of the details of cellular surface topography, whereas there are few studies on mammalian ova [37–41].

The zona pellucida is composed of fine granules and tended to thin during blastocyst expansion. Throughout blastocyst stages, the zona is loosely associated with the trophoblast cells. The trophoblast cells form a single continuous layer of low cuboidal cells lining the

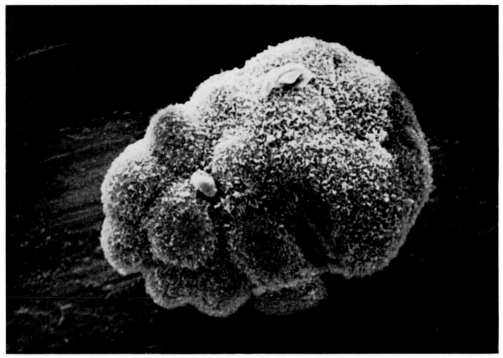

Fig. 8   Scanning micrography of a zona-free rat blastocyst ($\times$ 3,300).

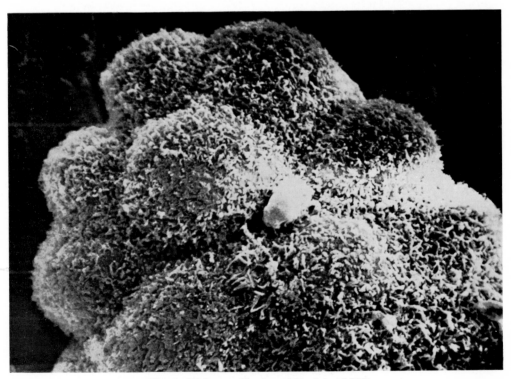

Fig. 9   High magnification of Fig. 8 ($\times$ 6,000).

zona and have a basal surface facing either on the cavity of the blastocyst or on the inner cell mass. Electron micrographs reveal relatively short, uniform microvilli which irregularly distribute and are formed by the cell membrane overlying the apical surface of the trophoblast cells. The trophoblast cells are united at their lateral borders by junctional complexes which consist of a region of close apposition and fusion of the cell membrane. Beneath the junctional complex, desmosomes are occasionally found. The basal surface of the trophoblast is formed by irregular projections of cytoplasm rather than microvilli. The organelles are found principally in the dense regions of cytoplasm, usually in a juxtanuclear and peripheral position. The presence of extensive inner cell mass cells is similar to that of other inner cell mass cells. The mitochondria with lamelliform cristae are numerous and the tuberous endoplasmic reticulum with associated ribosomes are common. The features of the nuclei in the inner cell mass cells are also similar to those in the trophoblast cells.

By the scanning electron microscopy, most of the blastocytes are spherical or elliptical in shape. The surface of the zona pellucida is rather rough and numerous minor cavities are observed. The blastocysts treated with pronase show the outer surface of trophoblast cells with numerous convexities corresponding to microvilli. The intercellular borders are not rather distinct but each trophoblast cell is bounded by grooves. In other experiment using rabbit blastocyst, the inner surface of the trophoblast is somewhat smooth with regular lining of cells like paving-stones and the individual cell has a large nucleus in the middle and several nucleoli. The proliferation and bulging of cells is distinct and no microvilli is seen on the surface of the inner cell mass.

At the blastomere stage of rabbit, the cytoplasmatically dense inner cell mass becomes distinguish from a less dense trophoblast cells. On day 4, the both cells have the same density, while on day 5–6, this difference is reversed [29]. The density is mainly due to not only the differences in the cytoplasmic ground-substance, but also the number of ribosomes in the cell.

In our data, the difference in density of both cells was not distinct and the distribution and structure of organelles were similar in both cells. However, it was observed that the characteristics of the inner cell were loose organization with numerous intercellular spaces which apparently communicated.

Changes in the cellular junction are interesting problem. At the first cleavage, the association of the two cells is rather loose, but in order to form blastocyst it is necessary to form tight junctional complexes around the border of the trophoblast cell [42]. In fact, the tight junctional complexes between trophoblast cells were observed in our results while the association of inner cell mass was loose. Since desmosomal structure becomes more common in the inner cell mass during the pre-implantation period, the tight junction would be supposed to be formed after implantation.

The organelles of the blastocysts are quite specific. Polyribosomes are considerably abundant, especially in the morula and early blastocyst stage. Granular endoplasmic reticulum appears in the later cleavage stages, but is sparse in the early blastocyst stage. ZAMBONI and MASTROIANNI [23] and KRAUSKOPF [43] found that the endoplasmic reticulum was closely associated with the mitochondria in the rabbit oocytes and blastomeres.

Although inclusions restricted to the blastocyst stage are less common, crystal-like inclusions have previously been seen in the trophoblast of other species besides the rabbit [28], such as in the mouse blastocyst [30], in the binucleate cell of early sheep blastocyst [44] and in the syncytial trophoblast of the implanting blastocyst of the bat [45]. The crystall-like inclusions in the rabbit blastocyst may represent a storage organelle for material synthesized by the trophoblast during development [46].

The ultrastructure of the zona surface is indistinguishable from that at earlier stages studied. Moreover, in order to delay or hasten the shedding by various hormonal conditions, the zona surface in the mouse remained unchanged [38].

An abembryonic shedding has been reported to prevail in the rat blastocyst [47, 48]. However, our data could not confirm the same findings. In the zona-free rat blastocyst, two types: blastocyts with and without abembryonic proliferation were observed in normal pregnancy. Abembryonic proliferation could be provoked by estrogen in ovariectomized animals [38]. POTTS and PSYCHOYOS [49] reported that microvilli are absent from the trophoblast surface but this is not correct as mentioned previously by BERGSTROM [38]. Our data also show numerous microvilli on the apical surface of trophoblast cells.

Ultrastructural studies including radioautography are much available on the morphology and function of mammalian ova. In particular, quantitative analysis in studies of blastocyst and endometrium will be worthwhile to be investigated for the more detailed information on the mechanism of implantation. Futhermore, in association with the functional aspects, interesting subjects, such as the initiation of the differenciation between trophoblast cells and inner cell mass cells and the timing of hormone production, remain as further investigations.

THE ULTRASTRUCTURAL OBSERVATIONS
ON THE AGED OVA

In mammals of most species, coitus is restricted to a relatively short time in the cycle when ripe follicles are present in the ovaries and the animal comes into estrus. Since spermatozoa and ova have only a brief of several after liberation, the relationship of this receptive phase to the time of ovulation is extremely important. In a wide variety of animals, anomalies in early stages of development and increased embryonic mortality were observed following aging of the gametes.

Recently FUGO and BUTCHER [50] reported that delayed ovulation of the ripening rat ova for two days by pentobarbital administrations showed an increase of developmental abnormalities. Similar studies on delayed insemination had been reported in the guinea pig [51, 52], rat [53, 54], rabbit [55, 56], and hamster [57]. WITSHI and LAGUENS [58] concluded that aged ova were an important cause of chromosomal nondisjunction during both meiosis and mitosis.

Even though there have been clarified the effects of aged ova on both mortality and anomalies in early stages of development among the offspring in a wide variety of animals, only a few papers have been reported about the fine structural changes occurring in the aging process of ova.

BACA and ZAMBONI [22] and ZAMBONI [59] observed double membrane vesicles in the perivitelline space in the human and mouse ova. They interpret these structures as "cell debris". On the other hand, HADEK [60] reported the presence of "segrosomes" in the perivitelline space of tubal ova in the hamster and rabbit. He suggested that they were formed by the association of multivesicular and foreign bodies which subsequently became surrounded by thin membranes originating from the vitelline surface.

Cortical granules have been observed in the growing oocytes and tubal ova of as diverse mammals as rabbits, guinea pigs, coypus, rats, mice, domestic pigs and rhesus monkeys. The disappearance of mammalian cortical granules following sperm penetration was thought to trigger the "zona reaction" through the release of a chemical that made the zona impermeable to succeeding sperm [61]. Other investigators have reported that cortical granules in mammals play an active role in the fertilization reaction. It is assumed that at the time of sperm penetration cortical granules become lodged in the perivitelline area, and after dissolution their membrane joins the disrupted cell membrane in an effort to patch up the hole caused by the penetrating sperm.

In several aged mouse ova fixed 16 hours after HCG injection, MERCHANT and CHANG [26] observed a considerable decrease in the number of cortical granules and evidence of extrusion of their contents into the peri-vitelline space. Our study also showed an obvious decrease in the number of them and their movement to the center of cytoplasm. In the aged hamster ova, YANAGIMACHI and CHANG [62] reported a release of the PAS-positive contents of the cortical granules. However, HADEK [63] found an accumulation of cortical granules in the aged rabbit ova recovered 60 hours after coitus. MERCHANT and CHANG [26] observed the accumulation of cortical granules in some regions near the vesicular aggregates and the presence of granular materials in the perivitelline space of tubal ova fixed 26 hours after the administration of human chorionic gonadotropin. This suggests that if the ova were not fertilized, the formation of cortical granules would be a continuous process.

Other morphological changes are loss of microvilli, and a high concentration of lamellae, vesicular elements and granular materials in the perivitelline space.

KONDO [64] reported that the ova recovered from the oviducts six or more hours after the expected ovulation, most of granulosa cells had been already denuded and it had been observed that diminishing fertility occurred when the corona radiata cells partially or completely separated from the ova. It has been demonstrated that ovulation without fertilization is followed by rapid degeneration and fragmentation of the vitellus. However, the subject of the final fate of the degenerated ova and the processes of the loss of fertility of these aged ova have not been sufficiently resolved for any mammals except the rat. When the aged ova were fertilized, it appeared occasionally that the cytoplasma of the fertilized ova had been degenerated or fragmented, while the zona pellucida was still kept in normal condition. The loss of fertility in the rabbit ova might be likely related to changes in the cytoplasma or cytoplasmic membrane of the vitellus which occur before the zona pellucida loses its physiological intergrity for sperm penetration.

Developmental defects which result from the overripening or aging of gametes before fertilization have been studied in great detail in a wide variety of animals and it has been demonstrated that when aged ova are fertilized, an increase in abnormalities and fetal loss has geen found.

BLANDAU [65] reported that even though 70 per cent of the greatly overriped rat ova might be penetrated by spermatozoa, various abnormalities of development resulted which were compatible with continued growth and development. Thus at the time of implantation only 4 per cent of the experimental rats were impregnated and the ova which did implant successfully were retarded in their development, and the majority died before the fetal period was reached.

It is considered that there may exist some biological differences between the overripeness and aging of the ova. BEATTY [66, 79] reported that delayed fertilization leading to ovum aging was one means of inducing suppression of the second polar body, polyspermy and fragmentation of the nucleus and blastomeres and these resulted in polyploidy. Recently SCHAVER and CARR [67] reported that triploidy was the commonest anomaly and was found in six instances from rabbits mated 8 and 9 hours after injection of gonadotropin.

Although the fine morphological changes of the aging rabbit tubal ova have been demonstrated in the present study, it is not yet clear what mechanism brings about the congenital anomalies caused by the aging ova. This problem is worthy of continued attention in the future, through the study of more biochemical method.

METABOLIC CHANGES IN THE PRE-IMPLANTATION
EMBRYOS

In the mouse embryo, it has been shown that there is a sharp increase in the synthesis of both RNA and protein in the morula and the rate continues to accelerate to the blastocyst stage. In the rat, polyribosomes appear at the eight cell stage and are a conspicuous component of the cytoplasm in the early blastocyst [42].

LOBEL et al. [68] showed that the uptake of ^{3}H-thymidine by rat blastocyst was observed in the early morning of day 5 of pregnancy. At this time the blastocyst was still enclosed with the zona pellucida. SYNYAL and MEYER [69] also reported the nuclei of blastocysts on day 5 showed active DNA synthesis in vitro and there was no significant difference between blastocysts with or without zona pellucida with respect to the total numbered nuclei and number of nuclei incorporated. Recently, MOHLA et al. [70] observed that the synthesis of DNA, RNA and protein in the rat blastocyst were evident on day 4 when the zona pellucida was still intact and concluded that the presence of the zona did not interfere with the incorporation of the precursors.

Our data showed that the pre-implantation blastocyst of the rat synthesized DNA, RNA and protein utilizing exogenous ^{3}H-thymidine, ^{3}H-uridine and ^{3}H-phenylalanine. Synthetic activity in the blastocysts was evident when the zona pellucida was still intact. In the delayed blastocyst, our results showed that moderate RNA and protein synthesis with minimal DNA synthesis were observed. PRASAD et al. [71] showed that in the delayed blastocyst minimal RNA synthesis could be found, but DNA and protein synthesis were not observed. Estrogen enhanced the synthesis of RNA, DNA and protein in the delayed blastocyst. It had been reported that the delayed blastocysts remained in a domant state without any appreciable increase in the number of cells and mitotic activity in the inner cell mass was completely inhibited. SANYAL et al. [72] showed that during delayed implantation the blastocysts had nuclei progressively increased in number and the number incorporated with ^{3}H-thymidine in vivo and in vitro declined as the period of delay was extended and estrogen administered thirty hours before autopsy markedly enhanced DNA synthesis both in vivo and in vitro. JACOBSON et al. [73] reported that the administration of subimplantation does of estrogen had no effect on the percentage of nuclei incorporated with ^{3}H-thymidine in vitro and the total number of nuclei in the blastocysts during delayed implantation. In our experiment, occasional mitosis were seen in the inner cell mass of the delayed blastocysts. Estrogen enhanced the synthesis of DNA, RNA and protein in the delayed blastocyst; forty-two hours after estrogen treatment, significant DNA synthesis was seen in the inner cell mass and RNA and protein synthesis were enhanced considerably eighteen hours after estrogen administration. DASS et al. [74] reported that estrogen treatment enhanced the synthesis of RNA in the delayed blastocyst and this was maintained up to eighteen hours. Estrogen also increased DNA synthesis in the delayed blastocyst by forty-two hours.

PRASAD et al. [71] studied the action of estrogen on the blastocyst and uterus in delayed implantation. They showed that minimal RNA and protein synthesis occurred in the uterus during delayed implantation, but eighteen hours after estrogen treatment, RNA and protein synthesis were considerably enhanced, while DNA synthesis was not observed in the uterus either during delayed implantation of forty-two hours after estrogen administration. DASS et al. [74] studied the time sequence of action of estrogen and concluded that estrogen had a differential time sequence of action on the uterus and blastocyst and that activation of the delayed blastocyst might be due to a direct action of estrogen on it. The implantation response was significantly higher when blastocysts treated with 10^{-8}M estradiol were transferred to foster mothers than in the case of untreated control blastocysts. She studied the incorporation of ^{3}H-estradiol by the blastocysts cultured in vitro and concluded that there was a direct relationship between the action of estradiol on the blastocyst and implantation.

The mechanism by which estrogen initiates implantation of blastocyst has not been fully investigated. However, it has been suggested that RNA synthesized under the influence of estrogen may mediate the necessary requirement for further cell differentiation of the blastocyst and invasion of the endometrium by the trophoblast cells.

Quantitative analysis of the precursors incorporated into the blastocyst and endometrial tissues in the normal pre-implantation stages and during delayed implantation will be worthy while to be investigated for the more detailed informations on the mechanism of implantation.

REFERENCES

1. SUZUKI, S. and MASTOIANNI, L.: Maturation of monkey ovarian follicular oocytes in vitro. Amer. J. Obstet. Gynec. **96**; 723, 1966.
2. SUZUKI, S.: In vitro cultivation of rabbit ova following in vitro fertilization in tubal fluid. Cytologia **31**;416, 1966.
3. SUZUKI, S. and MASTROIANNI, L.: The fertilizability of in vitro cultured monkey ovarian follicular oocytes. Fertil. Steril. **19**; 500, 1968.
4. SUZUKI, S. and MASTROIANNI, L.: In vitro fertilization of rabbit follicular oocytes in tubal fluid. Fertil. Steril. **19**; 716, 1968.
5. SUZUKI, S.: In vitro cultivation of early rat embryos. Cytologia **34**; 496, 1969.
6. SUZUKI, S.: Maturation of human ovarian follicular oocytes. Experientia **26**; 640, 1970.
7. SUZUKI, S.: Capacitation of gamete and survival in the female genital tracts. Symposium at the Seventh International Congress on Fertility and Sterility, Kyoto, 1971.
8. INOUE, M.: Nucleic acids and protein synthesis in the rat embryos and uterus in the pre-implantation stages. Acta obstet. gynec. Japonica **18**; 251, 1971.
9. SUZUKI, S., INOUE, M. and HAMADA, Y.: Nucleic acid synthesis in the developing rat embryos in the pre-implantation stages. At the Fourth Annual Meeting of the Society for the Study of Reproduction, Boston, 1971.
10. ITAKURA, K.: Electron microscopic studies on the aging process in rabbit tubal ova. Acta obstet. gynec. Japonica **19**; 154, 1972.
11. SUZUKI, S., INOUE, M., MIZUMOTO, H., HAMADA, Y., MITANI, H., KAMI, K. and HAMADA, M.: Autoradiographic studies on the rat embryo, in the pre-implantation stages. Experientia **29**; 84, 1973.
12. SUZUKI, S.: An Atlas of Mammalian Ova. Igaku Shoin, Tokyo, 1973.
13. SUZUKI, S.: Oogenesis. At the Thirty-sixth Symposium of the Japanese Medical Association, Hakone, 1974.
14. SUZUKI, S.: Scanning electron microscopy of the human oocyte. Workshop at the Eighth International Congress on Fertility and Sterility, Buenos Aires, 1974.
15. SEKI, K., SUZUKI, S., TOJO, R., HAMADA, M. and FUJIWARA, T.: Electron microscopical studies on the cultured human oocytes. At the Eighth International Congress on Fertility and Sterility. Buenos Aires, 1974.
16. ITO, T., SUZUKI, S., HAMADA, M. and FUJIWARA, T.: Scanning electron microscopic studies on pathologic conditions of human reproductive tracts. At the Eighth International Congress on Fertility and Sterility, Buenos Aires, 1974.
17. HAMADA, Y.: Electron microscopic studies on the mammalian blastocyst in the pre-implantation stages. Keio J. Med. **23**; 77, 1974.
18. SEKI, K.: Electron microscopic studies on the human follicular oocyte cultured in vitro. Keio J. Med. **25**; 22, 1975.

19. Rock, J. and Menkin, M. F.: In vitro fertilization and cleavage of human ovarian eggs. Science **100**; 105, 1944.

20. Edwards, R. G.: Maturation in vitro of human ovarian oocyte. Lancet **2**; 926, 1965.

21. Ingram, D. L.: In Ovary, Vol 1. Zuckerman, S. (ed.) Academic Press, New York, 1962, p. 247.

22. Baca, M. and Zamboni, L.: The fine structure of human follicular oocytes. J. Ultrastruct. Res. **19**; 354, 1967.

23. Zamboni, L. and Mastroianni, L.: Electron microscopic studies on rabbit ova. J. Ultrastruct. Res. **14**; 95, 1966.

24. Soupart, P. and Strong, P. A.: Ultrastructural observations on human oocytes fertilized in vitro. Fertil. Steril. **25**; 11, 1974.

25. Zamboni, L., Thompson, R. S. and Smith, D. M.: Fine morphology of human oocyte matured in vitro. Biol. Reprod. **7**; 425, 1972.

26. Merchant, H. and Chang, M. C.: An electron microscopic study of mouse eggs matured in vivo and in vitro. Anat. Rec. **171**; 21, 1971.

27. Larsen, P. F.: Electron microscopy of the implantation site of the rabbit. Am. J. Anat. **109**; 319, 1961.

28. Hadek, R. and Swift, H.: Nuclear extrusion and intracisternal inclusions in the rabbit blastocyst. J. Cell. Biol. **13**; 445, 1962.

29. Hesseldahl, H.: Ultrastructure of early cleavage stages and pre-implantation in the rabbit. Z. Anat. Entwickl-Gesch. **135**; 139, 1971.

30. Enders, A. C. and Schlatke, S. J.: The structure of the blastocyst: Some comparative studies. In: Pre-implantation Stages of Pregnancy. Wolstenholme, G. E. W. and O'Connor, M. (eds.) Churchill, London, 1965, p. 29.

31. Enders, A. C.: The structure of the armadillo blastocyst. J. Anat. **96**; 39, 1962.

32. Enders, A. C.: Electron microscopy of an early implantation stage with a postulated mechanism of implantation. Develop. Biol. **10**; 395, 1964.

33. Potts, M.: A method for locating specific histological features for electron microscopy. Jl. R. Microsc. Soc. **85**; 97, 1966.

34. Potts, M. and Wilson, I. B.: The pre-implantation comceptus of the mouse at 90 hours post coitum. J. Anat. **102**; 1, 1967.

35. Reinius, S.: Ultrastructure of blastocyst attachment in the mouce. Z. Zellforsch. **77**; 257, 1967.

36. Enders, A. C.: The uterus in delayed implantation. In: Cellular Biology of the Uterus. Wynn, R. M. (ed.), Appleton-Century-Crofts, New York, 1967, p. 151.

37. Waterman, R. E.: Use of the scanning electron microscope for observation of vertebrate embryos. Develop. Biol. **27**; 276, 1972.

38. Bergstrom, S.: Delay of blastocyst implantation in the mouse by ovariectomy or lactation. A scanning electron microscope study. Fert. Steril. **23**; 548, 1972.

39. Bergstrom, S.: Preparation of ova for scanning electron microscopy. Uppsala J. Med. Sci. **78**; 1, 1973.

40. Gould, K. G.: Preparation of mammalian gametes and reproductive tract tissues for scanning electron microscopy. Fert. Steril. **24**; 448, 1973.

41. Suzuki, S., Hamada, M., Ito, T., Seki, K. and Fujiwara, T.: Ova. Obst. and Gynec. **41**; 59, 1974. (in Japanese)

42. Schlafke, S. J. and Enders, A. C.: Cytological changes during cleavage and blastocyst formation in the rat. J. Anat. **102**; 13, 1967.

43. Krauskopf, C.: Elektronenmikroskopische Untersuchungen über die Struktur der Oozyte und des 2-Zellenstadiums beim Kaninchen. II. Blastomeren. Z. Zellforsch. **92**; 296, 1968.

44. Davies, J. and Wimsatt, W. A.: Observation on the fine structure of the sheep placenta. Acta Anat. **65**; 182, 1966.

45. Enders, A. C. and Wimsatt, W. A.: Formation and structure of the hemodichorial chorioallantoic placenta of the bat. Am. J. Anat. **122**; 453, 1968.

46. Steer, H. W.: The ultrastructure of the extraembryonic region of the preimplanted rabbit blastocyst before trophoblastic knob formation. J. Anat. **106**; 263, 1970.

47. Yasukawa, J. J. and Meyer, R. K.: Effect of progesterone and oestrone on the pre-implantation and implantation stages of embryo development in the rat. J. Reprod. Fertil. **11**; 245, 1966.

48. Kraicer, P. F.: Studies on the mechanism of nidation. XXIV. Isolation and study of intrauterine ova from the rat: technique and observation. Int. J. Fertil. **12**; 320, 1967.

49. Potts, M. and Psychoys, A.: L'ultrastructure des relations ova-endometriales au cours du retard de nidation chez la souris. C. r. hebd. Seanc. Acad. Sci. **264;** 956, 1967.

50. Fugo, N. W. and Butcher, R. L.: Ovarripeness and the mammalian ova. I. Overripeness and early embryonic development. Fert. Steril. **17;** 804, 1966.

51. Young, W. C. and Blandau, R. J.: Ovum age and the course of gestation in the guinea pig. Science **84;** 270, 1936.

52. Blandau, R, J, and Young, W. C.: The effects of delayed fertilization on the development of the guinea pig ovum. Am. J. Anat. **64;** 303, 1939.

53. Blandau, R. J. and Tordan, E. S.: The effect of delayed fertilization on the development of the rat ovum. Am. J. Anat. **68;** 275, 1941.

54. Austin, C. R. and Braden, A. W.: Polyspermy in mammals. Nature **172;** 82, 1953.

55. Hammond, J.: The fertilization of rabbit ova in relation to time. A method of controlling litter size, the duration of pregnancy and the weight of the young at birth. J. Exp. Biol. **11;** 140 1934.

56. Chang, M. C.: Fertilizability of rabbit ova and the effects of temperature in vitro on their subsequent fertilization and activation in vivo. J. Exp. Zool. **121;** 358, 1952.

57. Chang, M. C. and Fernandez-Cano, L.: Effects of delayed fertilization on the development of pronucleus and the segmentation of hamster ova. Anat. Rec. **132;** 307, 1958.

58. Witschi, E. and Laguens, R.: Chromosomal aberrations in embryos from overripe eggs. Devel. Biol. **7;** 605, 1963.

59. Zamboni, L.: Ultrastructure of mammalian oocytes and ova. Biol. Reprod. **2;** 44, 1970.

60. Hadek, R.: Mammalian Fertilization. Academic Press, New York, 1969.

61. Braden, A. W., Austin, C. R. and Dvaid, H. A.: The reaction of the zona pellucida to sperm penetration. Aust. Biol. Sci. **7;** 391, 1954.

62. Yanagimachi, R. and Chang, M. C.: Fertilizable life of golden hamster ova and their morphological changes at the time of losing fertilizability. J. Exp. Zool. **148;** 185, 1961.

63. Hadek, R.: Submicroscopic study on the sperm-induced cortical reaction in the rabbit ovum. J. Ultrastruct. Res. **9;** 99, 1963.

64. Kondo, Y.: The fertilization and implantation of the aged ovum in the rabbit. Acta Obstet Gynaec. Jap. **17;** 115, 1970.

65. Blandau, R. J.: The female factor in fertility. 1. Effects of delayed fertilization on the development of pronuclei in rat ova. Fertil. Steril. **3;** 349, 1952.

66. Beatty, R. A.: Polyploidy in Mammalian Development. Cambridge University Press, London, 1957.

67. Schaver, E. L. and Carr, D. H.: Chromosome abnormalities in rabbit blastocysts following delayed fertilization. J. Reprod. Fert. **14;** 415, 1967.

68. Lobel, B. L., Lery, E. and Shelesnyak, M. C.: Studies on the mechanism of nidation, XXXIV. Dynamics of cellular interactions during progestation and implantation in the rat. Acta Endocr. (Suppl. 123) **56;** 1, 1967.

69. Sanyal, M. K. and Meyer, R. K.: Deoxyribonucleic acid synthesis in vitro in preimplantation blastocysts of prepuberal rat ovulated with gonadotrophins. Endocrinology **85;** 585, 1969.

70. Mohla, S., Prasad, M. R. N. and Dass, C. M. S.: Nucleic acid and protein synthesis in the blastocyst and uterus during early pregnancy in the rat. Endocrinology **87;** 383, 1970.

71. Prasad, M. R. N., Dass, C. M. S. and Mohla, S.: Action of oestrogen on the blastocyst and uterus in delayed implantation: An autoradiographic study. J. Reprod. Fertil. **16;** 97, 1968.

72. Sanyal, M. K. and Meyer, R. K.: Effect of estrone on DNA synthesis in preimplantation blastocysts of gonadotrophin-treated immature rats. Endocrinology **86;** 967, 1970.

73. Jacobson, M. A., Sanyal, M. K. and Meyer, R. K.: Effect of estrone on RNA synthesis in preimplantation blastocysts of gonadotrophin-treated immature rats. Endocrinology **86;** 982, 1970.

74. Dass, C. M. S., Nigkam, S. and Prasad, M. R. N.: Time sequence of action of estrogen on nucleic acid and protein synthesis in the uterus and blastocyst during delayed implantation. Endocrinology **85;** 528, 1969.

75. Suzuki, S., Seki, K., Ito, T., Tojo, R., Hamada, M. and Fujiwara, T.: Morphological characteristics of human ova. In: Recent Advances in Human Reproduction. Campos de Paz, A., Drill, V.A., Hayashi, M., Rodrigues, W. and Schally, A.V. (eds.) Excerpta Medica, Amsterdam–Oxford, p. 275. 1976.

Fetal growth and intrauterine environment

Kotaro SUZUKI, M.D., Ph.D.

Department of Obstetrics and Gynecology, Harvard Medical School,
Beth Israel Hospital, Boston, Massachusetts

INTRODUCTION

In a strict sense of terminology fetal growth should be defined to be permanent enlargement or increase in total mass of the fetus excluding fluctuations, such as, excessive storage of fat or water. In this article, however, the definition is more conventional and is primarily meant to be an increase in anthropometric measures such as fetal weight or length. The fetal stage is generally considered to begin at around eight weeks post conception or ten weeks from the onset of the last menstrual period. By this time nearly all major structures have been formed and subsequent development consists in the growth and maturation of existing structures. Fetal growth is controlled by genetic and environmental factors. It is well known that diffrences in race, maternal stature, or sex of the fetus affect the birth weight. Abnormalities of genes or of the chromosomes are often associated with morphogenetic abnormalities and subsequent growth disturbances. For example, intrauterine growth retardation is often associated with the fetus with Down's Syndrome, 13–15 or 16–18 trisomy, or Turner's Syndrome. The environmental factor for fetal growth is mainly related to intrauterine nutrition, which, in turn, depends upon the placental transfer of various nutrients.

While the genetic factor must be considered in evaluation of fetal growth, its effect is either physiological (differences in race, fetal sex, or maternal height) or rare (fetal congenital anomalies), and always irreversible. Thus, it is less significant clinically than the intrauterine environment.

In the present article, I shall discuss fetal growth mainly in relation to the intrauterine environment, primarily, placental transfer. Clinical implications are indicated whenever appropriate. Emphasis is placed on the data derived from man, but where information is lacking or insufficient, the results of animal experiments are discussed.

NORMAL FETAL GROWTH

1. GROWTH PATTERN OF FETAL WEIGHT

The weight, length, and head circumference of the fetus grow in the fashion of sigmoid

Fetal growth curve

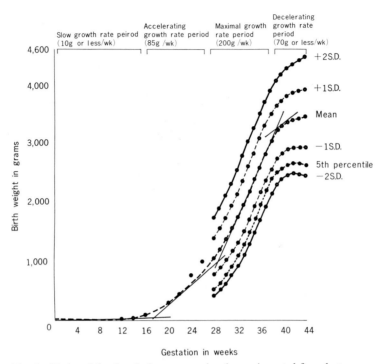

Fig. 1   Birth weights in relation to gestational ages (counted from last menstrual period). The mean growth curve can be divided into four distinct tangential lines, each depicting different growth rate. (Modified from GRUENWALD, P.: Amer. J. Obstet. Gynec. **94**; 1112, 1966, for data from 28 to 44 weeks; WALKER, J.: Cold Spring Harbor Symp. Ouant. Biol. **19**; 39, 1954 and STREETER, G.L.: Contrib. Embryol. **11**; 143, 1920 for data up to 28 weeks.)

curve as gestation advances. Fig. 1 shows changes in the fetal weight throughout human pregnancy. The fetal weight is the most sensitive indicator for abnormal growth in a sense that it is affected earlier than the length and head circumference by adverse intrauterine environment. Clinically, birth weight and gestational age have been used to define premature* or dysmature babies who are at high risk. (Dysmaturity is defined to be inappropriate maturity for gestational age, such as, abnormally light or heavy weight for length of gestation). For these reasons, the fetal weight is chosen for analysis of the fetal growth pattern. Since LUBCHENCO [2] first presented comprehensive fetal growth curve based upon liveborn birth weight data from Denver, Colorado in 1963, quite a few similar curves or figures of fetal weight as a function of gestational age have been reported from various parts of the world [3–12]. Despite the fact that the various known factors influencing the birth weight such as racial composition, socioeconomic status or altitude, to name a few, are not the same, they are quite consistent and a certain general pattern of fetal growth emerges (Fig. 1). The growth curve can be divided into four distinct tangential lines, each depicting different growth rate from preceding one, during normal pregnancy up to 42 weeks.

---

*   Premature infants have been traditionally defined to be those of birth weight of 2,500 g or less since the First World Health Assembly in 1948. Recently, however, it has been recommended by WHO that those infants with birth weight <2,500 g be called "low birth weight infants" with the implication that "prematurity" could better be defined by a gestational age of less than 37 weeks [1].

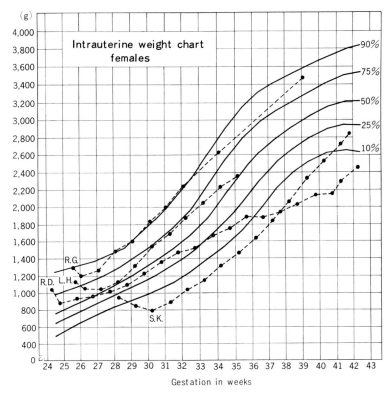

Fig. 2   Examples of the postnatal growth of selected premature infants. R.G., L.H., R.D., S.K. denote each patient. (From LUBCHENCO, L.O. et al.: Pediatrics **32**; 793, 1963.)

Slow growth rate period : This period lasts up to 15–16 weeks of gestation. The growth rate is minimal and 10 g or less per week.

Accelerating growth rate period: This period ranges from 16–17 weeks to 26–27 weeks of gestation. The growth rate accelerates to approximately 85 g per week.

Maximum growth rate period : This period starts at around 28 weeks and ends at around 37–38 weeks of gestation. The growth rate is maximum and in the order of about 200 g per week.

Decelerating growth rate period: This period is beyond 37–38 weeks of gestation. The growth rate decelerates to approximately 70 g per week or less. After 42 weeks the fetal weight grows very little, if any.

It can be seen that the first half of the time of pregnancy is spent in achieving the first ten percent of the ultimate term weight. During this period, however, not only organogenesis, but also further development and rearrangement of fetal structures are achieved. It is not until the first two thirds of pregnancy is passed before the fetus attains one third of the term weight. Around 28 weeks when the maximum growth rate period starts, the fetal weight reaches approximately 1,000 g, and only from this time on, the fetus has any significant chance for extrauterine survival. The conventional prematurity range as based by birth-weight alone (1,000–2,500 g) corresponds to most of the maximal growth rate period (28–35.5 weeks). During this crucial period, the fetal prognosis improves markedly with rise in birth weight. The importance of gaining time, even a few weeks, by suppressing premature labor with medications and bed rest would be recognized as a crucial point of

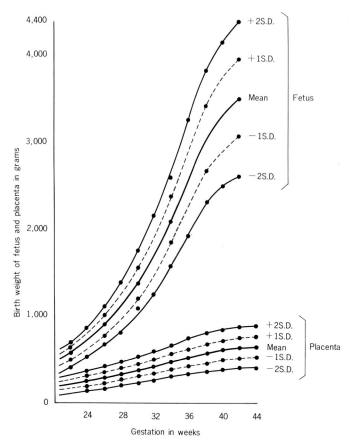

Fig. 3 Birth weights of fetus and placenta in relation to gestational ages (counted from last menstrual period). (Modified from HENDRICKS, C.H.: Obstet. Gynec. **24**; 357, 1964.)

obstetrical management. So called normal term weight of more than 2,500 g is attained only during the last four weeks of pregnancy.

Like many other biological parameters, the fetal weight at a given gestational age is normally scattered around the mean value. There are two ways to express distribution of fetal weights at a specific gestational age. One way is to express it with the median (50th percentile) and other percentiles [2, 6, 7, 11] (Fig. 2) and the other way is to depict it with the mean and standard deviations [3, 7] (Fig. 1,3). Generally, distribution is wider as pregnancy advances toward term. To define the "normal" range for clinical purposes is rather arbitrary. When the percentile curves are used, the tenth percentile curve has been used as the critical curve to designate the infants who have experienced retarded intrauterine growth. Excessively large babies, such as those born in diabetic pregnancy, are often above the 90th percentile. Thus, the normal range is implied to be from the 10th percentile to the 90th percentile. GRUENWALD [15] proposed to use the mean minus two standard deviations in each week of gestation for critical value to determine intrauterine growth retardation. In this method, the normal range is implied to be the mean ±2 standard deviations. Since approximately 95 per cent of the group should be included in the range of the mean ±2 standard deviations the mean −2 standard deviations represents 2.5 to 3 percentile. This may be too strict to include sufficient numbers of retarded infants and in a later publication

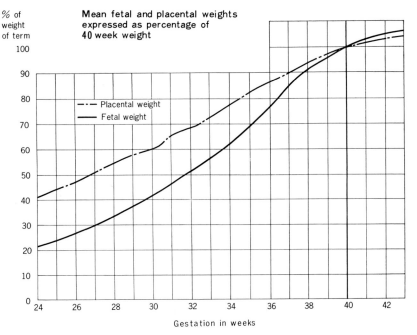

Fig. 4   Mean fetal and placental weights at various gestational ages expressed as percentage
of 40-week weight. (From HENDRICKS, C.H.: Obstet. Gynec. **24**; 357, 1964.)

[7] GRUENWALD suggested the fifth percentile instead of −2 standard deviations. Whether
percentiles or standard deviations are used, the intrauterine growth chart is very useful
clinically. The position of the newly-born infant on the growth chart should reflect considerably his performance in utero in response to his intrauterine environment. It may
reveal that his weight at birth is quite in proportion to his gestational age. Any deviations
from normal weight at specific gestational age is recognized and proper diagnostic and
therapeutic measures are instituted immediately, whenever possible. For follow-up of the
prematurely born infant the chart is useful in a sense that the post-natal growth can be
compared to the standards for intrauterine growth and that a perspective is obtained which
differs from that of comparing his growth to the post-natal growth of other infants in his
birth weight but different gestational age group. The intrauterine growth chart is useful in
determining when the prematurely born infant has regained the percentile zone standing
he had at birth. An example is seen in patient S.K. in Fig. 2.

Because of differences in the known factors influencing fetal growth rate, such as racial
and socioeconomic composition of the population and geography, the growth curves for
fetus cannot usually be expected to be identical in any two localities. Each institute of large
scale in every locality should construct its own fetal growth curves.

2.   INTERRELATIONSHIP BETWEEN FETAL AND PLACENTAL WEIGHT

Since placenta works as lungs, intestines, kidneys and endocrine gland for the fetus, it
would be natural to try to find out the interrelationship between fetal and placental growth.
The placental growth curve is less-well defined than the fetal one, but HENDRICKS [3]
presented detailed data in relation to fetal growth in the latter half of normal pregnancy
(Fig. 3). While the placenta continues to grow in terms of weight, its initial growth is much

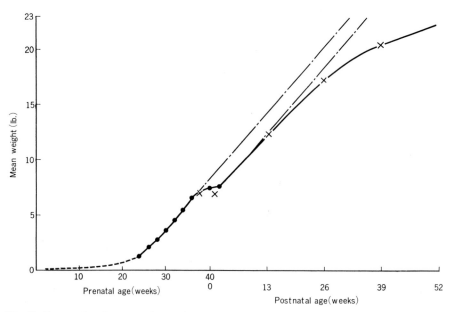

Fig. 5   Pre-natal and post-natal growth rates of singletons. (From MᴄKᴇᴏᴡɴ, T. and Rᴇᴄᴏʀᴅ, R.G.: J. Endocrin. **9**; 418, 1953.)

more rapid than that of the fetus. In fact, the placenta is heavier than the fetus until the 16th week of gestation [13]. And by the time (27 weeks) the placenta achieves 50 per cent of its 40-week weight, the fetus gains only 30 per cent of its term weight (Fig. 4). During the maximum growth rate period of the fetus, velocity of the fetal growth exceeds that of the placenta and especially after 38 weeks, slowing of the placental growth is more marked, while the fetal growth rate is also decelerated. The ratio of fetal to placental weight increases as pregnancy advances. The mean ratio of about 3.0 at 24 weeks rises to approximately 5.6 at 40 weeks*. MᴄKᴇᴏᴡɴ and Rᴇᴄᴏʀᴅ [16] noted reduction in the rate of growth of single fetuses after 36 weeks and compared pre-natal and post-natal growth rates of single births. They found that the weekly mean weight increment in single fetuses of 30 to 36 weeks gestation and that in singletons between birth and three months of age are almost identical (Fig. 5). Their findings seem to suggest that the reduction in the rate of growth of single fetuses during the last weeks of gestation (decelerating growth period) is due to restrictions imposed by the intrauterine environment, as in the case of multiple births, rather than to a change in the growth capacity of the fetus.

3.   CELLULAR GROWTH

On the cellular level, growth is due to an increase in the number of cells (hyperplasia) and/or in the size of individual cells (hypertrophy). Recently, Wɪɴɪᴄᴋ and his associates

---

*   However, the interpretation of the ratio between fetal and placental weight could be underestimated. In any two series of linearly increasing quantities (A, B) with slope values a and b, and initial ratio of A/B=r, the ratio A/B will increase linearly, if B increases with any b values which are less than 1/r a. As described before, the fetal growth curve can be broken doen into three straight lines between 24 and 40 weeks. The placental growth curve can also be broken down into three straight lines at nearly corresponding time to the lines of the fetal curve (Fig. 3). With these considerations, the fact that the fetal and placental weight ratio increases progressively means the rate of placental growth declines progressively twice at around 28 and 38 weeks in the later half of pregnancy, as compared with the rate of fetal growth.

have measured growth by determing the number and size of cells within an organ or whole body of rats [17, 18] and human placenta [19]. Since DNA is limited almost entirely to the nucleus of a cell and constant in quantity within the diploid nucleus of a given species, the amount of DNA should reflect the number of diploid nuclei. Determining the total DNA content of an organ and dividing it by the fixed amount of DNA in a single diploid nucleus (6.2 micromicrograms in the rat), the actual number of cells in that organ can be calculated. The weight, protein or RNA per cell, then is determined by dividing the total organ weight, protein or RNA by the number of cells in the organ. Exceptions where these calculations can not be applied are such tissues containing a significant number of non-diploid nuclei as liver or testis, or those containing many multinucleated cells, e.g., pancreas in the older animal. DNA content also doubles in all cells just prior to division. Such cells, however may be considered as two cells in all practical purposes, since they are about to divide. With these exceptions, DNA content should reflect cell number regardless of whether actual cell number is calculated. Weight/DNA or protein/DNA ratios should reflect the average weight or protein per cell in tissues where extracellular material is minimal. These ratios give an estimation of cell size and RNA/DNA ratio should reflect the average RNA content per cell. Based upon the data in rats which were obtained from serial measurements of the weight, DNA, RNA and protein content of various organs from ten days post-conception (about mid-pregnancy) until maturity [17], a certain insight into cellular growth of the fetus during the latter half of gestation may be obtained.

DNA : There is a progressive increase in DNA content both for whole fetus and for various organs.

Total weight : Although total organ weight increases throughout the latter half of pregnancy, weight/DNA ratio varies with development. Weight and DNA increase proportionally until near term, when weight increases more rapidly than DNA in the whole fetus and heart.

Protein : Total organ protein, like weight, increases throughout the latter half of pregnancy. Protein and DNA increase proportionally (hyperplasia), but near term protein increases more rapidly than DNA (hyperplasia and hypertrophy) in the whole fetus and heart. This disproportional increase in protein and DNA is a result of a decrease in the rate of DNA synthesis. The ratios in the kidney and lung, however, remain constant.

Cellular changes of the fetus and its organs before mid-pregnancy are probably dominated by hyperplasia though the data are lacking.

Together with post-natal growth, WINICK and NOBLE [17] recognize three phases of growth for the rat and most of its organs: 1) hyperplasia, 2) hyperplasia and hypertrophy, and 3) hypertrophy alone.

Regarding placental growth, the rat and human placentas seem to have the three phases of growth similar to other organs [18, 19]. In the human placenta, initially DNA, RNA, and protein rise proportionally (hyperplasia), then the rate of increase in DNA rapidly declines when the placenta reaches about 300 g and the fetus about 2,300 g (about 35 weeks). Thus, placental growth in the final month or so during pregnancy is due to hypertrophy without cell division.

These cellular growth patterns in the fetus and placenta have important implications from the standpoint of possible pathologic interference with cell growth by various factors. Interference during hyperplasia phase of cell growth in the fetus (probably throughout gestation) or in the placenta (first 35 weeks of gestation), e.g. nutritional deprivation, may not be readily overcome, and might result in permanent stunting. This time-dependent response was demonstrated in the organs of growing young rats exposed to undernutrition at various phases of the post-natal growth period. Early caloric restriction interfered with

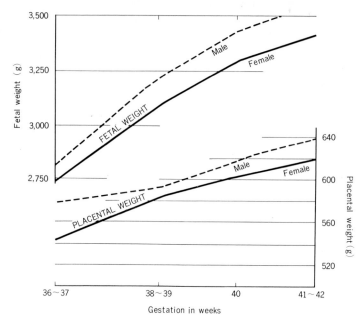

Fig. 6   Relation of sex of child to fetal and placental weight. (From HENDRICKS, C.H.: Obstet. Gynec. **24;** 357, 1964.)

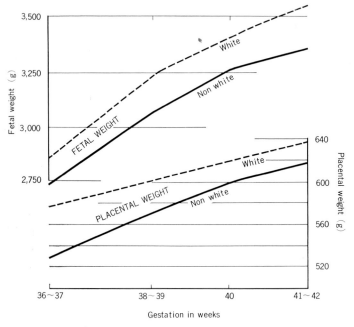

Fig. 7   Relation of ethnic group to fetal and placental weight. (From HENDRICKS, C.H.: Obstet. Gynec. **24;** 357, 1964.)

cell division and resulted in permanent growth failure. Later caloric restriction resulted in smaller cells, but they resumed normal size when the animal was adequately refed [20].

4. FACTORS RELATING TO NORMAL FETAL GROWTH

1) GENETIC FACTORS

Certain genetic factors are known to modify the mean birth-weight at any given stage of gestation. Sex of the fetus is best known among them. According to HENDRICKS' data from Cleveland, which are based on a series of over 11,000 births between 1956 to 1962 [3] the male infant at term is approximately 140 g heavier than the female infant, a difference of about 4 per cent (Fig. 6). Less well-known is the fact that the male placenta tends to be heavier than the female placenta, a difference of about 2 per cent at 40 weeks (Fig. 6). It is tempting to ascribe the difference to the effect of testosterone, inasmuch as it can be formed in the fetal testis as early as 10 weeks of age and is known to have anabolic effect in protein metabolism. Race is another factor. The report from Cleveland indicates that in average, the white fetus is 156 g heavier than the non-white fetus at 40 weeks (about 4.8%). The placenta of the white fetus is approximately 20 g heavier than that of the non-white fetus at 40 weeks (about 3.3%) (Fig. 7). Since socioeconomic factor is known to be another factor, relating to maternal nutritional condition, it might well be argued that the non-white might have occupied low socioeconomic group in more proportion than the white. And higher socioeconomic group tends to produce heavier babies than lower socioeconomic group. One way to judge the socioeconomic status of the patient is whether the patient is on the private service or the staff service in the United States. The former is generally considered to be financially and socially better off than the latter. Another known factor affecting birth weight, that is, parity must also be considered in this regard. The multipara tends to give birth to heavier babies than the primigravida. There might have been more primigravida in the non-white group than in the white group. Taking these variables into consideration and holding them at constant, HENDRICKS showed that there were still racial differences in the fetal and placental weight (Fig. 8–11). The mean weight of the white baby on the private service was 5.36 per cent greater than that of the non-white baby on the same service in multiparas, and 6.08 per cent in primigravidas. Likewise, the white baby on staff service was heavier in mean weight than the non-white baby on the same service by 3.77 per cent in multiparas and 8.72 per cent in primigravidas. Even the mean weight of the white baby on staff service was approximately 1 per cent greater than the non-white baby on private service in both multiparas and primigravida. Comparison of placental weight showed the similar pattern of difference due to races.

Other genetic factors suggested to influence fetal growth rate are stature [11] and birth weight [21] of the mother. Influence of each of these genetic factors upon fetal growth might be considered rather insignificant. Combined together with some other non-genetic factors, however, their influence becomes quite substantial since effects of these factors are often additive (Fig. 12, 13). They must be taken into consideration in determining the low birth-weight baby.

2) ENVIRONMENTAL FACTORS (FETAL NUTRITION)

The most significant and relevant factor influencing fetal growth is fetal nutrition which is dependent upon placental transfer function. Though intuition tells us the importance of supply of nutrients to fetal growth, this fact becomes assuringly impressive when it is expressed in the concrete formula. PAYNE and WHEELER [22] showed that the fetuses of mammalian and avian species, after an initial lag period, conform to a cubic law of growth as

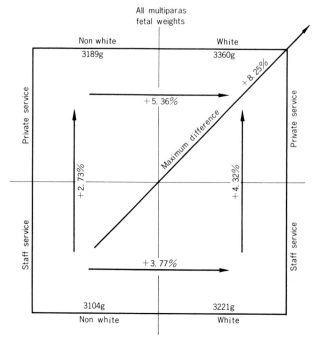

Fig. 8 Weights of infants of all multiparas with respect to ethnic group and service. (From HENDRICKS, C.H.: Obstet. Gynec. **24;** 357, 1964.)

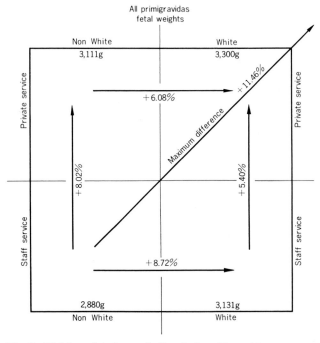

Fig. 9 Weights of infants of all primigravidas with respect to ethnic group and service. (From HENDRICKS, C.H.: Obstet. Gynec. **24;** 357, 1964.)

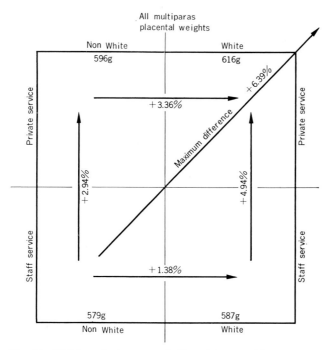

Fig. 10 Weights of placentas of all multiparas with respect to ethnic group and service. (From HENDRICKS, C.H.: Obstet. Gynec. **24;** 357, 1964.)

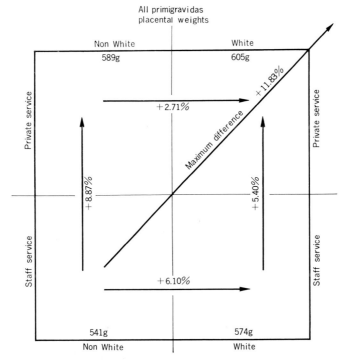

Fig. 11 Weights of placentas of all primigravidas with respect to ethnic group and service. (From HENDRICKS, C.H.: Obstet. Gynec. **24;** 357, 1964.)

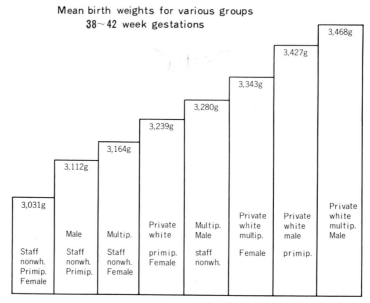

Fig. 12   Mean birth weights for various groups (38 to 42-week gestations). (From HENDRICKS, C.H.: Obstet. Gynec. **24**; 357, 1964.)

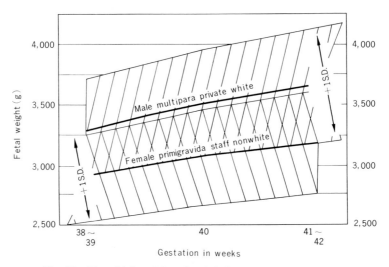

Fig. 13   Mean birth weights of male infants born to private, white, multiparous patients and of female infants born to staff, nonwhite, primigravid patients. (From HENDRICKS, C.H.: Obstet. Gynec. **24**; 357, 1964.)

related to time. The equation is :

$$W = a(t - t')^3$$

where W is the weight of the fetus in kilograms on any day of gestation, "a" is a constant denoting the rate of supply of nutrients per unit surface area of the fetus, "t" is the gestational age in days and "t'" is the lag period which lasts until the primitive streak appears

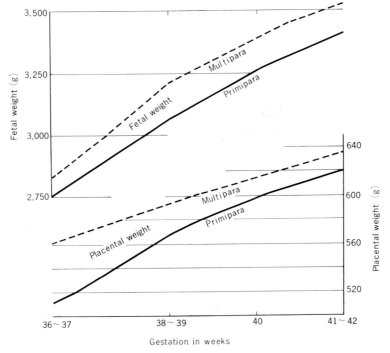

Fig. 14 Relation of parity to fetal and placental weight. (From
HENDRICKS, C.H.: Obstet. Gynec. **24**; 357, 1964.)

(this also corresponds to the period of time during which the placental function becomes established). For man, the value for a$=0.2 \times 10^{-6}$ and the value for t$'=36$ (when calculated from the first day of the last menstrual period rather than conception). Though the value for "a" should be slighly larger than 0.2×10^{-6} (around 0.24–0.25 times 10^{-6}) for better fit to recent data of the human fetal weight, this equation indicates that the fetal weight at any given time is determined by a constant "a", the rate of transport of nutrients per unit surface area of the fetus. A decrease in the value of "a" will result in intrauterine growth retardation, the effect of which becomes progressively marked as gestation advances.

Parity is known to affect birth weight. The second or third baby is usually heavier than the first one at birth in the same mother. The mean weight of the fetus and placenta born to the multipara is greater than that of the primigravida (Fig. 14). The fetal and placental difference is 3.4 and 2.5 per cent respectively at 40 weeks. The difference exists among the ethnic and socioeconomic group (Fig. 8, 9, 10, 11). Though we have no definitive explanation for this difference, it seems that after experiencing the first full pregnancy the uterine vasculature becomes more responsive to the succeeding stimuli of pregnancy and a more favorable environment is provided, thus, the larger placenta and better fetal nutrition being brought about.

Besides placental transfer function, intrauterine nutrition of the fetus is related to fetal metabolism and hormones, circulation, and maternal nutrition. Therefore, these related areas are briefly reviewed before placental transfer is discussed in the next section.

a) Fetal metabolism and hormones

The fetus is very active metabolically. Oxygen consumption of the mature fetus in the sheep and human has been reported to be about 5.0 ml/kg·min [23–26]. More recently the carbon dioxide production rate in the near-term monkey fetus was estimated to be about

11 ml/kg·min [27]. The metabolic activity of the primate fetus near term seems to be about equal [26] to or higher [27] than that of the mother.

Glucose is the primary source of energy for fetal metabolism and growth. There are two kinds of evidence to support this. One is the observation that the respiratory quotient of the immediate newborn infant is approximately 1.0 which indicates that carbohydrate is the fuel for metabolism [28]. Though the concentration of fructose, which is synthesized in the placenta, is higher in fetal blood than in maternal blood, it is not readily metabolized and much of plasma fructose is excreted in the urine after birth, at least in sheep [29, 30]. Thus, the direct contribution of fructose to fetal oxidative metabolism is trivial [31]. Another evidence is the fact that supply of free fatty acids to the human fetus is very much limited unlike that of glucose which is transferred rapidly across the placenta from the mother [32]. Those fatty acids which are transferred are probably utilized for the synthesis of lipids and most of them are stored as the future metabolic fuel in the newborn period. Thus, free fatty acids are not readily available as a metabolic fuel in the fetus.

In approximating the amount of glucose metabolized by the human fetus at term the difference in the glucose concentration between the umbilical venous and arterial plasma is reported to be approximately 12 mg/100 ml [33]. If we assume that near term a fetal plasma flow is about 180 ml/min and the fetal oxygen consumption is about 5 ml/kg·min, a fetus weighing 3,200 g will consume about 22 mg of glucose per minute and about 16 ml of oxygen. This amount of oxygen is just about necessary for complete oxidization of this amount of glucose. Since we do not know the exact umbilical plasma flow rate in man and the value seems to increase with more experience gained in the technique of measurement [31], the umbilical plasma flow rate, in actuality, may be higher than 180 ml/min near term. Then, glucose consumption by the fetus could be higher than 22 mg/min and probably more oxygen would have to be taken up by the fetus if all glucose were to be oxidized.

The fetus, like the adult, needs insulin for metabolism of glucose and it is generally agreed that in the human all of the effective insulin is secreted from the fetal pancreas. No significant quantities of maternal insulin cross the placenta. The fetal pancreas starts to secrete insulin as early as the 12th week, and the plasma insulin concentration increases progressively as the fetus matures. Since the fetus is in a constantly fed state, the fetal supply of glucose is relatively constant under normal conditions. Therefore, the responses of the pancreatic islets of the fetus to fluctuations of the glucose concentration are absent or at least blunted when compared with those in the adult [21]. The newborn of the diabetic mother, however, is more adult-like in insulin response to glucose, as if the intermittent episodes of hyperglycemia in utero had "conditioned" the fetal pancreas [32]. Fetuses of diabetic mothers are often accelerated in growth, and this is presumed to be due to recurring episodes of hyperglycemia and resultant hypersecretion of insulin. Insulin seems to be only one fetal hormone which regulates the rate of fetal growth. It is very likely that glucose and insulin are the most important determinant of the growth rate of the fetus. Concentrations of the fetal blood glucose are about 50–60 per cent of the maternal levels. This low fetal level is mainly due to the rapid utilization of glucose by the fetal tissues and extraction of glucose by the placenta during transfer for its own metabolism. The fetal glucose level is the net result of supply through the placenta, by glycogenolysis and gluconeogenesis in the fetus, and consumption by the fetal and placental tissues. With an adequate supply of oxygen, the fetus metabolizes glucose through pathways which differ in various organs. The cerebral cortex, for example, uses the glycolysis-Krebs cycle exclusively, whereas the adrenal gland uses the pentose pathway [34]. During asphyxia, the fetus resorts to anaerobic glycolysis with a large rise in blood lactate concentration and excess lactate is readily cleared through the placenta.

During the latter half of gestation the fetus accumulates large quantities of glycogen and fat. Large glycogen reserves are built up in the liver, heart, and skeletal muscles. These are utilized as metabolic fuel by the neonate right after birth when he is separated from his placental source of glucose. Accumulation of fetal liver glycogen seems to be under control of adrenocorticotropic hormone [35]. A term fetus has large lipid stores of both brown and white adipose tissues. Brown adipose tissue is primarily used for heat production, while white adipose tissue is a fat store. Under normal circumstances, however, it is unlikely that these potential energy sources are called upon, since the fetus is in a constantly fed state. The mechanism for rising hepatic glycogen during gestation remains to be elucidated. One would be tempted to ascribe it to changes in the activity of the liver enzymes concerned with glycogen synthesis and breakdown. But the correspondence between the hepatic enzyme activity in vitro and the pattern of glycogen accumulation in the liver is not exact, and no particular step in the enzyme chain has been identified as rate limiting [31]. Nonetheless, with increasing rate as gestation advances, the fetus synthesizes its own glycogen and fat from glucose and fatty acids which are transferred from the mother across the placenta. At term glycogen concentration in the liver is about 50 mg/g of liver [36], 27 mg/g of muscle, and 10 mg/g of heart [37]. Total lipid concentration at term becomes about 160 g/kg B.W. [38]. Unlike liver glycogen, muscle glycogen is not mobilized for metabolic use elsewhere during asphyxia, but is used rapidly with increased muscular activity after birth [31]. Another characteristic feature of the fetus is significant stores of glycogen in the epithelial tissues such as skin, lung and renal epithelia. These may play a role in carbohydrate homestasis in the fetus [21].

For the most part, the fetus synthesizes its own tissue proteins from the essential amino acids which are transferred from the mother across the placenta. Amino acid concentrations in the fetal blood are higher than in the maternal blood. The normal fetal to maternal ratio is about 1.8 in average [39]. Fetal tissues, like trophoblasts, tumors, and regenerating tissues, take up amino acids more avidly than do adult normal tissues. Each tissue concentrates the amino acids to a different degree [40].

When all essential amino acids are available to the fetus in appropriate proportions and all energy needs are met, protein synthesis by the fetus should proceed at normal rates for any period of growth. It is unlikely that amino acids are utilized for net oxidation or net gluconeogenesis [21].

Fetal weight gain does not seem to be regulated by fetal production of the hormones which are necessary after birth, perhaps with exception of insulin. Growth hormone is formed in the fetal pituitary gland at 12 weeks of gestation. The concentration is higher in the umbilical arterial blood than in the umbilical and maternal venous blood, indicating that the fetal pituitary is secreting growth hormone quite actively. However, growth hormone does not seem to be necessary for normal fetal growth. Maternal growth hormone and chorionic growth hormone-prolactin do not reach the fetus in appreciable amounts. Idiopathic pituitary dwarfs [41] and anencephalic apituitary fetuses have normal birth weights. Destruction of the fetal hypophysis by intra-uterine decapitation in rats and rabbits do not appreciably affect the body weight at term [42]. However, when development of particular organs is considered, there is some evidence of the action of growth hormone in utero, at least in rats. It was demonstrated that injection of purified bovine pituitary growth hormone into pregnant rats, while it did not change fetal weight, caused an increase in brain weight of 30 per cent, an increase of total DNA per brain, and a rise in cerebral cortical cell density of 63 per cent in the offspring [43]. Timing of the injection (7th to 20th day of gestation) corresponds to the period during which neurons are proliferating rapidly in this species. Fetal thyroid gland can form thyroxine by 12 weeks of gestation. Fetal thyroid hormone does not appear to regulate fetal growth as evidenced by the mean birth weight in one series of 49 cretins being 3.6 kg [44]. More recent reports also show normal birth weight and length in cretins, indicating no important role played by thyroid hormones in fetal growth [45, 46]. Maternal thyroid stimulating hormone, thyroxine, and triiodothyronine do not seem to cross the placenta in any significant rate. In sheep, abolition of fetal adrenal glands does not affect birth weight at term [47]. Anencephalic fetuses have atrophy of the fetal adrenal cortex, and yet reach normal birth weights. Thus, as described previously, fetal insulin appears to be only one hormone directly related to fetal growth among all the fetal hormones. Beginning at 12 weeks the fetal pancreas secretes insulin and its concentration is comparable to that found in the newborn. In rats the injection of fetuses with insulin for three days prior to term resulted in higher fresh weight, dry weight, total lipids, and total nitrogen [48]. It must be understood, however, that insulin itself only acts as a growth regulator in the presence of adequate quantities of glucose and that inasmuch as the maternal supply seems to be flow limited rather than diffusion limited, the final determinant of fetal growth may well be the rates of maternal blood flow and fetal blood flow which perfuse the total area of diffusing surface in the placenta.

Human placental lactogen (human chorionic somatomammotropin, chorionic growth hormone-prolactin), though it is produced in the placenta and mainly secreted into maternal circulation, is related to fetal growth indirectly since it alters maternal metabolic processes in such a way that favors carbohydrates supply to the fetus. GRUMBACH, KAPLAN, SCIARRA and BURR [49] ascribed a variety of maternal changes to this hormone. They are: 1) an increased mobilization of fat stores with an increase in the plasma free fatty acids; 2) an increased resistance to insulin; 3) a rise in circulating insulin with an increase in the insulin response to glucose loads and islet cell hyperplasia; 4) the accretion of nitrogen, which will promote conservation of maternal protein; 5) mammary growth and initiation of the phase of lactation. This hormone can be detected in the serum of pregnant women as early as the sixth week of gestation and its concentration increases steadily during the entire period of gestation. The concentration in the blood is not affected by blood glucose level. The syncytiotrophoblast of the placenta has been implicated as the site of its synthesis. The net result of these maternal changes by human placental lactogen is a sparing of glucose and gluconeogenic precursors and a shift toward the utilization of lipids as a source of energy, namely, changes similar to the fasting state. Thus, human placental lactogen appears to have many properties in common with the pituitary growth hormone. Although its growth promoting action is far weaker than that by comparable doses of pituitary growth hormone (1/100), its production rate is great and its concentration in maternal plasma at term pregnancy is 1,000 times as great as that of pituitary growth hormone. Because of the unique feature that there are no known feedback mechanisms in placental hormone secretions, effects of human placental lactogen on maternal metabolism are unremitting and progressive. Thus, the mother utilizes lipids progressively and relies less upon carbohydrates. Since lipids are not transferred to the fetus in large amounts and carbohydrates are main metabolic fuels for the fetus, this maternal condition favors the fetal nutrition.

Whenever oxidative degradation of organic substrates takes place, heat is produced. The fetus, who is in a state of active energy metabolism, is producing heat constantly. Indeed, it was found by ADAMSONS and TOWELL [50] that the temperature of the fetus is about 0.5 °C higher than that of the maternal colon, and approximately 0.3 °C above that of the uterine wall, and about 0.2 °C above that of the amniotic fluid. The fetus has two principal sites for heat exchange. One is external body surface including that of the umbilical cord and placenta, and the other is the surface of villous capillaries in the placenta. The latter is more important than the former for thermal homeostasis since the thermal diffusion capacity of villous capillaries considerably exceeds that of the body surface. High thermal diffusion capacity implies that at a given caloric output by the fetus, the difference in temperature between the fetus and mother is determined by the rate and direction of the blood flow of the mother and fetus in the placenta. An increase in the fetal-maternal temperature gradient is the result of the increased ratio of heat output by the fetus to placental blood flow. Interference with heat dissipation would result when fetal or maternal blood flow in the placenta is reduced, or fails to increase corresponding to rise in heat production by the fetus.

b)   Fetal circulation

Growth and development of all organ systems of the fetus depend upon its adequate circulation. Most of the knowledge about the fetal circulation has been derived traditionally from the sheep experiment [31, 51–53], mainly because of easy accessibility to the fetus of this animal and unavailability and technical difficulty of the primate fetus. Recently, some information on fetal circulation in the primate has become available [54, 55]. The general circulatory features of the mature lamb fetus appear to be similar to that of the mature primate fetus. Transport of sufficient oxygen to various fetal tissues is one of the primary functions of the fetal cardiovascular system. Certain fetal tissues which have higher oxygen consumption or greater growth or development demand more oxygen than others and require preferential perfusion. These arrangements must be made under low partial pressure and content of oxygen in the fetal blood. In order to accomplish this task, the fetus has unique features in his circulatory pattern and circulating blood. Because of the shunts between the left side and right side of the heart, the ventricles of the fetal heart, unlike those of the adult, work in parallel rather than in series. The cardiac output is extremely high, and, according to ASSALI and associates [52], it amounts to about 220 ml/kg. min, which is approximately three times the cardiac output of the adult. This high cardiac output is accomplished partly by the fast heart rate. The high concentration of hemoglobin and greater affinity of fetal hemoglobin in intact red cells with oxygen result in higher oxygen carrying capacity of the fetal blood and greater oxygen content at a given partial pressure of oxygen than the maternal blood. These features are responsible for sufficient oxygenation of the fetal tissues despite the low oxygen partial pressure in the fetal blood.

Well oxygenated, nutrient rich blood from the placenta is carried by a single umbilical vein in the cord, and reaching the fetus, it is carried by the abdominal portion of the umbilical vein. It enters the liver and forms many branches. Some branches join the hepatic veins mainly for the left side of the liver and others carry the umbilical vein blood to the intrahepatic portal circulation, mainly for the right side of the liver. A major branch connecting directly the umbilical vein and the inferior vena cava is the ductus venosus. It is about half as wide as the umbilical vein, and usually gives no branches to the hepatic substance as the hepatic branches of the umbilical and portal veins do. Presence of a sphincter-like structure of the ductus venosus at its junction with the umbilical vein, which is innervated by vagal branches, has been reported [53, 56], but recently its distinct anatomical identity and functional significance has been challenged [57]. The oxygen content of the blood in the ductus venosus is identical with that in the umbilical vein, and greater than that in the hepatic artery, and much greater than that in the portal vein, so it is unlikely that the hepatic arterial or the portal venous bloods normally enter the ductus venosus. Thus, it is generally believed that the ductus venosus shunts well oxygenated blood directly from the umbilical vein to the inferior vena cava. However, the magnitude of this shunt is not definitely known, and the factors controlling the blood flow through it are not known at all. One recent investigation estimates that 43 per cent of the umbilical venous flow normally passes through the ductus venosus in the sheep fetus [58]. The blood which perfused the liver parenchym is drained into the inferior vena cava via the hepatic vein. The caudal portion of the inferior vena cava carries the venous return of the caudal part of the fetal body. Thus, the blood flowing to the fetal heart through the inferior vena cava is an admixture of the well-oxygenated blood from the ductus venosus and less-oxygenated blood from most of the veins below the level of the diaphragm. As a result, the oxygen saturation of blood going to the heart from the inferior vena cava is reduced compared with that in the umbilical vein (from 80% down to 67% in mature fetal lambs), but greater than that from the superior vena cava (31%) (Table 1).

Table 1 Mean oxygen saturation (%) in circulating blood in various fetal vessels in six mature lambs [59].

Umbilical vein, ductus venosus		80
Portal vein		27
Inferior vena cava	above diaphragm	67
	below diaphragm	26
Superior vena cava		31
Brachiocephalic artery, ascending aorta		62
Ductus arteriosus		52
Descending aorta, umbilical artery		58

After centuries of controversy whether the two blood flows from the inferior and superior vena cava mix or cross each other in the right atrium, it is now well accepted that two vena caval blood streams cross each other with small portion of the inferior vena caval blood mixing with the superior vena caval blood in the right atrium [54, 55]. This crossing is made possible because of the anatomical position of the foramen ovale that it opens directly off the inferior vena cava so that the inferior vena caval blood stream is mostly deflected by the crista dividens (interatrial septum) through the foramen ovale into the left atrium [31, 54]. Also, a small portion of the superior vena caval flow seems to mix with the inferior vena caval flow [54, 55]. Crossing of two vena caval blood streams with partial mixing in the heart of the intrauterine primate fetus is shown in Fig. 15–20. The exact magnitude of each flow distribution is not known. The preferential flow of blood from the inferior vena cava through the foramen ovale to the left atrium, then into the left ventricle, permits ejection of the more highly oxygenated blood from the left ventricle to the ascending aorta for perfusion of two vital organs, heart and brain. Dilution with a small portion of the superior vena caval blood and pulmonary venous blood is minimal. The less-oxygenated blood from the superior vena cava together with a small portion of the inferior vena caval blood flows into the right atrium, then into the right ventricle, from where it is ejected into the pulmonary trunk. The majority (about 70%) of the blood in the main pulmonary trunk is shunted through the ductus arteriosus into the descending aorta. Thus, only a small volume of the blood, about 10–15 per cent of the combined cardiac output, perfuses the fetal lung. This is due to high pulmonary vascular resistance and pressure of the fetus. The fetal right ventricle must work against this high pulmonary resistance and pressure, and it is considerably more developed in thickness and contour than the left ventricle, contrary to the adult heart. It appears that right ventricular cardiac output is either slightly greater than or at least, equal to left ventricular output [52].

The ductus arteriosus has a diameter close to that of the fetal ascending aorta. Since the ductus arteriosus plays a major role in both the systemic and pulmonary hemodynamics before and immediately after birth, it is the most important vascular shunt in the fetal circulation. ASSALI and associated [52] studied dynamics of ductus arteriosus circulation of

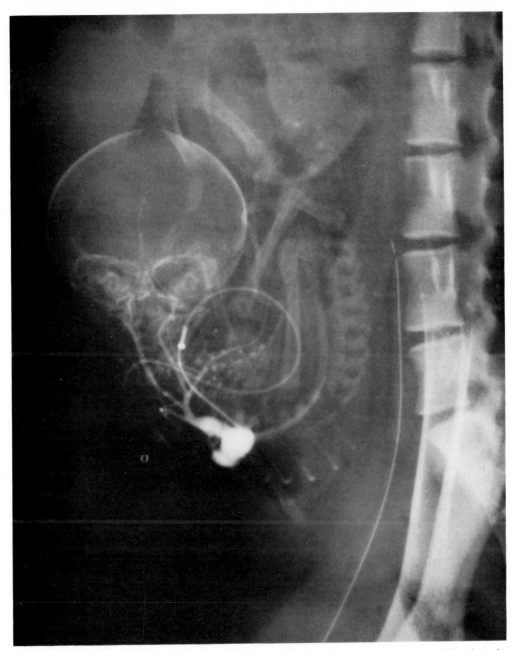

Fig. 15 Fig. 15–17 are three representative films taken following injection of contrast medium into the inferior vena cava of the monkey fetus in utero in the third trimester of pregnancy. A catheter was placed through the right internal jugular vein, passed through the right atrium down to a site in the inferior vena cava, just below the crista dividens of the fetal heart. Contrast medium, 3 cc, was injected over three seconds. Fig. 15 was taken 2.5 seconds after start of injection. The contrast medium filled the left side of the heart, the aortic arch, and the neck vessels densely with ventricular systole. The right atrium just began to be visualized partly. (From Suzuki, K. et al.: J. Reprod. Med. **7**; 65, 1971.)

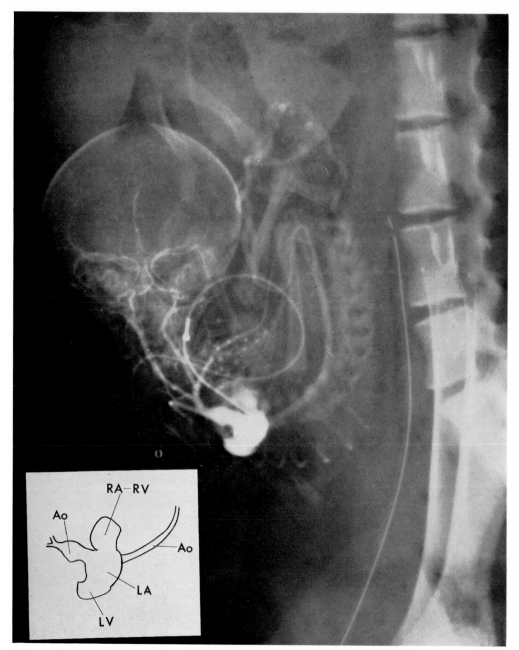

Fig. 16 This was taken three seconds after start of injection. The left side of the heart, aortic arch, and the neck vessels were clearly visualized while the right side of the heart became outlined palely. (From SUZUKI, K. et al.: J. Reprod. Med. **7;** 65, 1971.)

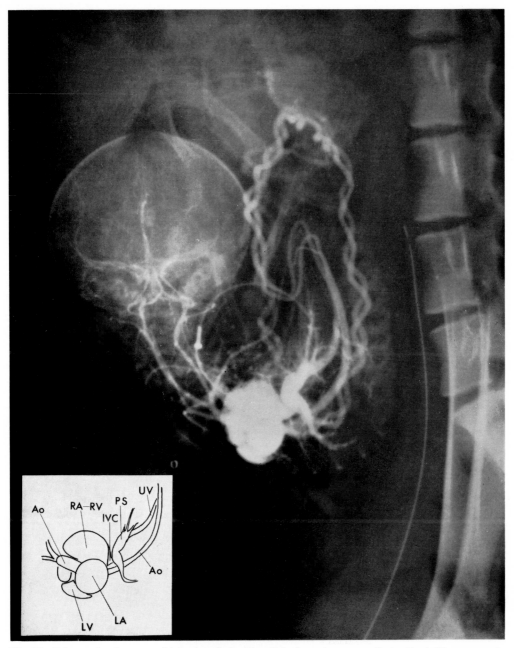

Fig. 17 6.5 seconds after start of injection. Both sides of the heart became well visualized. The retrograde filling of the inferior vena cava, portal sinuses, hepatic vessels, and abdominal portion of the umbilical vein were seen. (SUZUKI, K. et al.: J. Reprod. Med. **7**; 65, 1971.)

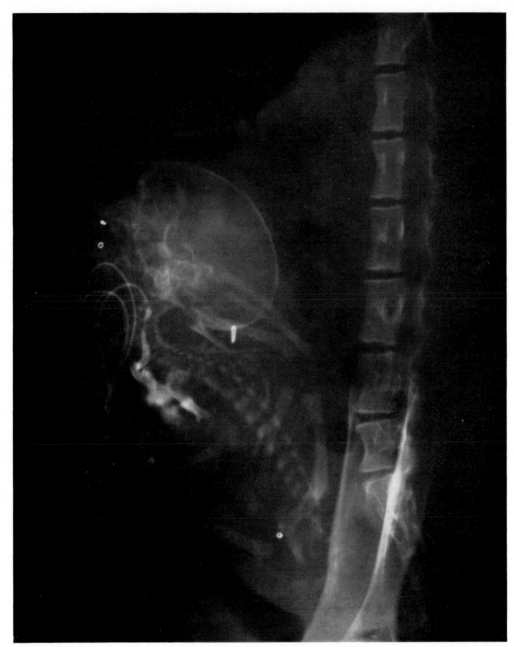

Fig. 18 Fig. 18–20 are three representative films taken following injection of contrast medium into the left external jugular vein of the monkey fetus in utero in the third trimester of pregnancy. A catheter was placed in the left external jugular vein and contrast medium, 1.5 cc, was injected over 1.5 seconds. Fig. 18 was taken two seconds after start of injection. The right side of the heart was densely outlined while the left side was also palely visualized. (SUZUKI, K. et al.: J. Reprod. Med. **7;** 65, 1971.)

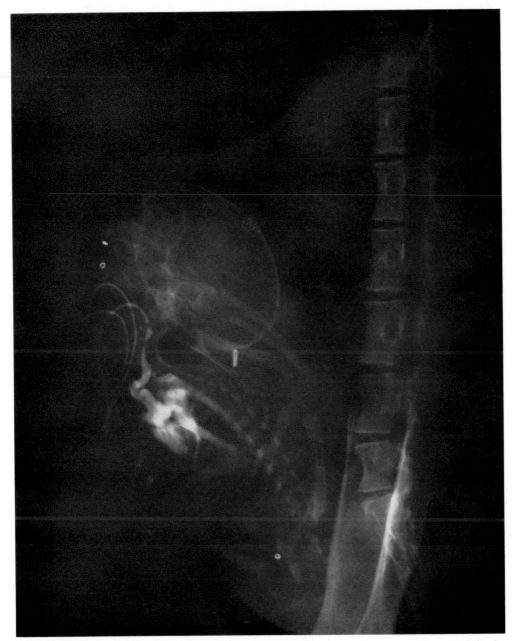

Fig. 19 Three seconds after start of injection. The main pulmonary trunk, ductus arteriosus, and the descending aorta were visualized while the ascending aorta, the aortic arch, and the neck vessels were not opacified at all. (Suzuki, K. et al.: J. Reprod. Med. 7; 65, 1971.)

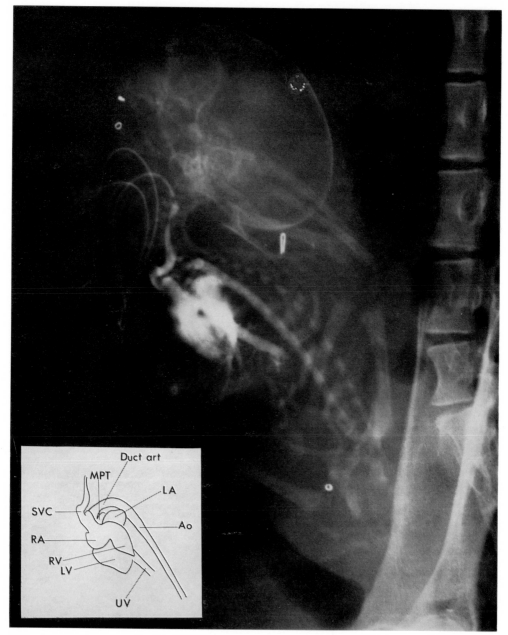

Fig. 20 Four seconds after start of injection. Characteristic shunting became more prominent. MPT: main pulmonary trunk, Duct art.: ductus arteriosus. (SUZUKI, K. et al.: J. Reprod. Med. **7**; 65, 1971.)

the fetal lamb extensively and found that the ductus flow is influenced by the right ventricular output, the oxygen tension of the blood passing through the ductus, and the pressure gradient between the pulmonary and systemic circuits. Especially, P_{O_2} of the blood in the ductus was inversely and reversibly correlated with the ductus blood flow rate. When the blood P_{O_2} rises to 50 to 60 mmHg, the ductus flow begins to decrease, which increases again when P_{O_2} drops. The constricting effect of oxygen is direct on the vessel walls and does not require the presence of the nervous system. The reverse is true in the pulmonary vascular bed. Low oxygen tension causes vasoconstrictive effects on the pulmonary vessels. With the first breath at birth, the oxygen tension rises in the blood and this closes the ductus arteriosus and dilates the pulmonary vessels. In this regard, the low oxygen tension of the blood which normally present in the fetus, is an absolute necessity for the proper functioning of the fetal circulation.

The blood stream which passes through the aortic arch and that passing through the ductus arteriosus join to form the descending aorta. A minor fraction of the descending aorta is distributed to the trunk, the various viscera, and lower extremities. The large portion, 60 to 65 per cent of the combined cardiac output, returns to the placenta through the two umbilical arteries. The oxygen saturation in the blood of the descending aorta and umbilical arteries becomes about 58 per cent compared with those of about 62 per cent in the aortic arch blood and about 52 per cent in the ductus arteriosus blood, in the mature fetal lamb (Table 1).

Angiocardiographic studies in the human fetus in the mid-trimester of gestation by LIND and his associates [54] and in the monkey fetus in the third trimester by SUZUKI and his associates [55] indicate that the blood supply to the head, heart, liver and upper extremities is much greater than that to the gastrointestinal tract, kidneys and lower extremities in the primate fetus.

Mainly because of presence of low vascular resistance system, the umbilicoplacental circulation, the overall systemic arterial pressure of the fetus is low. The fetal arterial pressure seems to increase progressively throughout gestation, reaching a maximum at term. Though not essential for fetal survival, a considerable degree of nervous control on fetal circulation is normally established by the end of gestation.

c)   Maternal nutrition

The effects of experimental restriction of maternal nutrition upon the fetus have been investigated in lower species of animals than the primate. These animals are usually polytocous and the ratio of the total weight of the litter to the maternal weight is large, compared with that in the primate. In these animals, especially in sheep, undernutrition has a marked effect on birth weight of the fetus. These studies have usually been limited to a reduction in total food intake rather than reduction in specific food constituents, making it difficult to see the differential effects of, for example, caloric and protein restriction. Because of the interrelationship among various food constituents and their conversion to energy, interpretation becomes difficult, even when a certain food constituent is restricted. Generally, restricted diet during pregnancy in animals reduces the number of fetuses, the survival rate, postnatal growth, as well as the size of each fetus. Furthermore, deficiencies in intellectual function and metabolic activities of a permanent nature have been described [60, 61].

Regarding effects of maternal nutrition on the human fetus, information is limited. As far as the birth weight is concerned, however, the effect of maternal undernutrition is clearly seen, though in less degree than in animals. Weight gain during pregnancy, which could be considered as one indication of nutrition, shows a strong positive association with birth weight. The fetal outcome in terms of birth weight and neonatal performance is considerably better when the total maternal weight gain is more than 11.8 kg [62]. There are also three sets of data derived from severe food deprivation periods during World War II. There was a state of severe generalized undernutrition in the urban areas of Northwest Holland during the six months prior to the liberation in May, 1945. During this time, the average neonatal birth weights fell by about 250 g and the premature rate rose [63]. In Leningrad in 1942 a more severe food deprivation occurred, and the mean birthweight decreased by 500 to 600 g. The prematurity rate increased to 41 per cent [64]. In evaluating the effect of food deprivation upon birth weights in a population, it is necessary to compare weights for comparable gestational ages, eliminating the effect of increased prematurity rate. GRUENWALD and associates [9] compared the fetal growth rate in Japan during the year of greatest food deprivation (1945–1946) with that of a prosperous year (1963–1964). Fig. 21 shows the result. The effect is persistently seen in the order of 200 g at least after 35 weeks of pregnancy. At 40 weeks the mean difference is 285 g. Though these differences might appear small, it could be related to differences in functional maturity. Thus, it seems justified to state that available data, incomplete as they are, indicate nutritional restriction of the mother during pregnancy may have adverse effects upon fetal growth and development, especially when restriction is severe.

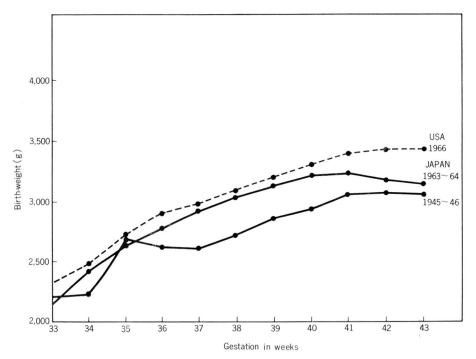

Fig. 21 Fetal growth curves during two periods in Japan. American curve is shown for comparison. (Modified from GRUENWALD, P. et al.: Lancet, **1;** 1026, 1967.)

Here, one must delineate maternal undernutrition from maternal malnutrition, in which the total caloric intake may be adequate or even excessive but serious deficiencies of specific nutriments may exist. Severe malnutrition may well increase the frequency of such obstetrical complications as prematurity, abruptio placentae, megaloblastic anemia or iron deficiency anemia, preeclampsia and eclampsia. These conditions, in turn, could retard the fetal growth.

Recently, the subject of maternal nutrition during pregnancy has aroused great interest among obstetricians. Pertinent review is presented by PITKIN, KAMINETZKY, NEWTON and PRITCHARD in a recent article [65]. They speculate that the common obstetric practice of routinely limiting caloric intake to restrict weight gain during pregnancy could be partially responsible for the number of low birth weight babies who contribute a disproportionate share to infant mortality. In normal pregnancy an increase in caloric intake of approximately 10 per cent over non-pregnant requirements is reported to be necessary to meet the necessary adjustments in maternal physiology and provide for fetal growth and development. An average total weight gain of 10 to 12 kg is thought to be optimal, the normal pattern of gain consisting of minimal gain (approximately 1 kg) in the first trimester and accumulation of 0.3 to 0.4 kg/wk during the second and third trimesters. They warn that there is no scientific justification for routine restriction of weight gain to amounts less than those stated above and that severe caloric restriction is potentially harmful to both mother and fetus. In evaluating excessive weight gain during pregnancy, these authors emphasize the importance of differentiating between fluid retention and tissue accumulation. There is no definitive evidence that excessive weight gain due to tissue deposition is related to toxemia or to any other obstetric complications. It may, however, lead to the patient's obesity if not lost after delivery. Regarding sodium intake by the mother, the routine restriction of sodium intake in normal pregnancy is of uncertain value, possibly harmful.

While maternal physiologic changes are taking place in various organ systems for fetal growth and development, the maternal homeostasis must be maintained. In maternal sodium metabolism, the sodium homeostasis is preserved by the renin-angiotensin-aldosterone system when sodium loss due to increased glomerular filtration rate and the natriuretic effect of pregesterone occurs during pregnancy [66]. However, experimental data in pregnant rats indicate that sodium restriction stresses the physiologic mechanism of sodium conservation sufficiently to cause the system to break down, so that blood volume cannot be expanded and hyponatremia develops in fluids and tissues [67]. Thus, sodium restriction might cause maternal electrolyte imbalance in man. Another possible adverse effect of severe sodium restriction is elimination of essential nutritional components in diet, either because they contain high sodium levels or because limiting salt impairs taste preference. Supplemental ferrous iron, 30 to 60 mg daily, should be given to every pregnant woman during the second and third trimesters and through lactation, or two or three months postpartum in non-breast feeding women. The value of routine vitamin supplementation, at least in developed countries, is dubious, and probably neither beneficial nor harmful as long as excessive intakes of vitamins, especially A and D are avoided [65].

PLACENTAL TRANSFER

Among various factors relating to fetal growth and development, placental transfer functions are the most important and influential factor. Adequate supply of nutrients from the maternal circulation to the fetal circulation and proper disposal of the metabolic waste products in the opposite direction are essential for normal fetal growth and metabolism. In most substances, transmission of molecules of substances across the placenta is bidirectional, i.e. transfer from mother to fetus and that from fetus to mother, and the difference between these two transfers is the net transfer. In this sense, the commonly used words "placental transfer", which connotes unidirectional transport, should be termed as placental exchange. The order of magnitude of the exchange rate, therefore, is not related to the

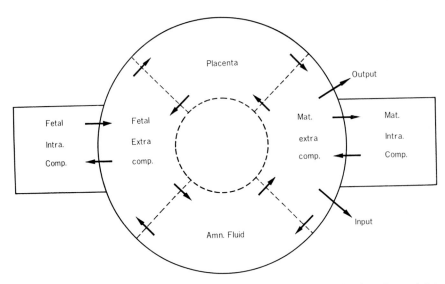

Fig. 22 Six compartments and the 14 exchanges which may affect the distribution of materials in the pregnant organism. The fetal and maternal intracellular compartments are shown at the sides of the circle. The fetal and maternal extracellular compartments (which include the respective blood volumes) are shown in relation to the placenta and amniotic fluid. "Output" and "input" represent the activities of the maternal lungs, kidneys, skin, and gastrointestinal tract. (From PAGE, E.W.: Amer. J. Obstet. Gynec. **74;** 705, 1957.)

net transfer rate. On molecular levels placental exchange is a kinetic phenomenon and each endogenous substance which exists as compartment or pool in the maternal and fetal blood in a steady state, i.e. in a constant total amount in each blood for a given period of time, is in a dynamic equilibrium with each other for that period of time, like any body constituents in other parts of living animals. Each blood compartment of a certain substance across the placenta is, in turn, in dynamic equilibrium with other compartments of this substance, for example, those in the intracellular space, amniotic fluid, and placenta (Fig. 22). It follows that complete and precise knowledge of kinetics of the placental exchange requires the use of tracer methods (usually isotopes as tracers) and analysis of multicompartmental systems. With the use of the tracer method, each bi-directional transfer rate of a substance among various compartments can be determined without need for blood flow measurement, and the net transfer rate between any two compartments is the difference between two transfer rates in opposite directions. The tracer method has been introduced rather recently by FLEXNER and associates [68, 69], and extensively used in the study of placental exchange of various substances by PLENTL and associates [27, 70–78]. The reader is referred to the detailed description of tracer methods in the placental transfer study by PLENTL [79]. Traditional and most widely used method in the placental transfer study has been mainly concerned with direct determination of the net transfer rate. This method involves measurement of concentration differences of a substance either between uterine artery and vein or between umbilical artery and vein, and determination of uterine or umbilical blood flow rate. Then, the transfer rate of the substance to the whole pregnant uterus from the maternal blood is determined by multiplying the uterine arteriovenous difference of concentration by the uterine blood flow rate. The transfer rate to the fetus is measured as product of the umbilical arteriovenous concentration difference and the umbilical blood flow rate. When diffusion is applicable as transfer mechanism for a substance, for example, oxygen, Fick's diffusion equation has been used sometimes to calculate

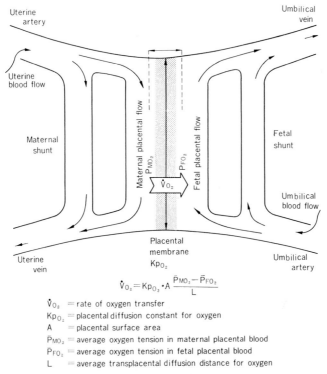

$$\dot{V}_{O_2} = Kp_{O_2} \cdot A \frac{\bar{P}_{MO_2} - \bar{P}_{FO_2}}{L}$$

$\dot{V}_{O_2}$ = rate of oxygen transfer
Kp_{O_2} = placental diffusion constant for oxygen
A = placental surface area
$\bar{P}_{MO_2}$ = average oxygen tension in maternal placental blood
$\bar{P}_{FO_2}$ = average oxygen tension in fetal placental blood
L = average transplacental diffusion distance for oxygen

Fig. 23 Schematic diagram of placenta and its circulations using oxygen diffusion as an example. Maternal and fetal circulations both contain "shunts" through which blood flows without participating in gas exchange. Gas transfer occurs between the placental streams according to the laws of gas diffusion. Geometric relationship between the maternal and fetal blood streams is depicted here as countercurrent flow for illustrative purposes, but in reality the human placenta probably has a complex multivillous stream system (From METCALFE, J. et al.: Physiol. Rev. **47**; 782, 1967.)

the transfer rate by determining the concentration difference of a substance between the maternal and fetal blood and estimating the placental surface area, thickness, and diffusion constant for the substance (Fig. 23). Since accurate measurement of either uterine or umbilical blood flow rate is extremely difficult, results with the use of the former method are often no more than estimates. The use of the latter method in diffusion is encountered with almost insurmountable problems. Besides extreme difficulty in estimating surface area and functional thickness of the placenta, one must determine concentration of a substance under study in both the maternal intervillous space blood and the fetal villous capillary blood. The uterine and umbilical vessel blood samples are not real representatives of the maternal and fetal blood at the exchange site of the placenta since there exist shunts in both sides of the placenta, which carry the blood not participating the exchange at the placenta. With these reservations, however, numerous studies have been conducted and a considerable amount of information has been gathered regarding placental transmission of various substances. BARRON and associates [80–87] have been mostly responsible for a large amount of data with use of these traditional methods. Especially data obtained from chronic preparations in ewes have enabled one to obtain umbilical venous and arterial blood under near-ideal, physiologic conditions over weeks and contributed a great deal to further knowledge of placental transfer [86].

For practical purposes, what matters is naturally the net transfer rate. Therefore, in this section the net transfer is mainly discussed. The words "placental transfer" is meant for the net placental transfer. A small net transfer rate, however, by no means indicates slow exchange across the placenta. For example, the concentrations of urea in the maternal and fetal blood are nearly the same, and as the major metabolic end product of fetal nitrogen metabolism, urea must be produced in the fetus constantly and transferred to the mother, the fetal production rate being the net transfer rate. But the concentration gradient between the fetus and mother is so small that it is hardly measurable. Thus, one may well think the net transfer rate is very small based on the diffusion mechanism. Indeed, the net transfer rate of urea from the fetus to mother, calculated with the tracer method using C^{13} and C^{14} labeled urea, is small, but it seems to be only a fraction of the total placental exchange [75].

Another important consideration in the placental transfer is the fact that virtually any substances could cross the placenta. We know that even fetal red cells can traverse to the maternal circulation normally. What matters is the placental transfer rate. Any transfer rates which are physiologically significant to the fetus concern us. When the transfer rate of a substance is so slow that its effects upon the fetus is not significant physiologically, it is often treated as non-permeable to the placenta.

1. MECHANISMS OF PLACENTAL TRANSFER

Several different mechanisms commonly exist for transport of substances across the placenta, namely, simple diffusion, facilitated diffusion, active transport and pinocytosis. These mechanisms are not peculiar to the placenta, but common to other epithelial membranes, such as the gastrointestinal or renal tubular epithelium.

1) SIMPLE DIFFUSION

Simple passive diffusion is movement of molecules by random thermal motion from an area of high concentration to one of low concentration. It takes place in response to chemical or electrochemical gradients of substances across a membrane which passes these substances. When these gradients cease to exist, then the rate of exchange across the membrane becomes the same in both directions, and a net transfer ceases. It is a passive process involving no energy or work by the membrane and continues "downhill" until uniform concentration or electrochemical equilibrium is reached. It is generally agreed that oxygen and carbon dioxide cross the placenta by simple diffusion alone.

The rate of simple diffusion across the placenta is described by FICK's diffusion equation [88]:

$$\frac{dQ}{dt} = \frac{KA}{L}\Delta C$$

where dQ/dt = net transfer rate (quantity transferred per unit of time), K = placental diffusion constant for the substance in question, A = surface area of exchange in the placenta, L = functional thickness of the placenta, and ΔC = concentration difference of the substance across the placenta. In a strict sense, it is the difference of chemical activity of the substance rather than the concentration itself that is important in driving the substance across the placental membrane (e.g. free form of a substance vs. protein bound substance). For diffusion of gases, where the concentration is proportional to the partial pressure, ΔC in the above equation can be replaced by ΔP = partial pressure difference but K becomes a function of the solubility of the gas in question in the placental membrane.

2) FACILITATED DIFFUSION

The rate of transfer in some substances, typically glucose, is faster than would be predicted on simple diffusion. The kinetics deviate from FICK's principle as evidenced by a decreased transfer rate at very high concentration and competition of transfer between substances with similar molecular spatial configuration with the resultant decrease in the transfer rate. Facilitated diffusion does not take place against an electrochemical gradient and does not require energy or work by the placental membrane. The exact mechanism is not established. It is assumed that a given substance combines chemically with a "carrier" in the trophoblast membrane of the placenta. This carrier-substrate complex, then traverses the membrane at a rate faster than that of the substrate alone (Fig. 24). For example, the placental transfer rate of naturally occuring D-xylose is faster than that of the L-isomer [89].

3) ACTIVE TRANSPORT

This mechanism of transport requires expenditure of metabolic energy. Active transport usually takes place "uphill" against an electrochemical gradient. Though the exact mechanism has not been established, the simplest working hypothesis again involves a membrane "carrier" that combines chemically with the substance (Fig. 25). It is believed that the carrier or the substrate-carrier complex undergoes endergonic chemical alteration and is linked to an adenosine triphosphate (ATP) energy source [90].

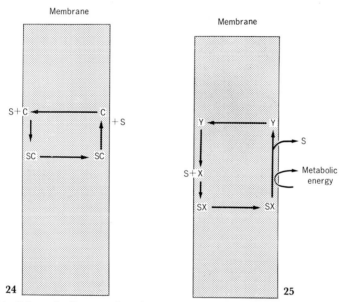

Fig. 24 Schematic diagram of carrier mediated facilitated diffusion. The carrier, C, has the same affinity for the substance on both sides of the membrane. The substrate-carrier complex, S.C., diffuses across the membrane more rapidly than does the substrate alone. (From LONGO, L.D.: Placental transfer mechanisms—An overview. In: Obstetrics and Gynecology Annual. Wynn, R.M. (ed.) Appleton-Century-Crofts, New York, 1972.)

Fig. 25 Schematic diagram of a carrier system capable of active transport. An important difference between this system and that illustrated in Fig. 24 is that the carrier undergoes a change at the inner surface of the membrane from a form X, with a relatively high affinity for the substance, to a form Y, which has a relatively low substrate affinity. Energy is required in the reversible transformation of the carrier between X and Y forms. It is generally assumed to be supplied at the inner surface of the membrane. (From LONGO, L.D.: Placental transfer mechanisms—An overview. In: Obstetrics and Gynecology Annual. Wynn, R.M. (ed.) Appleton-Century-Crofts, New York, 1972.)

In addition to such features common to the carrier system, like those in facilitated diffusion, as (a) decreased transfer rate at very high concentration of substrate (saturation of the carrier system); (b) competition for the transfer by molecules with similar structural or molecular configuration; and (c) presence of stereo-specificity in the transport process; active transfer is characterized by the following features; (d) net transfer in the direction opposite to the concentration or electrochemical gradient; (e) presence of a chemical or electrochemical gradient at equilibrium in the opposite direction to net transfer, in the absence of any other factors affecting transfer, such as protein binding or Gibbs-Donnan equilibrium; and (f) inhibition of transfer by metabolic poisons which reduce the available energy. Substances actively transported by the placenta are amino acids, probably the water-soluble vitamins and ions such as calcium.

4) PINOCYTOSIS

This process consists of invaginations of cell membranes, engulfing by these cell membranes of tiny droplets of solute and water which appear as vacuoles within the cytoplasm, transportation across the cell and discharge of these microdroplets on the other side. Pinocytosis has been observed chiefly with electron microscopy, but macropinocytosis may be observed with light microscopy. Though commonly seen in a variety of cells, the process is poorly understood. Energy dependence is suggested by histochemical studies demonstrating that the pinocytotic vesicles are surrounded by high concentrations of ATPase.

While the rate of transfer in this process may be relatively slow, this process is considered to be of importance in the placental transfer of immune globulins, lipoproteins, phospholipids and other molecules whose large size precludes the placental transfer by any other process.

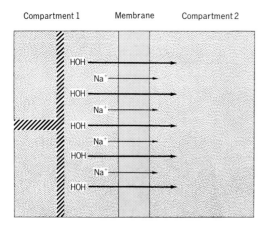

Fig. 26 Schematic diagram of bulk-flow or ultrafiltration. Increased hydrostatic pressure, indicated by the piston in compartment 1, results in more solvent's crossing the membrane into compartment 2 than would be predicted by the laws of diffusion. Ions such as sodium may be carried along with the solvent, so-called solvent drag. Osmotic pressure, caused by a higher concentration of solute in compartment 2 than in compartment 1, may have a similar effect. (From Longo, L.D.: Placental transfer mechanisms—An Overview. In: Obstetrics and Gynecology Annual. Wynn, R.M. (ed.) Appleton-Century-Crofts, New York, 1972.)

5) MISCELLANEOUS MODES OF TRANSPORT

A "bulk" flow of water may occur in response to minor or intermittent changes either of hydrostatic or osmotic pressure gradients, and when this occurs, water movement will carry dissolved solutes (solvent drag) (Fig. 26). This will result in a more rapid rate of transfer of water and solutes than predicted on the basis of simple diffusion.

Microscopic breaks in the placental villi may explain the passage of intact fetal red blood cells into the maternal circulation. Though the significance of minute leaks in normal circumstances is not known, they are important as the initial step for sensitizing the Rh negative mother to Rh positive fetal red cells. Some cells, e.g. maternal leukocytes, or organisms, e.g. treponema pallidum, may cross the placenta under their own power. A large number of viruses may infect the fetus though relatively few are known to do so, and the precise mechanism of their transport across the placenta is not known. A few viral particles might be transported in the pinocytotic process and then multiply rapidly within fetal cells [21].

Finally, it should be pointed out that a given substance may be transferred by more than one of these mechanisms simultaneously. For instance, while amino acids are actively transferred by the membrane carrier, some of the amino acids may be transported by simple diffusion and some by micropinocytosis.

2. PHYSICOCHEMICAL FACTORS INFLUENCING PLACENTAL TRANSFER

From Fick's diffusion equation previously described, it is obvious that *placental diffusion constant* (K), *placental surface area for exchange* (A), *average transplacental diffusion distance* (L), and *concentration gradient* (ΔC) or *partial pressure gradient* (ΔP) affect the placental transfer rate in simple diffusion. Permeability of the placental membranes to various diffusible solutes can be compared by determining diffusion constant (K) that is the quantity of solutes transferred per unit time per unit concentration difference per unit distance and surface area of the placenta, or *permeability constant* (K/L) that is the quantity of solutes transferred per unit time per concentration difference per unit surface area of the placenta. Also permeability of various placental membranes to the same solute can be compared with K or K/L. The larger the values of K are, the more rapid diffusion exists. These values have been determined in vitro using chorion and amnion. Since the functional area and thickness of the exchange surface of the placental membranes are almost impossible to be measured in vivo, *diffusing capacity* (KA/L) of the placenta for specific solutes have been measured. In this expression the area and thickness become part of the constant and it describes the quantity transferred per unit time per unit concentration difference. It can be determined in vivo for the same purposes as K or K/L.

Regarding placental surface area for exchange, AHERNE and DUNNILL [91] reported that the mean chorionic villous surface area of the normal human placenta increases from about 5 m² at 28 weeks to about 11m² at 40 weeks, measured by a morphometric technique. They also found that the value of the villous surface area corresponded closely to that of surface area of fetal placental capillaries, which is the actual placental surface area for exchange of substances. As expected, they found a close positive correlation between the chorionic villous surface area and the infant birth weight at all gestational ages, whether the pregnancy was normal, complicated by hypertension, or an abnormally small fetus (Fig. 27).

As for the average transplacental diffusion distance, current estimates of the average distance between maternal and fetal blood depend on electron microscopic measurements. AHERNE and DUNNILL [92] reported a mean value of 3.5μ in the human placenta at term. Since there are differing opinions among anatomists about the functional cross section of the channels in the intervillous space in which the maternal blood flows, estimation of the mean diffusion distance is extremely difficult.

Several other physicochemical factors are known to affect the rate of diffusion across the placenta. They are as follows:

Molecular size : In general, substances of smaller molecular size diffuse more rapidly across the placenta than larger molecules. For substances with molecular weights below

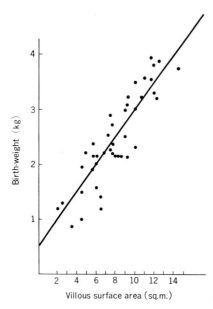

Fig. 27 Infant birth weight plotted against chorionic villous surface area in normal, hypertensive and normotensive small fetus pregnancies. (From AHERNE, W. and DUNNILL, M.S.: J. Path. Bact. **91**; 123, 1966.)

250 such as oxygen and D-glucose, the Graham-Exner relation (diffusivity is inversely proportional to the square root of the molecular weight) is found to hold fairly well in many cell membranes [90]. While most substances below a molecular weight of 700 appear to cross the placenta by diffusion, there is a difinite difference in the transfer rate of uncharged molecules depending on molecular size [94]. In fact, small, uncharged lipid-soluble molecules diffuse so rapidly that their concentrations equilibrate during a single capillary transit [94, 95]. Substances with molecular weights more than 700 to 1,000 such as polypeptides and proteins cross the placenta more slowly, if at all.

Ionization : Electrical charge influences the transfer rate across most biologic membranes including those of the placenta. Uncharged molecules cross more rapidly across the placenta than do ionized molecules of similar size. For example, Na^+, K^+, and HCO_3^- cross the placenta more slowly than water, urea, and CO_2.

Lipid solubility: Lipid soluble substances cross the placenta more easily than water soluble substances. This phenomenon is also found in many other biologic membranes. The large lipid content of the cell membrane seems to be the reason. Lipid soluble substances appear to diffuse through the entire cell membrane while water soluble substances seem to cross cellular membranes through water-filled pores between cells [96]. As one example, lipid soluble, unconjugated bilirubin crosses the placenta much more easily than water soluble, conjugated bilirubin.

Protein binding: Small solutes bound to protein no longer contribute to chemical gradients. Only free or unbound forms of compounds are available for placental transfer. Thus, changes in the affinity or binding constant of the protein for certain compounds and concentration or total amount of the protein in both maternal and fetal blood affect the placental transfer rate and total concentration of such compounds in maternal and fetal bloods at equilibrium or in the steady state. One example of such compounds is cortisol. Fetal cortisol concentration is about one-third the maternal one, closely paralleling differences in concentration of transcortin, the plasma protein binding specifically cortisol [97].

Gibbs-Donnan equilibrium: This phenomenon exists across partially semipermeable mem-

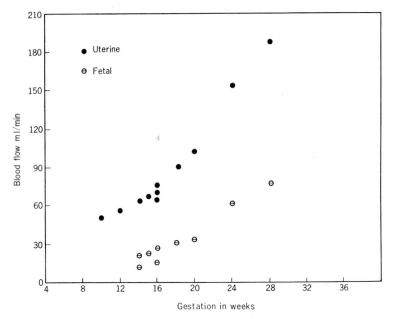

Fig. 28 Total uterine and umbilical blood flows in the human pregnancy are related to gestational ages. Both flows increased progressively and in a parallel fashion. However, the uterine blood flow was consistently higher than the fetal blood flow. The major portion of the total uterine blood flow is believed to perfuse the intervillous space. (From ASSALI, N.S. et al.: Amer. J. Obstet. Gynec. **79**; 86, 1960.)

branes and it is the redistribution of permeable solutes across this membrane to restore electrochemical equilibrium that has been disturbed due to the inability of other charged solutes to cross the membrane. For example, in early pregnancy the chloride anion concentration is higher and protein concentration is lower in the amniotic fluid than in the maternal or fetal serum while major cations are in identical concentrations in the three spaces. Probably, in order to preserve electrochemical neutrality, an increased amount of chloride anion crosses the membranes into the amniotic fluid to compensate for the relative inability of the negatively charged protein molecules to diffuse into this fluid.

Peculiar to facilitated diffusion or active transport involving the membrane carrier transport system is *stereospecificity*. It has been demonstrated that naturally occurring forms of optical isomers are more rapidly transferred across the placenta than the other optical isomers. Natural L-histidine crosses the placenta more rapidly than its D-isomer [77, 98]. Natural D-glucose is transferred more rapidly than L-glucose [99].

Placental enzymes affect transfer of certain substances by altering them during their passage through the placenta. Examples are various amines. Ordinary amounts of tyramine, 5-hydroxy-tryptamine (serotonin), and probably epinephrine are deaminated by the high content of monoamine oxidase and rendered harmless. The same is true of histamine because of the high content of diamine oxidase in the placenta. Also various precursors for steroid hormones, cholesterol, pregnenolone, and dehydroisoandrosterone, are converted to progesterone or estrogen by various enzymes in the placenta.

Perhaps the most important factor influencing the placental transfer rate or rapidly diffusible substances is the *rate of maternal and fetal blood flow* perfusing the placenta, since transfer of these substances is limited by blood flow rather than by diffusion. For example, the transfer rate of oxygen, carbon dioxide, or glucose is most strongly influenced by the

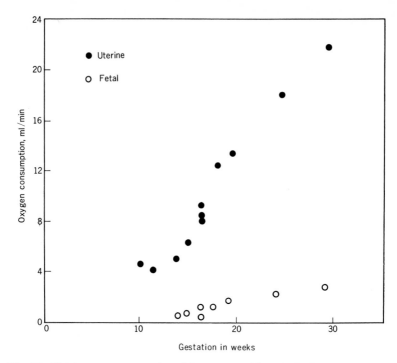

Fig. 29   Total oxygen consumption of the uterus and fetus in the human pregnancy. Although both increased progressively during pregnancy, the uterine oxygen consumption increased at a much faster rate than the fetal oxygen consumption, particularly after the 16th week of gestation. Placenta is believed to consume the major portion of this difference. (From AssALI, N.S. et al.: Amer. J. Obstet. Gynec. **79**; 86, 1960.)

blood flow rate of uteroplacental and umbilicoplacental circulation. For these substances, only such a small barrier to rapid diffusion exists in the placental membranes that the transfer rate is mainly dependent upon the amount of supply of these substances to the placenta per unit time, which, in turn, is regulated mainly by the amount of blood perfusing the placenta per unit time. On the other hand, for substances which cross the placenta with difficulty, that is, those with small transfer rate, the supplied quantity is depleted so slowly that the membrane barrier to diffusion (thus, concentration gradient across the membrane) becomes the main determinant of placental transfer rates.

AssALI and associates [100] measured uterine and umbilical blood flow rates from 10 to 28 weeks of human pregnancy. They showed that the uterine and umbilical blood flow rate increased progressively as pregnancy advanced during this period of gestation (Fig. 28). Uterine and fetal oxygen consumption also increased progressively during the same period, primarily due to the progressive rise in the uterine and umbilical blood flow (Fig. 29). However, when the values were expressed on the basis of unit weight of pregnant uterus and fetal weight, both blood flow (Fig. 30, 31) and oxygen consumption remained constant during the course of gestation.

3. PLACENTAL TRANSFER OF SPECIFIC SUBSTANCES

Detailed description of placental transfer of specific substances is beyond the scope of the current article and the reader is referred to various review articles [90, 93, 101–108].

Concentration gradients of various substances between the maternal and fetal blood are

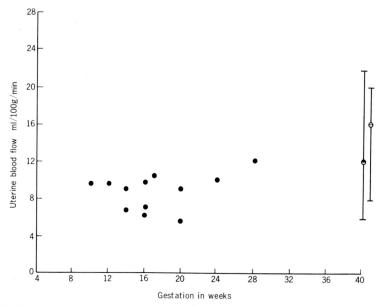

Fig. 30   Uterine blood flow expressed as milliliters per 100 grams of pregnant uterus per minute in various gestational ages. The values at 40 weeks are from data by MET-CALFE et al. (J. Clin. Invest. 34: 1632, 1955, depicted as 0) and ASSALI et al. (Amer. J. Obstet. Gynec., depicted as θ). The blood flow per unit weight of pregnant uterus remains fairly constant throughout the course of gestation. (From ASSALI, N.S. et al.: Amer. J. Obstet. Gynec. **79**; 86, 1960.)

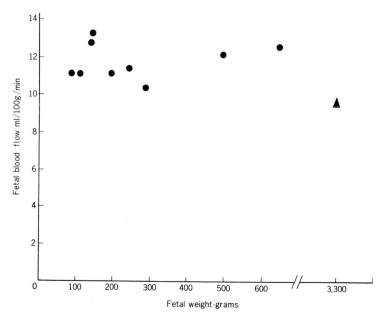

Fig. 31   Fetal umbilical vein blood flow expressed as milliliters per 100 grams of fetus per minute in various gestational ages. Blood flow per unit of fetal weight remains constant throughout gestation and averaged 11 ml/100 g min. (From ASSALI, N.S. et al.: Amer. J. Obstet. Gynec. **79**; 86, 1960.)

Table 2 Concentration gradient of substances across the placenta.*

Higher in fetal blood	About equal	Highter in maternal blood
CO_2	Sodium	O_2
Amino acids	Potassium	Total proteins
Fructose	Chloride	α and β globulins
Meso-inositol	Urea	γ-A and γ-M immuno globulin (IgA and IgM)
Sorbitol	Uric acid	Fibrinogen
Iron	Creatine	β-lipoprotein
Calcium	Creatinine	Glucose
Inorganic phosphate	Magnesium	Total lipids
Lactate	α-lipoprotein	Phosholipids
Iodine	γ-G immunoglobulin (IgG)	Cholesterol
Vitamins B group and C		Fatty acids
		Cortisol
		Vitamins A and E

*From PAGE, E.W.: Physiology and Biochemistry of the Placenta. In: Obstetrics. Greenhill, J.P. (ed.), 13th ed. Chapter 3, W.B. Saunders, Philadelphia, 1965.

shown in Table 2. Those substances present in about equal concentrations in both maternal and fetal blood should not be considered slow in transfer. In fact, many of those substances are rapidly diffused across the placenta in both directions, but concentration differences are too small to be detected by the currently available technique. For example, the maximal rate of endogenous urea production in the fetus (i.e. the net transfer rate of urea from the fetus to mother) amounts to less than 10 per cent of the total placental exchange of urea [75].

RESPIRATORY GASES

Placental transfer of oxygen has been studied extensively by many investigators. Minimal data required for determination of placental oxygen transfer are blood flow rates and arteriovenous oxygen contents on maternal and fetal sides of the placenta. Exact values for these parameters, especially blood flow rates, have not been determined mainly due to technical difficulties. Most of data have been obtained from sheep and goats. Only a few human data are available from studies by ASSALI and associates [100, 109] and METCALFE and associates [26, 110]. The kinetics of diffusion are illustrated in Fig. 23. A counter-current flow in the figure between the maternal and fetal blood streams is only for illustrative purposes because, in reality, it is not applicable for the human placenta which has probably a complex multivillous stream system. Vascular geometry, whether the two blood streams are counter-current, concurrent or multivillous streams becomes an important determinant on respiratory gas transfer since oxygen or carbon dioxide transfer is "flow limited" rather than "diffusion limited". An extensive and detailed review on gas exchange in the pregnant uterus was recently made by METCALFE, BARTELS, and MOLL [107]. While the rate of fetal oxygen utilization is rapid, about 15 cc/min for a 3 kg human fetus, the total oxygen extracted by the pregnant uterus near-term is small, about 24 cc/min, and there are no known mechanisms by which the fetus can increase its oxygen stores. Therefore, an uninterrupted oxygen supply is of vital importance for fetal survival. Irreversible brain damage is known to appear after 7–8 minutes of oxygen deprivation in monkeys. Out of 24 cc of oxygen transferred to the near-term pregnant uterus per minute, about 60 per cent is usually utilized by the fetus and 40 per cent by the uterus and placenta. Placental transfer

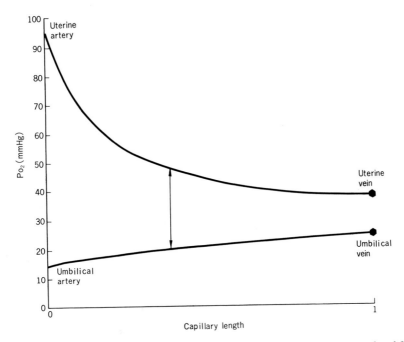

Fig. 32 Diagramatic representation of the time course of change in O_2 tensions in maternal and fetal bloods during a single transit in placnetal exchange vessels, assuming that the PO_2 values in the uterine and umbilical veins are the same as those of the maternal and fetal end capillaries. This assumption is probably incorrect, however. A combination of O_2 consumption by placental tissue, vascular shunts in the uterine and umbilical circulations, and nonuniform distribution of maternal to fetal placental flows probably accounts for the PO_2 difference between uterine and umbilical veins. The arrow indicates the average maternal to fetal PO_2 difference of about 25 mmHg. (From LONGO, L.D.: Placental transfer mechanisms—An overview. In: Obstetrics and Gynecology Annual. Wynn, R.M. (ed.) Appleton-Century-Crofts, New York, 1972.)

of oxygen is determined by several factors, namely, 1) placental diffusing capacity, 2) the uterine and umbilical arterial oxygen tensions, 3) the characteristics of maternal and fetal oxyhemoglobin dissociation curves, 4) the maternal and fetal placental hemoglobin flow rates (the blood flow rate corrected by the ratio of the hemoglobin level to a standard hemoglobin concentration 15 g/100 cc. It is expressed as the product of the actual flow rate and Hb/15.), 5) the pattern of maternal to fetal blood flows, and 6) the amount of carbon dioxide exchanging (by Bohr effect). Each of these determinants is, in turn, a function of other factors.

Oxygen diffusing capacity of the placenta (DpO_2) is defined, as previously described, as the rate of oxygen transfer for a given partial pressure between maternal and fetal blood and expressed as:

$$DpO_2 = \frac{KpO_2 \cdot A}{L}$$

where $KpO_2 =$ placental diffusion constant for oxygen, $A =$ placental surface area, and $L =$ average transplacental diffusion distance for oxygen (Fig. 23). From Fick's diffusion equation in Fig. 23, it can be expressed as:

$$DpO_2 = \frac{\dot{V}_{O_2}}{P_{MO_2} - P_{FO_2}}$$

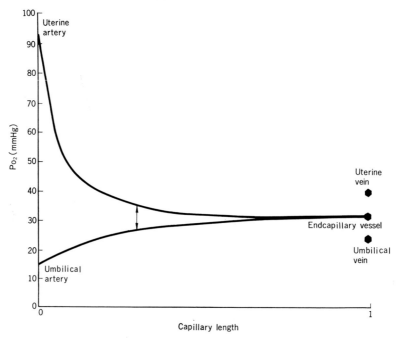

Fig. 33 The time course of change of PO_2 values in maternal and fetal bloods during a single transit in placental exchange vessels, assuming the O_2 diffusing capacity calculated from studies using carbon monoxide. In this instance the O_2 tensions in maternal and fetal blood reach equilibrium. Typical PO_2 values of uterine and umbilical venous blood are indicated by closed hexagons. The arrow indicates the "true" maternal to fetal mean PO_2 difference of about 6 mmHg. (From LONGO, L.D.: Placental transfer mechanisms—An overview. In: Obstetrics and Gynecology Annual. Wynn, R.M. (ed.) Appleton-Century-Crofts, New York, 1972.)

where $\dot{V}_{O_2}$ = rate of oxygen transfer (cc/min) and $\overline{P}_{MO_2}$-$\overline{P}_{FO_2}$ = the average oxygen tension difference between maternal and fetal placental blood (mmHg) $\dot{V}_{O_2}$ is estimated to be about 15 cc/min for a 3 kg fetus. The average PO_2 in the maternal intervillous space blood is estimated to be about 40 to 50 mmHg (Fig. 32) and that in the fetal placental blood to be 20 to 25 mmHg. A mean difference is, thus, estimated to be about 23 mmHg. Therefore, the placental oxygen diffusing capacity would be about 15/23=0.65 cc/min·mmHg for a 3 kg human fetus. However, neither the mean nor the end-capillary oxygen tensions in the placental exchange vessels can be determined with any precision from the oxygen tensions in the uterine and umbilical bloods as have been usually done so far, since placental tissues consume a considerable amount of oxygen [111, 112], and there are probably vascular shunts on both sides of the placenta (Fig. 23) [113, 114], and nonuniform distribution of maternal to fetal placental blood flows [115] may limit oxygen transfer, producing some of the uterine-to-umbilical vein PO_2 difference. Although the placental diffusing capacity is often considered as a convenient index of the efficiency of placental transfer of respiratory gases, this may be somewhat misleading since the diffusing capacity may vary in different areas of the placenta and be large or small according to the ability of fetal blood to carry oxygen away from the exchange site. Thus, it is actually the ratio of the diffusing capacity to transport capacity of the fetal blood (fetal placental hemoglobin flow rate) that is critical in determining whether oxygen exchange proceeds to equilibrium and is a useful measure of the diffusional limitation existing in the placenta [116]. LONGO and associates assessed placental diffusing capacity and the mean maternal-fetal PO_2 difference more accurately by measurement of carbon monoxide exchange [117]. Their studies indi-

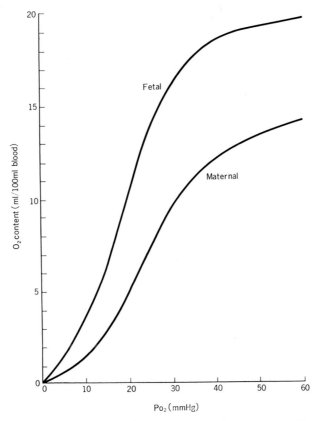

Fig. 34 Relation of O_2 content to O_2 partial pressure for maternal and fetal blood, assuming O_2 capacities of 12 and 16 g/ml, respectively. (From LONGO, L.D.: Placental transfer mechanisms—An overview. In: Obstetrics and Gynecology Annual. Wynn, R.M. (ed.) Appleton-Century-Crofts, New York, 1972.)

cate that the "true" maternal to fetal P_{O_2} difference is about 5 to 6 mmHg (Fig. 33), and that the "true" oxygen diffusing capacity of the placenta is about 2 cc/min·mmHg for a 3 kg fetus. With the use of this small value for P_{O_2} difference and certain other values, calculation reveals that oxygen tensions in the maternal and fetal blood would equilibrate at about 32 mmHg at the end of a single transit in the exchange vessels of the placenta (Fig. 33) [118]. It should be, however, emphasized that under normal conditions the placental transfer of oxygen is not limited by the resistance to diffusion of the placental membrane, but rather by the maternal and fetal blood flow rates [107, 119].

The oxygen transfer rate across the placenta and the resulting end-capillary P_{O_2} are also critically dependent upon values of P_{O_2} of uterine and umbilical arterial blood. Uterine P_{O_2} can decrease 10 to 20 mmHg from a normal value of 95 mmHg without significantly affecting placental oxygen transfer, but when it falls below about 75 mmHg, oxygen transfer will decrease sharply [119]. It has been known that fetal oxyhemoglobin dissociation curve lies to the left of the maternal curve under normal conditions, that is, the fetal blood has a higher affinity for oxygen. Figure 34 depicts oxygen contents of maternal and fetal blood as a function of P_{O_2}, assuming concentration of maternal hemoglobin = 12.0 g/100cc and fetal hemoglobin 16.0 g/100cc. It can be seen from Fig. 34 that when oxygen is diffusing from maternal blood with P_{O_2} of 40 mmHg to fetal blood with P_{O_2} of 25 mmHg, oxygen is actually moving against a concentration gradient.

Since most of the oxygen transported to and from the placenta is combined with hemo-globin, it is useful to consider the blood flow rate corrected for hemoglobin concentration. This corrected blood flow rate is termed as hemoglobin flow rate (F_{Hb}) and is related to the actual blood flow rate (F) by the equation: $F_{Hb} = F(Hb/15)$ and is expressed as cc/min (a standard hemoglobin concentration of 15 g/100cc is used).

Placental transfer of carbon dioxide has been far less extensively studied than that of oxygen. The exchange of carbon dioxide across the placenta is extremely rapid and the net transfer is from the fetal to maternal blood by passive diffusion. Its transfer is affected by the same factors that influence oxygen transfer though their relative importance differs. The movement of carbon dioxide in placental blood normally involves the reaction:

$$HCO_3^- + H^+ \rightleftharpoons H_2CO_3 \leftrightarrows CO_2 + H_2O$$

It proceeds to the right in fetal placental blood and to the left in maternal placental blood. Normally, the reaction $CO_2 + H_2O \rightleftharpoons H_2CO_3$ is catalyzed by the enzyme carbonic anhy-drase in the red blood cells. Recently, it has been shown that the enzyme concentration in fetal erythrocytes is sufficient to maintain normal carbon dioxide transfer despite its lowered concentration [90]. Also theoretical calculations indicate that the mean fetal to maternal P_{CO_2} difference is less than 1 mmHg in the placental exchange vessels and that the P_{CO_2} difference of less than 1 mmHg occurs within the first 5 per cent of a capillary transit [90].

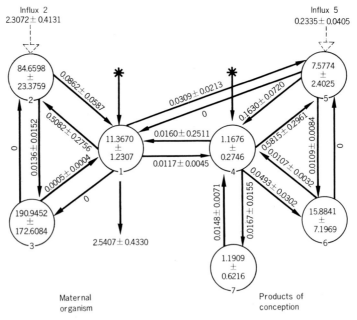

Fig. 35 Exchange and distribution of carbon dioxide in the model of seven compartmental system in the pregnant Rhesus monkey near term. Compartments 1,4, and 7 are maternal and fetal blood compartments and amniotic fluid compartment of CO_2 respectively. Compartments 2,3, and 5,6 are maternal and fetal extravascular compartments respectively. Both mother and fetus have their own characteristic production rate of CO_2 (Influx rate). Numbers along the arrows are fractional transfer rates, in fractions per minute. Numbers within the circles are compartment sizes of CO_2, in millimoles of CO_2. For example, size of com-partment (A) times fractional transfer rate from compartment A to B will be the amount of CO_2 (millimoles) transferred from compartment A to B per minute. Influx into compartments 2 and 5 and loss of CO_2 from compartment 1 to outside the system are expressed in millimoles CO_2 per minute. All values represent mean ± 1 S.D. for four pregnant monkeys. (From SUZUKI, K. et al.: J. Clin. Invest. **48**; 1967, 1969.)

The normal umbical to uterine vein P_{CO_2} difference of 4 to 5 mmHg is probably due to a combination of placental production of carbon dioxide, vascular shunts, and uneven distribution of fetal to maternal placental blood flows, as noted in oxygen transfer.

As previously noted, since exchange of any substances in the pregnant organism involves many other compartments besides the maternal and fetal blood streams, multicompartmental analysis of exchange is necessary, if it is possible, in order to understand the placental exchange of substances more precisely and integrally. This is extremely difficult mainly because of inaccessibility of many compartments and complexity in analysis of data. Nevertheless, with the aid of a general purpose computer program, multicompartmental analysis of carbon dioxide exchange has been done in pregnant Rhesus monkeys near term [27]. The result is shown in Fig. 35. One can see rapid exchange of carbon dioxide (CO_2 in Fig. 35 denotes the total CO_2 which exists in various forms in the monkey, such as the physically dissolved CO_2, carbonic acid, bicarbonate, and carbamino compounds, and which can be measured as acid-volatile CO_2) between fetal and maternal blood across the placenta, between the blood compartment and some extravascular subcompartment in both mother and fetus and slow exchange between fetal blood and amniotic fluid, and no appreciable exchange between maternal blood and amniotic fluid. In this study the mean net production of CO_2 by fetus (net transfer of CO_2 from fetus to mother) was 0.476 ± 0.0402 (S.D.) mmoles/kg·min, and that by mother was 0.373 ± 0.0279 mmoles/kg·min, difference being significant statistically ($P < 0.01$). This suggests that the primate fetus near term has a higher metabolic rate per unit mass than its mother.

Table 3 Normal values of oxygen, carbon dioxide, and pH in human maternal and fetal blood [90].

	Uterine artery	Uterine vein	Umbilical vein	Umbilical artery
P_{O_2} (mmHg)	95.0	40.0	27.0	15.0
O_2Hb (% saturation)	98.0	76.0	68.0	30.0
O_2 concent. (ml/100ml)	15.8	12.2	14.5	6.4
Hemoglobin	12.0		16.0	
O_2 capacity (ml O_2/100ml)	16.1		21.4	
P_{CO_2} (mmHg)	32.0	40.0	43.0	48.0
CO_2 concent. (mM/L)	19.6	21.8	25.2	26.3
HCO_3^- (mM/L)	18.8	20.7	24.0	25.0
pH	7.40	7.34	7.38	7.35

Table 3 shows, normal values of oxygen, carbon dioxide and pH in major vessels of both sides of the placenta in man.

WATER AND ELECTROLYTES

Water is exchanged across the placenta more rapidly than any other known substances. The net transfer is an infinitesimal fraction of the total exchange. Despite numerous studies, the mechanisms and pathways of water transfer are not definitely known. Combination of simple diffusion and bulk flow due to small or intermittent gradients in hydrostatic or osmotic pressure seems to be involved, though relative importance of each mechanism is not known. Amnion, chorion, umbilical cord, and fetal skin in the first half of pregnancy are all freely permeable to water. Whatever mechanisms and pathways involved may be, extremely rapid exchange of water molecules among maternal, fetal, and amniotic fluid compartments have been demonstrated repeatedly, in vivo and in vitro, by HELLMAN et al. [69], VOSBURGH et al. [120], PLENTL et al. [73, 78, 121–123], GRAY et al. [124], HUTCHINSON et al. [72, 125], and FRIEDMAN et al. [71]. Exchange rates among these three compartments were calculated in the monkey [71] and in the human [72]. At term of human pregnancy, the exchange rate of water between mother and fetus, probably across the placenta, is very rapid reaching values of 3 to 4 liters per hour. Much slower rate of exchange occurs between amniotic fluid and mother or fetus. Some of the exchange routes of water between amniotic fluid and fetus are well known. The human fetus near term swallows about 500 cc of amniotic fluid per day [126] and urinates probably similar amount of hypotonic urine into the fluid daily [127]. On the other hand, turnover rate of the amniotic fluid is estimated to be much faster, about 500 cc/hr. Therefore, fetal swallowing and urination account for only 4 per cent of total turnover rate of the amniotic fluid. Fetal lung fluid is also considered to be one source of the amniotic fluid, though the flow rate of this fluid is not known in the human. Umbilical cord is also known to be a site for rapid water exchange [122].

Water exchange between the amniotic fluid and fetal circulation across the amnion on the fetal surface of the placenta or into fetal vessels between chorion laeve and amnion have been postulated [128]. Anyway, there must be some other sites for water exchange in the fetus than swallowing and urination, since 25 per cent, possibly more than 50 per cent of the transfer of water from the amniotic fluid takes place via the intermedium of the fetus [122].

PLENTL and associates contributed to the understanding of kinetics of water exchange and a new concept of "circulation of amniotic fluid" emerged, the net flow is directed from mother to fetus, fetus to amniotic fluid, and then amniotic fluid to mother. A gradual rise in water exchange rates among maternal, fetal, and amniotic fluid compartments were described as gestation advanced from 12 weeks to term [73].

Large quantities of sodium and other electrolytes cross the placenta rapidly. Though high exchange rates are known to exist, little information is available on the net transfer rates in vivo. Most of body cell membranes actively pump sodium out of and potassium into the cell, but this active process has not been demonstrated in trophoblastic cells. However, possibility of presence of active transport for these ions in these cells cannot be ruled out [90]. General assumption is that most univalent ions such as sodium, potassium, chloride cross the placenta by simple diffusion and to some degree by "solvent drag" (Fig. 26). They reach equal levels in fetal and maternal blood. When the exchange amount of sodium is compared with its net increments in the growing fetus during a given time, it is evident that far larger amount of sodium is exchanged than is retained.   FLEXNER and associates [68] termed this ratio the "fetal safety factor." It was about 160 at 12 weeks of gestation and rose to 1,130 at term. Similar but larger "safety factor" was noted in water transfer [69]. This safety factor was not apparent with phosphorus [129, 130] and iron [131], at least in guinea pigs and rabbits. This suggests that a general reduction in placental transfer function might produce specific deficiencies.

Higher fetal concentration of phosphate, calcium and iron is maintained in a steady state. Inorganic phosphate readily crosses the placenta against concentration gradient in various species of animals. Active transport of this ion is suggested. A considerable fraction of calcium is transported in the blood in protein bound form. Since the exact information of fetal serum binding capacity for this ion is lacking, active transport process from mother to fetus, though suggestive, has not been definitely demonstrated [132]. Considerable fraction of serum iron is also bound to a specific iron-binding protein, transferrin. The iron-binding capacity of fetal blood is about equal to that of maternal blood and thus, the two to threefold higher concentration of fetal serum iron than that of maternal serum indicates the higher unbound fetal serum iron concentration than maternal one. Active transport process is probably involved.

CARBOHYDRATES

Glucose, the main metabolic fuel for the fetus, has been investigated in many placental transfer studies, but the precise rate of glucose supply to the human fetus is not known. Lack of precise quantitative information is mainly due to lack of precise values of the umbilical blood flow rate, the fact inherent to almost all transfer studies which rely upon the blood flow rate for the net uptake of substances by the fetus. Estimates, however, have been made for the net transfer rate of glucose from mother to fetus and values range from 18 [90] to 22 mg/min in the human fetus near term (see the previous section "Fetal metabolism and hormones," pp. 29–33). WIDDAS [133] demonstrated that a carrier mediated facilitated diffusion would be required to account for the observed rapid transfer rate of glucose in the sheep. Existence of facilitated diffusion with carrier system is further supported by findings in various animals and human that naturally occurring D-glucose [99] or D-xylose [89] is transferred more rapidly than L-form of these sugars (stereospecificity), and that glucose (aldohexose) is transferred more rapidly than fructose (ketohexose) or other sugars with similar molecular weights [134–139] (competitive transfer). Glucose concentration in the human uterine venous blood is higher than that in the umbilical venous blood. The transplacental glucose gradient is in the range of 20–25 mg/100 cc [140, 141]. Similar gradient was reported in the Rhesus monkey [142]. Probably part of the maternal to fetal glucose concentrations gradient is due to placental metabolism of glucose [136].

The human placenta contains large amounts of glycogen, most of which is synthesized from maternal glucose. Its physiologic role in carbohydrate metabolism in the fetus is not clear. It has been shown in in-vitro study by VILLEE [143] that placental glycogen concentration declines as pregnancy advances, from a maximum concentration at 8 weeks (fertilization age) to the lowest at term. In contrast, glycogen concentration in the fetal liver increases after 9 weeks of age as gestation proceeds. It is suggested that the placenta acts to regulate the blood glucose level of the fetus in early part of pregnancy until the fetal liver is able to assume this function. There is a continuous exchange of glucose between maternal glucose, placental glycogen, and fetal glucose.

It is known that in ungulates (cattle, sheep, and goats) fructose is the main carbohydrate in fetal blood and continuously produced by the placenta from maternal glucose with production rate independent of glucose concentration [144], and that the placenta contains only small amounts of glycogen. Although fructose is present in small amounts in human fetal blood (less than 5 mg/100 cc), its concentration is still somewhat higher than that in the maternal blood, and the human placenta is capable of producing fructose from maternal glucose [145]. However, its role in fetal metabolism is not known. Other monosaccharides, sorbitol [90] and meso-inositol [146] are also present in higher concentrations in fetal than maternal blood. While sorbitol can be produced by the placenta from glucose, the placenta does not transfer or synthesize inositol. Their role in fetal metabolism is unknown.

In-vitro permeability studies show some correlation between molecular weight of carbohydrates and their ability to cross the chorion. While pentoses, hexoses, sucrose and other sugars with molecular weight up to about 700 all cross this membrane readily, inulin (M.W. 991) and various dextrans (M.W. 10,000) do not cross it [93].

PROTEINS

The fetus synthesizes most of its proteins from amnio acids transferred across the placenta from the maternal circulation with the one possible exception of the gamma globulins. It has been confirmed that free amino acids concentrations in fetal blood are higher than in maternal blood [89, 147–151]. The fetal to maternal ratio in normal pregnancy at term ranges from 1.2 to 4.0 with a mean ratio of about 1.8 [39]. The amino acids are transferred by carrier-mediated active transport against concentration gradients. This is evidenced by following facts: 1) naturally occurring L-histidine crosses the placenta more rapidly than D-histidine [77, 98]; 2) competition exists between amino acids such as histidine and glycine for transfer [147]; 3) the transport system becomes saturated at high concentration [89]; 4) the transfer rate is decreased in the presence of poisons for oxidative metabolism such as sodium cyanide or 2,4-dinitrophenol [152].

Polypeptides cross the placenta very slowly or not at all. Insulin crosses only slowly and in physiologically insignificant amount [153]. Fetal adrenal hypoplasia develops in an anencephalic fetus and normal thyroid development fails in decapitated animal fetuses [154, 155] indicating the inability of maternal ACTH and TSH to cross the placenta.

Proteins are selectively transported across the placenta in varing amounts. Large amounts of gamma G immuno globulin (M.W. 165,000) is transported to the fetus, while smaller amounts of albumin (M.W. 65,000), acid glycoprotein (M.W. 44,000), and transferrin (M.W. 90,000) are also transferred across the placenta. Only small amounts of fibrinogen (M.W. 350,000) and macroglobulin (M.W. 1,000,000) appear in the fetal blood [156]. The fetal plasma concentration of gamma G immuno globulin (IgG) becomes about the same with the maternal one after 26 weeks of gestation [156]. This fact offers one evidence of transfer of protein from mother to fetus, for the fetus cannot synthesize gamma globulin.

Because of the large molecular size of these proteins and the membrane specificity in their transfer, it is thought that they cross the placenta by pinocytosis. Unlike the rodents, the primate probably transfers proteins directly across the placenta, not via amniotic fluid and fetal gastrointestinal tract [93, 108].

Urea, nitrogenous end-product of amino acids and protein metabolism is found to be in equal concentration in maternal and fetal blood at term, but in much higher concentration in the amniotic fluid. There is a rapid exchange of urea between the maternal and fetal blood and an appreciably slower exchange with the amniotic fluid [75].

LIPIDS AND STEROIDS

Fetal lipids probably originate from both free fatty acids transferred across the placenta and fetal synthesis from carbohydrate and acetate [157, 158]. Free (unesterified) fatty acids such as linoleic, margaric, palmitic, and stearic acids and acetate are rapidly exchanged across the placenta by simple diffusion [159–161]. There was no significant difference in the transfer rate of fatty acids whether they were saturated or unsaturated, whether the carbon chain length was in even or odd number, or whether they were given singly or as a group in perfused guinea pig placenta [159]. Cholesterol passes the placenta slowly, the maternal cholesterol accounting for only about 10 to 20% of the fetal cholesterol in the rat [157]. This might be explained by placental consumption of maternal cholesterol as precursor for the very active steroid synthesis [93]. It is generally thought that no phospholipids cross the placenta intact from mother to fetus, and that phospholipids present in the fetus are synthesized de novo in fetal tissues [158]. Maternal phospholipids are probably metabolized in the placenta during transfer with enzymatic hydrolysis of the phosphate group, yielding free phosphate to fetal circulation, or new fetal phospholipids are resynthesized in the placenta and released to the fetus [158, 162]. Relatively high levels of estrogens, progesterone, and other steroids exist in both maternal and fetal bloods. High levels of estrogens and progesterone are mainly due to synthesis of these hormones by the feto-placental unit. Many steroids undergo enzymatic alteration during transit through the placenta and such alteration may affect their transfer. Such precursors from mother and fetus as cholesterol, pregnenolone, pregnenolone sulfate, dehydroisoandrosterone sulfate and its 16 α-hydroxylated form are converted to progesterone and estrogens in the placenta, and then released into maternal and fetal circulation. Cortisol readily crosses the placenta from mother to fetus [163], and the maternal to fetal concentration gradient is 3:1 which parallels the maternal to fetal concentration gradient of cortisol binding globulin (transcortin), but cortisone does not readily cross the placenta [164].

In general, the naturally occurring steroids are lipid soluble and are almost completely bound to protein in circulating plasma. They are made water soluble in the liver by conjugation with glucuronide or sulfate. These conjugated compounds can then be excreted in bile and urine. As described previously, the water soluble or conjugated form of steroids do not cross the placenta very easily. On the contrary, the free or unconjugated, lipid soluble steroids cross the placenta easily. In addition, protein binding capacities of the maternal and fetal bloods influence the final steady state concentrations of steroids in the two blood compartments.

Immature glucuronyl transferase activity in the fetal liver appears to be beneficial for the fetal disposition of bilirubin. Most of the fetal bilirubin cannot be conjugated with glucuronide, and unconjugated bilirubin is lipid soluble and thus can be transferred to the mother across the placenta quite easily.

VITAMINS

Contrary to the general rule that lipid soluble solutes cross the placenta more readily than water soluble ones, water soluble vitamins (the B-group and C) exist in the fetal blood in higher concentration than in the maternal blood. Thus, active transport by the placenta has been assumed for their transfer mechanism, but there is no definitive evidence for active transport. Some of these vitamins are metabolized in the placental cells during exchange. In addition, protein binding capacity may be greater in the fetal blood, resulting in greater total concentrations while the concentrations of unbound vitamin may be equal in the maternal and fetal circulations. Flavin adenine dinucleotide, a riboflavin precursor, is transported to the placenta, and there it is converted to free riboflavin (Vitamin B_2) and released to the fetal circulation. While the concentration of the total riboflavin in the fetal blood was only slightly higher than that in the maternal blood, the fetal concentration of free riboflavin was about five times greater than the maternal one [165]. These findings suggest either active transport, or placental metabolism of the precursor and low permeability of the placenta to back diffusion of the free riboflavin. L-ascorbic acid (vitamin C) is present in the fetal blood in two to three times higher concentration than in the maternal blood. The suggested mechanism again involves conversion of the permeable precursor to impermeable vitamin C. The precursor, dehydroascorbic acid, readily crosses the guinea pig placenta [166] and its concentration is about equal in the maternal and fetal plasma. This precursor is readily converted to L-ascorbic acid, the active vitamin that crosses the placenta slowly if at all [166].

The concentrations of lipid soluble vitamins (A, D, E, and K) in the fetal blood are less than or equal to those in the maternal blood. Regarding vitamin A, it is reported that carotene is probably the form of the vitamin that is transferred by the placenta and that the fetal liver resythesizes it into vitamin A [167].

ABNORMAL FETAL GROWTH

Abnormal fetal growth is discussed here briefly, since it has considerable clinical implications.

1. FACTORS AFFECTING ABNORMAL FETAL GROWTH

Abnormality in any one of previously described factors affecting fetal growth would result in deviations in fetal growth. Thus, *deranged fetal metabolism* caused either by genetic abnormalities or by acquired disorder results in deviated fetal growth. A primordial dwarf or various congenital anomalies of the fetus, or chronic fetal infections are associated with low birth weight, which is caused by decreased rate of utilization of nutrients by the fetus per unit weight. The obverse is true for diabetic pregnancy. The fetus in the uncontrolled diabetic pregnancy responds with increased secretion of insulin to fetal hyperglycemia which is caused by maternal hyperglycemia. Fetal hyperinsulinism is responsible for excessive birth weight of the newborn in uncontrolled diabetic pregnancy because of lipotrophic and protein anabolic action of insulin. *Maternal undernutrition and/or malnutrition* will result in a reduced concentration of some essential nutrient in the uterine artery and thus intrauterine growth retardation. It may also affect fetal growth indirectly by producing some placental lesions. Among all the factors, genetic and environmental, the most important one is *disturbances in placental transfer function* because of its high incidence, severe effects and possibility for clinical management. It follows that disturbances in any factors affecting placental transfer would cause fetal growth retardation. Above all, disturbance in uterine and umbilical blood flow perfusing the placenta will be the most influential, since transfer of rapidly diffusible substances such as respiratory gases or glucose, which are vital for normal metabolism and growth of the fetus, are "flow limited" rather than "diffusion limited" as described previously. *A chronic reduction in the uterine blood flow rate* is probably the most common cause for retarded fetal growth. This condition can be caused by various diseases such as renal disease, preeclampsia, cardiac disease with reduced cardiac output, chronically increased uterine tonus of the mother. Though definitive cause is unknown, it is known that cigarette smoking mothers generally produce lighter babies than non-smoking mothers. A recent report [168] indicates that the uterine blood flow rate dropped by 25 to 50 per cent in the pregnant monkey when pharmacologic dose of nicotine was administered to the mother in that species. Thus, smoking is probably one of causes for reduced uterine blood flow. This would explain slow fetal growth in maternal smoking. Fetal growth retardaion was experimentally produced in the rat by ligation of one uterine artery [169]. *A chronic reduction in the umbilical flow rate* would certainly decrease the fetal growth rate. However, definitive information on the control of umbilical blood flow in human pregnancy is lacking and most of knowledge is limited to data derived from acute experiment in sheep. DAWES [31] observed vasoconstriction in the umbilical circulation in fetal lamb near term during hypoxemia which was produced by administering 10% O_2 to the ewe. He considers this umbilical vasoconstriction might be due in part to reflex vasoconstriction on the intraabdominal portion of the umbilical vessels which are only part of the umbilical vessels definitely known to have innervation, and partly due to liberation of fetal catecholamines from adrenals and their effect upon the extraabdominal portion of the umbilical vessels. However, degree of vasoconstriction was small though hypoxemia was severe enough to cause the femoral arterial Po_2 to fall from 25 to 8 mmHg. There was only a minor degree of umbilical vasoconstriction or none in response to extreme hypoxemia in younger fetal lambs. DAWES concludes that the umbilical vessels in vivo are so unreactive to changes in blood gas tensions. Valuable as they are, these observations are based on acute experiments where alteration in a few variables (blood gas and catecholamines) are made in one species of animal (sheep). Until we obtain more information from chronic experiments with alteration in various variables known to cause vasoconstriction or dilatation in addition to blood gas and catecholamines (e.g. nicotine, estrogen) in various species of animals including subhuman primate, we should consider that a chronic reduction in the umbilical blood flow might be responsible for some fetal growth retardation. The devastating effect of the reduced umbilical flow is demonstrated in the case of monozygotic twins with vascular anastomoses, through which one member has unequally exchanged blood with his partner, resulting in discordant twins. *A decrease in the exchange surface area of the placenta* occurs in such clinical situations as placental infarction or intervillous space coagulation. *An increase in the total surface area of the fetus* as seen in multiple pregnancy usually retard fetal growth. Most twins deviate their growth rate subnormally during late gestation, but they have an accelerated rate of growth after birth, reaching median levels for single-born infants by one year of age [170], thus indicating that unfavorable intrauterine environment rather than genetic factors is primarily responsible for the subnormal growth of twins in late fetal life. Tissue abnormalities in twins at birth also suggest malnutrition is the main cause of their subnormal growth. According to NAEYE [171], in twins whose birth weights are 75 per cent or more of single-birth standards, the weight deficit is mainly due to a subnormal cytoplasmic content of cells in various body organs. Thus, placental transfer function cannot often meet the increased fetal demand, and relative placental insufficiency occurs in late twin pregnancy. In triplets or quadruplets growth retardation will worsen. *A reduced rate of active transport function of the placenta* would certainly retard the fetal growth since amino acids are transported to the fetus by this mechanism. In preeclamptic pregnancy a loss of the ability to concentrate amino acids in the fetal plasma occurs [21].

In actuality, however, these factors known to cause abnormal fetal growth are often not recognizable at birth of infants with retarded growth, mainly because some of the main factors such as "placental insufficiency" often occur without clinically recognizable maternal diseases and escape the obstetrician's surveillance. At present we have no reliable methods to determine fetal weight. Fetal cephalometry with ultrasonography has been extensively used recently and it is quite accurate for determining the gestational age, but in predicting birth weight of the fetus whose biparietal diameter is measured by this technique shortly before birth, it is disappointing. What concerns us most is not merely size or weight of the fetus, but functional maturity. The reason why we are so concerned about fetal weight is the fact that the fetal weight increases, in general, in parallel with functional maturity. In this respect, newly developed technique by GLUCK and associates [172] to determine phospholipids in the amniotic fluid for fetal lung maturity has brought about profound excitement in clinical obstetrics and is being used in various institutes. It has been known in various animals that the fetal lung secretes fluids and that this fluid appears to flow into the amniotic fluid. Since lecithin is the major component of the surface-active alveolar-lining layer, lecithin biosynthesis should reflect the status of alveolar stability. As fetal lung matures, lecithin concentration in the lung fluid should increase, and that in the amniotic fluid should also increase, if the lung fluid really flows into the amniotic fluid. GLUCK showed this is true. There was a sharp spurt in concentration of lecithin in the amniotic fluid at 35 weeks of human pregnancy while another phospholipid, sphingomyelin concentration remained the same. Since amniotic fluid volume is quite variable among individual patients, a ratio of lecithin and sphingomyelin concentration was used and originally it was reported that this ratio of 4 or above indicates the mature fetal lung of at least 35 weeks of gestation. Recently this ratio has been lowered to 2 or above, but it seems to be well accepted by various investigators. Criterion upon which reliability of this test depends is its ability to predict whether the newborn develops respiratory distress syndrome or not. So far the result has been excellent. However, strict control study has not been reported yet. And we have no information how much fluid is secreted from the fetal lung to the amniotic fluid in primates. When these studies are done, and when they prove that this test accurately reflects fetal lung maturity, not gestational age, then this method will be established as a tremendous test for determining fetal lung maturity. Thus, as far as fetal lung is concerned, detection of maturity seems very promising. But what about maturity of the central nervous system, or the cardiovascular system, or the whole fetus? We have no way to detect maturity in these systems.

However, since fetal growth and maturity are primarily dependent upon placental function, reliable tests on placental function would give us valuable information about the present and future performance of the fetus regarding growth and maturity. Two tests are available to us. One is estriol assay in urine or plasma of the mother, and is currently in routine use in many institutes. Since the fetus plays an important role in contributing precursors for the synthesis of estriol, some fetal function as well as placental function would be detected by monitoring maternal estriol level serially, though day-to-day variation of estriol in the urine is quite wide in the same normal pregnant woman. Though the clinical usefulness of this test as corroborative evidence of fetal death is well established when estriol value drops truely below the normal range, it remains to be proved whether a clinically useful, early detection of placental malfunction or abnormal condition of the fetus is possible by this test. We need the control study which provides evidence that treatment based on maternal estriol assay has improved fetal salvage more than that achieved by the equivalent treatment without estriol assay. However, prospect for value of this test is very promising. Another test for placental function is new and used in relatively few institutes. It is oxytocin challenge test (stress test) [173]. Basic concept behind this test is that in the clinical condition of so-called "chronic utero-placental insufficiency" there is reduced margin of fetal reserve, so that the fetus is less able to withstand the stresses of pregnancy and labor. As the temporary and innocuous stress, uterine activity produced by the mini- mumly necessary amount of oxytocin is used to decrease intervillous space blood flow. While stress is applied, fetal heart rate and uterine activity are monitored electronically on the maternal abdomen. The stress would exceed the fetal margin of reserve if the reserve were low, and the fetus would respond with certain specific fetal heart rate changes in relation to the uterine activity. These specific responses are persistent late deceleration of fetal heart rate occurring repeatedly with most uterine contractions [173], which are early indicators of fetal compromise. Thus, the test is positive and immediate delivery of the fetus, often by cesarean section is indicated if the fetus is judged to be mature enough to have better chance for extra-uterine survival. If the margin of fetal reserve were adequate, no fetal response would occur. Then, the test could be repeated a few days later or what- ever intervals as deemed necessary depending on high risk obstetrical situations. This test is attractive since it offers an individual test for each fetus without comparing the test result to any normal range or standards. However, it is qualitative test, positve or negative. How early in the chronic process of placental insufficiency the test becomes positive, to what degree the fetus is compromised when it is positive, how long after the positive test the fetus grows on without the stress, the test will not tell us. But what clinically matters in the end is to get better fetal salvage rate with this kind of test than without it. For this

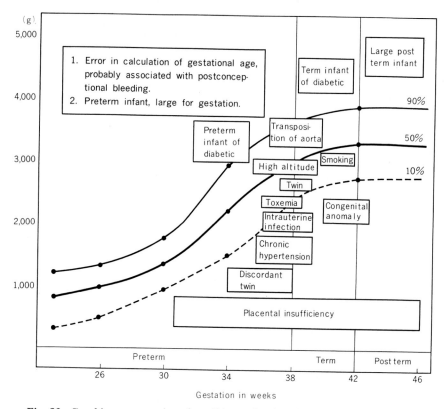

Fig. 36 Graphic representation of conditions related to deviations of fetal growth. The boxes roughly approximate birth weight (except for placental insufficiency and preterm large-for-gestational age babies 1 and 2) and gestational age when the condition is likely to occur. (Modified from LUBCHENCO, L.O. et al.: Factors influencing fetal growth. In: Nutricia Symposium—Aspects of Praematurity and Dysmaturity. Jonxis, J.H.P., Visser, H.K.A., and Troelstra, J.A. (eds.) H.E. Stenfert Kroese N.V., Leiden, 1968.)

reason this stress test also needs strict control study, which it has not had yet, before it is fully established as a diagnostic measure for chronic placental insufficiency.

2. CLINICAL CONDITIONS RELATED TO ABNORMAL FETAL GROWTH

Various conditons related to deviations of fetal growth (dysmaturity) are presented in Fig. 36. There are two categories in dysmaturity, large-for-gestational age babies and small-for-gestational age babies, the latter being far more common. Recently LUBCHENCO and her associates [174] have presented detailed anthropometric analyses of newborns with abnormal intrauterine growth.

1) LARGE-FOR-GESTATIONAL AGE BABIES
a) Preterm large babies
There are two kinds of large babies of short gestation. One group is true preterm babies who have grown to unusually heavy weight for the gestation age up to the time of birth. These babies after birth have the difficulties associated with preterm birth in proportion to the degree of prematurity [174]. BATTAGLIA and associates [6] suggest that these babies

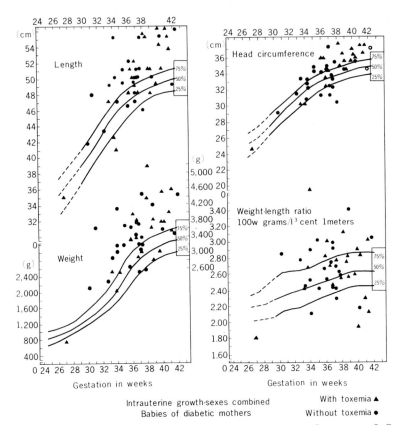

Fig. 37 Intrauterine growth of infants of diabetic mother. (From LUBCHENCO, L.O. et al.: Factors influencing fetal growth. In: Nutricia Symposium—Aspects of Praematurity and Dysmaturity. Jonxis, J.H.P., Visser, H.K.A., and Troelstra, J.A. (eds.) H.E. Stenfert Kroese N.V., Leiden, 1968.)

probably represent a form of pathophysiology characterized by an excessive growth rate. Another group is preterm large babies who are much larger than the 90th percentile and who behave like term infants. Possibly the mothers of these babies had menstrual-like bleeding after conception and mistook such a bleeding as her last normal menstrual period, thus gestational age being calculated erroneously. This episode of bleeding possibly would carry with it a poor infant prognosis regardless of its true gestational age at the time of birth [6].

Hence, these preterm large babies, whether they blong to one group or another, are at high risk and this fact is readily recognized by ERHARDT and associates' [4] data based on enormous number of 650,000 deliveries in New York City from 1958 to 1961 which indicate these babies have much higher perinatal mortality than term babies of the same weight.

b)   Post-term large infants

Some fetuses continue to grow progressively even post-term, presumably because of adequate placental transfer function [7]. Because of increased chance of birth trauma these babies are at high risk.

c)   Babies of mothers with diabetes mellitus (Fig. 37)

Diabetic and prediabetic mothers are known to often produce heavy babies for their gestational age. Their length and head circumference are also large for gestational age. The ratio of weight and length, however, scatter above and below the median curve, indicating that weight is not consistently excessive for length. They are at increased risk whether they are born preterm, term, post-term. These babies face various complications, such as respiratory distress syndrome, prematurity, and hypoglycemia in case of preterm delivery; death in utero, birth trauma, and hypoglycemia in case of term or post-term delivery.

Since incidence of intrauterine fetal death in diabetic pregnancy in general becomes high after 36 to 37 weeks of gestation, no diabetic pregnancy should be allowed to last beyond term. Timing of delivery must be individualized depending upon severity of diabetes and maturity and condition of the fetus.

d) Babies with transposition of the aorta

Unlike other congenital anomalies of the fetus, transposition of the aorta of the fetus is associated with heavy birth weight. The birth weight of 117 infants with complete transposition of the great vessels was reported to have tendency of being higher than the average birth weight of normal infants, difference in average being about 300 g [175]. The mechanism is unknown, but high incidence of diabetes mellitus in families of patients with transposition of the great vessels was noted [175].

2) SMALL-FOR-GESTATIONAL AGE BABIES

a) Babies with intrauterine undernutrition

Intrauterine undernutrition is meant to include a variety of conditions which result in decreased supply of nutrients to the fetus due to placental insufficiency and/or inadequate uterine blood flow. Placental insufficiency is a vague term, but generally used to refer to the insufficient placental function as the result of pathologic changes in the placenta, such as gross infarction, avascularity of the chorionic villi, excessive deposition of fibrin in the intervillous space, and so forth. The net effect of these lesions is to reduce the effective surface area for placental exchange, but it is extremely difficult to separate the effect of these changes from the effect of a reduced uterine blood flow to the placenta. Hence, it would be more appropriate to use the term "uteroplacental insufficiency" [21].

Truely post-term babies (those born beyond 42 weeks of gestation) are often considered postmature. They sometimes experience intrauterine undernutrition due to placental insufficiency. The nutritional deprivation is brief but may be severe. While such fetuses grow in length and head circumference, they lose weight. Their morbidity is due to chronic hypoxia in utero leading to passage of meconium into the amniotic fluid. They may have hypoglycemia. Respiratory distress and cerebral hypoxia develop sometimes. Placental insufficiency may also occur in term and preterm babies and mild or brief (near term) growth retardation in weight usually occurs while length and head circumference are not affected.

Undernutrition of the fetus after 33 to 35 weeks of gestation is generally seen in twin pregnancies. Fig. 38 shows median growth of twins in comparison with growth curves for single-born infants. Intrauterine growth retardation begins as early as 29 weeks of gestation in monochorionic twins and at 33 weeks in dichorionic twins. By 42 weeks the median weight for the former falls below 10th percentile [176]. Weight, length, and head circumference are all significantly reduced. In case of discordant twins, the larger of twins is not significantly different from the singleton in intrauterine growth, but the smaller twin is markedly retarded in growth in all dimensions.

Chronic cardiovascular disease, hypertensive disorders with pregnancy, small heart size, and smoking in the mother often result in small-for-gestational age babies. The common factor in these conditions seems to be a reduced uterine blood flow. Fig. 39 shows the intrauterine growth pattern in pregnancy complicated with hypertensive cardiovascular disease.

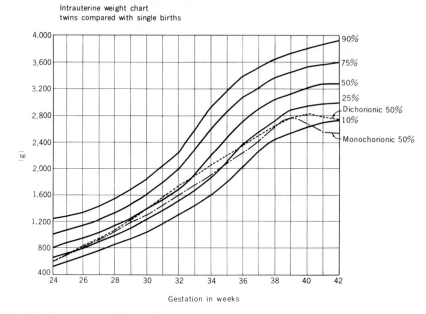

Fig. 38   Comparison of the median weight of twins with Lubchenco's intrauterine growth curves for singletons. (From Naeye, R.L. et al.: Pediatrics **37**; 409, 1966.)

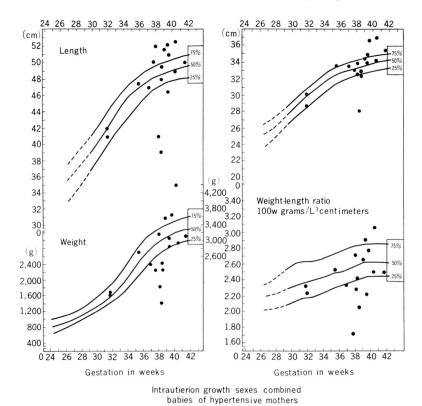

Intrautierion growth sexes combined
babies of hypertensive mothers

Fig. 39   Intrauterine growth of infants born to mothers with hypertension. (From Lubchenco, L.O. et al.: Factors influencing fetal growth. In: Nutricia Symposium—Aspects of Praematurity and Dysmaturity. Jonxis, J.H.P., Visser, H.K.A., and Troelstra, J.A. (eds.) H.E. Stenfert Kroese N.V., Leiden, 1968.)

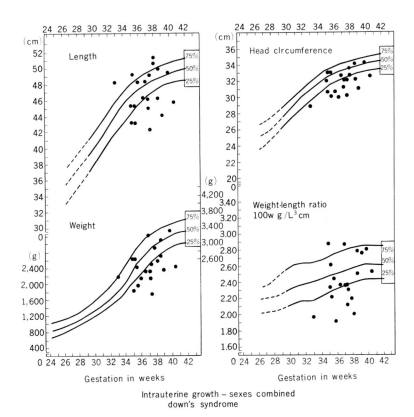

Fig. 40 Intrauterine growth of infants with Down's syndrome. (From LUBCHENCO, L.O. et al.: Factors influencing fetal growth. In: Nutricia Symposium—Aspects of Praematurity and Dysmaturity. Jonxis, J.H.P., Visser, H.K.A., and Troelstra, J.A. (eds.) H.E. Stenfert Kroese N.V. Leiden, 1968.)

Many are normally growing, but one-third of the fetuses are very light weight for gestation. Fewer have growth retardation in length and only one shows a head circumference below 10th percentile.

Another condition affecting fetal growth retardation, though moderate, is high altitude. Chronic maternal hypoxia might be working as a growth-limiting factor to some extent. Weight, length, and head size of newborns in Lake County, Colorado (10,000 ft above sea level) were all reduced as compared with those of babies born elsewhere in U.S.A. [177].

Recently, prenatal diagnosis and management of the small-for-gestational age fetus has been described practically [178], reflecting growing concern in clinical obstetrics for this relatively new, but important entity, intrauterine growth retardation.

b)   Babies with congenital abnormalities

Various congenital anomalies of the fetus are known to be associated with growth retardation. The majority of them progress to term. These anomalies include Down's syndrome or other trisomy, Turner's syndrome, congenital heart disease other than transposition of the aorta, osteogenesis imperfecta, dwarfism, and so forth [174]. Fig. 40 shows the position on the intrauterine growth chart of newborn babies with Down's syndrome. These babies are light at all gestational ages. Though their lengths are normal, head sizes are significantly reduced.

c)   Intrauterine infections

Various intrauterine infections often result in fetal growth retardation. They include

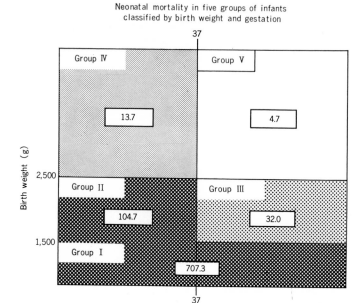

Fig. 41 Neonatal mortality in five categories of infants classified by birth weight and gestational age. Data are based on large number of single white live-born infants in New York City in a three-year period 1957–1959. (From YERUSHALMY, J.: J. Pediatr. **71**; 164, 1967.)

such diseases as extended rubella syndrome, cytomegalic inclusion disease, toxoplasmosis, and syphilis. It is said that in congenital rubella, the median birth weight is below the 10th percentile, median length between the 25th and 50th percentile, and that median head circumference is between the 10th and 25th percentile [174].

It is extremely important to differentiate dysmaturity from prematurity. Low birth weight infants do not represent a homogeneous group and they consist of premature babies who were born before 37 weeks of gestation with birth weight less than 2,500 g, and dysmature babies who were born at, or near, full term and yet weight less than 2,500 g at birth. The low birth weight in dysmature babies is presumed to reflect intrauterine growth retardation. These two groups of infants with low birth weight has quite different neonatal mortality, the dysmature infants having lower mortality but a higher incidence of severe congenital anomalies than the premature infants. Fig. 41 shows difference in neonatal mortality in five groups of infants classified by birth weight and gestational age.

CONCLUSION

It seems clear that the fetal growth is regulated by many factors which are interrelated with each other intimately. A dominant factor, however, is fetal nutrition which is primarily dependent upon placental transfer function. Though numerous studies have been done on placental transfer, little is known about exact transfer mechanisms, exact magnitude of each factor influencing placental transfer, and transfer rates of nutrients in the primate. Without definitive information about these basic matters it is natural that we do not possess reliable means to assess the fetal growth and functional maturity, and that we are so often confronted with dysmature babies who might have grown and matured normally if we had known the growth retarding processes and employed corrective measures if available. Regarding other factors relating to fetal nutrition, information about fetal metabolism and hormones is also insufficient. Knowledge on fetal circulation is far from complete, especially on regional organ blood flows. Recent emphasis on maternal nutrition in pre-natal care is healthy sign that we have turned more of our attention to fetal nutrition than before. Traditionally medical school curricula have paid little attention on fetal growth and maternal nutrition. It is about time for every medical student, obstetrician-gynecologist, and pediatrician to become familiar with fetal growth pattern and related factors and to get full knowledge on maternal nutrition.

Through evolutional processes the fetus has attained marvellous adjustments to survive and grow in the intrauterine environment. Low fetal partial pressure of oxygen is necessary for integrity of his circulation, and yet the fetal tissues are not hypoxic by virtue of increase in cardiac output, oxygen carrying capacity and affinity of hemoglobin to oxygen. Adequate rate of constant feeding of the fetus with glucose through the placenta is probably the main feature of the fetal homeostasis to secure main metabolic fuel and maintain constantly the adequate rate of insulin secretion. Since the fetus is growing and doing so even with different growth rates, fetal homeostasis must be maintained at different levels, successively.

The fetus also has remarkable autonomy. The fetus synthesizes, in a rate set by his own genetic program, his own protein, fat, and glycogen from amino acids, fatty acids, and glucose supplied from the mother through the placenta, provided these nutrients are supplied in an adequate rate.

The fetus is capable of maintaining adequate homeostasis and autonomy if all the growth related factors, especially placental transfer function, are within normal limits. However, there is a certain limit in the growth related factors beyond which maintenance of adequate fetal homeostasis and autonomy are no longer possible. For example, relentlessly repetitive hyperglycemia in the fetus in the maternal diabetes would result in hypersecretion of the fetal insulin, which, in turn, would promote fat and protein synthesis and cause the abnormally large fetus. The severely reduced uterine blood flow in the hypertensive pregnancy would limit supply of nutrients to the fetus to such a degree that he can no longer maintain adequate growth. The crucial point is to determine the limit of each growth relating factor beyond which fetal homeostasis and autonomy cannot be adequately maintained and deviations in the fetal growth result. This determination of normal limits is possible only when every factor is quantitatively and accurately determined.

Finally, it is extremely important for each large institute to construct its own normal fetal growth curves, whether percentile or standard deviation method, and use them for identifying the position of every newborn infant in the normal growth curves. Those infants whose standings are found to be outside 10th–90th percentile (or, perhaps, 5th to 95th percentile) should be treated as high risk dysmature babies.

ACKNOWLEDGEMENT

The author is grateful to many investigators and publishers who kindly gave me permission to use their figures and tables for this article.

REFERENCES

1. World Health Organization, Expert Committee on Maternal and Child Health: Public health aspects of low birth weight. WHO Technical Report. Series No. 217, Geneva, 1961.
2. LUBCHENCO, L. O., HAUSMAN, C., DRESSLER, M. and BOYD, E.: Intrauterine growth as estimated from liveborn weight data at 24 to 42 weeks of gestation. Pediatrics 32; 793, 1963.
3. HENDRICKS, C. H.: Patterns of fetal and placental growth: The second half of normal pregnancy. Obstet. Gynec. 24; 357, 1964.
4. ERHARDT, C. L., JOSHI, G. B., NELSON, F. G., KROLL, B. H. and WEINER L.: Influence of weight and gestation of perinatal and neonatal mortality by ethnic group. Amer. J. Public Health 54; 1841, 1964.
5. ANCTIL, A. O., JOSHI, G. B., LUCAS, W. E., LITTLE, W. A. and CALLAGAN, D. A.: Prematurity: A more precise approach to identification. Obstet. Gynec. 24; 716, 1964.
6. BATTAGLIA, F. C., FRAZIER, T. M. and HELLEGERS, A. E.: Birth weight, gestational age, and pregnancy outcome, with special reference to high birth weight—low gestational age infant. Pediatrics 37; 417, 1966.
7. GRUENWALD, P.: Growth of the human fetus. Amer. J. Obstet. Gynec. 94; 1112, 1966.
8. VAN DEN BERG, B. J. and YERUSHALMY, J.: The relationship of the rate of intrauterine growth of infants of low birth weight to mortality, morbidity, and congenital anomalies. Pediatrics 69; 531, 1966.
9. GRUENWALD, P., FUNAKAWA, H., MITANI, S., NISHIMURA, T. and TAKEUCHI, S.: Influence of environmental factors on foetal growth in man. Lancet 1; 1026, 1967.
10. YERUSHALMY, J.: The classification of newborn infants by birth weight and gestational age. J. Pediatr. 71; 164, 1967.
11. THOMSON, A. M., BILLEWICZ, W. Z. and HYTTEN, F. E.: The assessment of fetal growth. J. Obstet. Gynaec. Brit. Cwlth. 75; 903, 1968.
12. USHER, R. and McLEAN, F.: Intrauterine growth of live-born Caucasian infants at sea level: Standards obtained from measurements in 7 dimensions of infants born between 25 and 44 weeks of gestation. J. Pediatr. 74; 901, 1969.
13. WALKER, J.: Weight of the human fetus and of its placenta. Cold Spring Harbor Symp. Quant. Biol. 19; 39, 1954.
14. STREETER, G. L.: Weight, sitting height, head size, foot length, and menstrual age of the human embryo. Contrib. Embryol. 11; 143, 1920.
15. GRUENWALD, P.: Chronic fetal distress and placental insufficiency. Biol. Neonat. 5; 215, 1963.
16. McKEOWN, T. and RECORD, R. G.: The influence of placental size on foetal growth in man, with special reference to multiple pregnancy. J. Endocrin. 9; 418, 1953.
17. WINICK, M. and NOBLE, A.: Quantitative changes in DNA, RNA, and protein during prenatal and postnatal growth in the rat. Develop. Biol. 12; 451, 1965.
18. WINICK, M. and NOBLE, A.: Quantitative changes in ribonucleic acids and protein during normal growth of rat placenta. Nature 212; 34, 1966.
19. WINICK, M., COSCIA, A. and NOBLE, A.: Cellular growth in human placenta. 1. Normal placental growth. Pediatrics 39; 248, 1967.
20. WINICK, M. and NOBLE, A.: Cellular response in rats during malnutrition at various ages. J. Nutrition 89; 300, 1966.
21. PAGE, E. W., VILLEE, C. A. and VILLEE, D. B.: Human Reproduction. W. B. Saunders, Philadelphia, 1972.
22. PAYNE, P. R. and WHEELER, E. F.: Growth of the foetus. Nature 215; 849, 1967.
23. DAWES, G. S., MOTT, J. C. and WIDDICOMBE, J. G.: The foetal circulation in the lamb. J. Physiol. 126; 563, 1954.
24. ACHESON, G. H., DAWES, G. S. and MOTT, J. C.: Oxygen comsumption and the arterial oxygen saturation in foetal and new-born lambs. J. Physiol. 135; 623, 1957.
25. DAWES, G. S. and MOTT, J. C.: The increase in oxygen consumption of the lamb after birth. J. Physiol. 146; 295, 1959.
26. ROMNEY, S. L., REID, D. E., METCALFE, J. and BURWELL, C. S.: Oxygen ultilization by the human fetus in utero. Amer. J. Obstet. Gynec. 70; 791, 1955.

27. SUZUKI, K., PLENTL, A. A. and ADAMSONS, K.: Exchange of carbon dioxide in the pregnant Rhesus monkey: Multicompartmental analysis of carbon dioxide kinetics. J. Clin. Invest. **48;** 1967, 1969.

28. SMITH, C. A.: The Physiology of the Newborn Infant. Charles C Thomas, Springfield, Illinois, 1959.

29. DAWES, G. S. and SHELLEY, H. J.: Fate of glucose in newly delivered foetal lambs. Nature **194;** 296, 1962.

30. ALEXANDER, D. P., BRITTON, H. G. and NIXON, D. A.: Maintenance of the isolated foetus. Brit. Med. Bull. **22;** 9, 1966.

31. DAWES, G. S.: Foetal and Neonatal Physiology. Year Book, Chicago, Illinois, 1968.

32. PAGE, E. W.: Human fetal nutrition and growth. Amer. J. Obstet. Gynec. **104;** 378, 1969.

33. THOMAS, K., DE GASPARO, M. and HOET, J. J.: Insulin levels in the umbilical vein and in the umbilical artery of newborns of normal and gestational diabetic mothers. Diabetologia **3;** 299, 1967.

34. VILLEE, C. A. and LORING, J. M.: Alternative pathways of carbohydrate metabolism in foetal and adult tissues. Biochem. J. **81;** 488, 1961.

35. JOST, A. and JACQUOT, R.: Recherches sur les facteurs endocriniens de la change en glycogene du foie foetale chez le lapin (avec des indications sur le gycogene placentaire). Ann. Endocrinol. **16;** 849, 1955.

36. SHELLEY, H. J. and NELIGAN, G. A.: Neonatal hypoglycaemia. Brit. Med. Bull. **22;** 34, 1966.

37. SHELLEY, H. J.: Carbohydrate reserve in the newborn infant. Brit. Med. J. **1;** 273, 1964.

38. WIDDOWSON, E. M.: Chemical composition of newly born mammals. Nature **166;** 626, 1950.

39. YOUNG, M. and PRENTON, M. A.: Maternal and fetal plasma amino acid concentrations during gestation and in retarded fetal growth. J. Obstet. Gynaec. Brit. Cwlth. **76;** 333, 1969.

40. NOALL, M. W., RIGGS, T. R., WALKER, L. M. and CHRISTENSEN, H. N.: Endocrine control of amino acid transfer; distribution of an unmetabolizable amino acid. Science **126;** 1002, 1957.

41. ROOT, A.: Growth hormone. Pediatrics **36;** 940, 1965.

42. JOST, A.: Hormonal factors in the development of the fetus. Cold Spring Harbor Symp. Quant. Biol. **19;** 167, 1954.

43. ZAMENHOF, S., MOSLEY, J. and SCHULLER, E.: Stimulation of the proliferation of cortical neurons by prenatal treatment with growth hormone. Science **152;** 1396, 1966.

44. LOWREY, G. H., ASTER, R. H., CARR, E. A., RAMON, G., BEIERWALTES, W. and SPAFFORD, N. R.: Early diagnosistic criteria of congenitial hypothyroidism. Am. J. Dis. Child. **96;** 131, 1958.

45. ANDERSON, H. J.: Studies of hypothyroidism in children. Acta. Paediat. Scandinav. **50;** Suppl. 125, 1961.

46. ANDERSON, H. J.: The influence of hormones on human development. In: Human Development. Falkner, F. (ed.) W. B. Saunders, Philadelphia, 1966.

47. LIGGINS, G. C., KENNEDY, P. C. and HOLM, L. W.: Failure of initiation of parturtion after electrocoagulation of the pituitary of the fetal lamb. Amer. J. Obstet. Gynec. **98;** 1080, 1967.

48. PICON, L.: Effect of insulin on growth and biochemical composition of the rat fetus. Endocrinology **81;** 1419, 1967.

49. GRUMBACH, M. M., KAPLAN, S. L, SCIARRA, J. J. and BURR, I. M.: Chorionic growth hormone-prolactin (CGP): Secretion, disposition, biologic activity in man, and postulated function as the "growth hormone" of the second half of pregnancy. Ann. N. Y. Acad. Sci. **148;** 501, 1968.

50. ADAMSONS, Jr., K. and TOWELL, M. E.: Thermal homeostasis in the fetus and newborn. Anesthesiology **26;** 531, 1965.

51. BARCROFT, J.: Researches on Prenatal Life. Blackwell, Oxford, 1944.

52. ASSALI, N. S., BEKEY, G. A. and MORRISON, L. W.: Fetal and neonatal circulation. In: Biology of Gestation, Vol. II. Assali, N. S. (ed.) Academic Press, New York, 1968.

53. BARCLAY, A. E., FRANKLIN, K. J. and PRICHARD, M. M. L.: The Foetal Circulation and Cardiovascular System, and the Changes that They Undergo at Birth. Blackwell, Oxford, 1944.

54. LIND, J., STERN, L. and WEGELIUS, C.: Human Foetal and Neonatal Circulation. Charles C Thomas, Springfield, Illinois, 1964.

55. SUZUKI, K., HORIGUCHI, T. and PLENTL, A. A.: Radiographic study of intrauterine fetal circulation in the Rhesus monkey. J. Reprod. Med. **7;** 65, 1971.

56. BARRON, D. H.: The "sphincter" of the ductus venosus. Anat. Rec. **82**; 398, 1942.

57. LIND, J.: Discussion of Section 2 "Physiological adjustments in the newborn". In: The Heart and Circulation in the Newborn and Infant. Cassels, D. (ed.) Grune and Stratton, New York, 1966.

58. POWER, G. G. and LONGO, L. D.: Fetal circulation times and their implications for oxyge-nation. Presented at the twentieth annual meeting of the Society for Gynecologic Investigation, Atlanta, Georgia, March 30, 1973.

59. BORN, G. V. R., DAWES, G. S., MOTT, J. C. and WIDDICOMBE, J. G.: Changes in the heart and lungs at birth. Cold Spring Harbor Symp. Quant. Biol. **19**; 102, 1954.

60. CALDWELL, D. F. and CHURCHILL, J. A.: Learning ability in the progeny of rats administered a protein-deficient diet during second half of gestation. Neurology **17**; 95, 1967.

61. CHOW, B. F. and SHERVIN, R. W.: Fetal parasitism Arch. Environ. Health **10**; 395, 1965.

62. SINGER, J. E., WESTPHAL, M. and NISWANDER, K.: Relationship of weight gain in pregnancy to birth weight and infant growth and development in the first year of life. Obstet. Gynec. **31**; 417, 1968.

63. SMITH, C. A.: Effects of maternal undernutrition upon newborn infants in Holland (1944–1945). J. Pediatr. **30**; 229, 1947.

64. ANTONOV, A. N.: Children born during the siege of Leningrad in 1942. J. Pediatr. **30**; 250, 1947.

65. PITKIN, R. M., KAMINETZKY, H. A., NEWTON, M. and PRITCHARD, J. A.: Maternal nutrition: A selective review of clinical topics. Obstet. Gynec. **40**; 773, 1972.

66. WATANABE, M., MEEKER, C. I., GRAY, M. J., SIMS, E. A. H. and SOLOMON, S.: Secretion rate of aldosterone in normal pregnancy. J. Clin. Invest. **42**; 1619, 1963.

67. PIKE, R. L., MILES, J. E. and WARDLAW, J. M.: Juxtaglomerular degranulation and zona glomerulosa exhaustion in pregnant rats induced by low sodium intakes and reversed by so-dium load. Amer. J. Obstet. Gynec. **95**; 604, 1966.

68. FLEXNER, L. B., COWIE, D. B., HELLMAN, L. M., WILDE, W. S. and VOSBURGH, G. J.: The permeability of the human placenta to sodium in normal and abnormal pregnancies and the supply of sodium to the human fetus as determined with radioactive sodium. Amer. J. Obstet. Gynec. **55**; 469, 1948.

69. HELLMAN, L. M., FLEXNER, L. B., WILDE, W. S., VOSBURGH, G. J. and PROCTOR, N. K.: The permeability of the human placenta to water and supply of water to the human fetus as deter-mined with deutrium oxide. Amer. J. Obstet. Gynec. **56**; 861, 1948.

70. NESLEN, E. D., HUNTER, C. B., and PLENTL, A. A.: Rate of exchange of sodium and potassium between amniotic fluid and maternal system. Proc. Soc. Exper. Biol. Med. **86**; 432, 1954.

71. FRIEDMAN, E. A., GRAY, M. J., HUTCHINSON, D. L. and PLENTL, A. A.: The role of the monkey fetus in the exchange of the water and sodium of the amniotic fluid. J. Clin. Invest. **38**; 961, 1959.

72. HUTCHINSON, D. L., GRAY, M. J., PLENTL, A. A., ALVAREZ, H., CALDEYRO-BARCIA, R., KAPLAN, B. and LIND, J.: The role of the fetus in the water exchange of the amniotic fluid of normal and hydramniotic patients. J. Clin. Invest. **38**; 971, 1959.

73. PLENTL, A. A.: The dynamics of the amniotic fluid. Ann. N. Y. Acad. Sci. **75**; 746, 1959.

74. FRIEDMAN, E. A., GRAY, M. J., GRYNFORGEL, M., HUTCHINSON, D. L., KELLY, W. T. and PLENTL, A. A.: The distribution and metabolism of C^{14}-labeled lactic acid and bicarbonate in pregnant primates. J. Clin. Invest. **39**; 227, 1960.

75. HUTCHINSON, D. L., KELLY, W. T., FRIEDMAN, E. A. and PLENTL, A. A.: The distribution and metabolism of carbon labeled urea in pregnant primates. J. Clin. Invest. **41**; 1745, 1962.

76. PLENTL, A. A. and FRIENDMAN, A. A.: Isotope tracer studies on the carbon dioxide exchange in pregnant primates. Amer. J. Obstet. Gynec. **84**; 1242, 1962.

77. KELLY, W. T., HUTCHINSON, D. L., FRIEDMAN, E. A. and PLENTL, A. A.: Placental transmis-sion of tritium and carbon-14 labeled histidine enantiomorphs in primates. Amer. J. Obstet. Gynec. **89**; 776, 1964.

78. PLENTL, A. A.: Formation and circulation of amniotic fluid. Clin. Obstet. Gynec. **9**; 427, 1966.

79. PLENTL, A. A.: Placental transfer—The use of tracer methods for the study of placental trans-mission. In: Biology of Gestation, Vol. I. Assali, N. S. (ed.) Academic Press, New York, 1968.

80. BARRON, D. H.: The oxygen pressure gradient between the maternal and fetal blood in the pregnant sheep. Yale J. Biol. Med. **19**; 23, 1946.

81. BARRON, D. H.: Some aspects of the transfer of oxygen across the syndesmochorial placenta of the sheep. Yale J. Biol. Med. **24;** 169, 1951.

82. BARRON, D. H. and MESCHIA, G.: A comparative study of the exchange of the respiratory gases across the placenta. Cold Spring Harbor Symposia Quant. Biol. **19;** 93, 1954.

83. BARRON, D. H. and BATTAGLIA, F. C.: The oxygen concentration gradient between the plasmas in the maternal and fetal placental capillaries of the rabbit. Yale J. Biol. Med. **28;** 197, 1955.

84. BARRON, D. H.: Oxygen Supply to the Human Fetus. Charles C Thomas, Springfield, Illinois, 1959.

85. BARRON, D. H.: The placenta as the fetal lung. In: Placenta and Fetal Membranes. Villee, C. A. (ed.) Williams and Wilkins, Baltimore, 1960.

86. MESCHIA, G., COTTER, J. R., BREATHNACH, C. S. and BARRON, D. H.: The hemoglobin, oxygen, carbon dioxide and hydrogen ion concentrations in the umbilical bloods of sheep and goats as sampled via indwelling plastic catheters. Quart. J. Exper. Physiol. **50;** 185, 1965.

87. MESCHIA, G., COTTER, J. R., MAKOWSKI, E. L. and BARRON, D. H.: Simultaneous measurement of uterine and umbilical blood flows and oxygen uptakes. Quart. J. Exper. Physiol. **52;** 1966.

88. FICK, A.: Über diffusion. Poggendorffs Ann. Physic (Ser. 2) **94;** 59, 1855.

89. DANCIS, J., OLSEN, G. and FOLKART, G.: Transfer of histidine and xylose across the placenta and into the red blood cell and amniotic fluids. Amer. J. Physiol. **194;** 44, 1958.

90. LONGO, L. D.: Placental transfer mechanism—An overview. In: Obstetrics and Gynecology Annual. Wynn, R. M. (ed.) Appleton-Century-Crofts, New York, 1972.

91. AHERNE, W. and DUNNILL, M. S.: Quantitative aspects of placental structure. J. Path. Bact. **91;** 123, 1966.

92. AHERNE, W. and DUNNILL, M. S.: Morphometry of the human placenta. Brit. Med. Bull. **22;** 5, 1966.

93. SEEDS, A. E.: Placental transfer. In: Intra-uterine Development. Barnes, A. C. (ed.) Lea & Febiger, Philadelphia, 1968.

94. LONGO, L. D., DELIVORIA-PAPADOPOULOS, M., POWER, G. G., HILL, E. P. and FORSTER II, R. E.: Diffusion equilibration of inert gases between maternal and fetal placental capillaries. Amer. J. Physiol. **219;** 561, 1970.

95. MESCHIA, G., BATTAGLIA, F. C. and BRUNS, P. D.: Theoretical and experimental study of transplacental diffusion. J. Appl. Physiol. **22;** 1171, 1967.

96. PAPPENHEIMER, J. R.: Passage of molecules through capillary walls. Physiol. Rev. **33;** 387, 1953.

97. MIGEON, C. J., BERTRAND, J. and GEMZELL, C. A.: The transplacental passage of various steroid hormones in mid-pregnancy. Recent Progr. Hormone Res. **17;** 207, 1961.

98. PAGE, E. W., GLENDENING, M. B., MARGOLIS, A. and HARPER, H. A.: Transfer of D- and L-histidine across the human placenta. Amer. J. Obstet. Gynec. **73;** 589, 1957.

99. LONGO, L. D. and KLEINZELLER, A.: Transport of monosaccharides by placental cells. Fed. Proc. **29;** 802 Abs., 1970.

100. ASSALI, N. S., RAURAMO, K. and PELTONEN, T.: Measurement of uterine blood flow and uterine metabolism. VIII. Uterine and fetal blood flow and oxygen consumption in early human pregnancy. Amer. J. Obstet. Gynec. **79;** 86, 1960.

101. PAGE, E.W.: Transfer of materials across the human placenta. Amer. J. Obstet. Gynec. **74;** 705, 1957.

102. HAGERMAN, D. D. and VILLEE, C. A.: Transport function of the placenta. Physiol. Rev. **40;** 313, 1960.

103. DANCIS, J.: Placental function and fetal nutrition. In: The Placental and Fetal Membranes. Villee, C. A. (ed.) Williams and Wilkins, Baltimore, 1960.

104. STERNBERG, J.: Placental transfers: Modern methods of study. Amer. J. Obstet. Gynec. **84;** 1731, 1962.

105. DANCIS, J.: The placenta in fetal nutrition and excretion. Amer. J. Obstet. Gynec. **84;** 1749, 1962.

106. FREDA, V. J.: Placental transfer of antibodies in man. Amer. J. Obstet. Gynec. **84;** 1756, 1962.

107. METCALFE, J., BARTELS, H. and MOLL, W.: Gas exchange in the pregnant uterus. Physiol. Rev. **47;** 782, 1967.

108. ASSALI, N. S., KIRSCHBAUM, T. and GROSS, S.: Placental transfer—Transport systems and transfer of substances. In: Biology of Gestation, Vol. I. Assali, N. S. (ed.) Academic Press, New York, 1968.

109. ASSALI, N.S., DOUGLAS, Jr., R.A., BAIRD, W.W., NICHOLSON, D.B. and SUEMOTO, R.: Measurement of uterine blood flow and uterine metabolism. IV. Results in normal pregnancy. Amer. J. Obstet. Gynec. 66; 248, 1953.

110. METCALFE, J., ROMNEY, S.L., RAMSEY, L.H., REID, D.E., and BURWELL, C.S.: Estimation of uterine blood flow in normal human pregnancy at term. J. Clin. Invest. 34; 1632, 1955.

111. FRIEDMAN, E.A., LITTLE, W.A. and SACHTLEBEN, M.R.: Placental oxygen consumption in vitro. II. Total uptake as an index of placental function. Amer. J. Obstet. Gynec. 84; 561, 1962.

112. CAMPBELL, A.G.M., DAWES, G.S., FISHMAN, A.P., HYMAN, A.I., and JAMES, G.B.: The oxygen consumption of the placenta and foetal membranes in the sheep. J. Physiol. 182; 439, 1966.

113. METCALFE, J., MOLL, W., BARTELS, H., HILPERT, P., and PARER, J.T.: Transfer of carbon monoxide and nitrous oxide in the artificially perfused sheep placenta. Circulation Res. 16; 95, 1965.

114. RANKIN, J.H.G. and PETERSON, E.N.: Application of the theory of heat exchangers to a physiological study of the goat placenta. Circulation Res. 24; 235, 1969.

115. POWER, G.G., LONGO, L.D., WAGNER, Jr., H.N., KUHL, D.E. and FORSTER II, R.E.: Uneven distribution of maternal and fetal placental blood flows, as demonstrated using macroaggregates, and its response to hypoxia. J. Clin. Invest. 46; 2053, 1967.

116. POWER, G.G., HILL, E.P. and LONGO, L.D.: Analysis of uneven distribution of diffusing capacity and blood flow in the placenta. Amer. J. Physiol. 222; 740, 1972.

117. LONGO, L.D., POWER, G.G. and FORSTER II, R.E.: Respiratory function of the placenta as determined with carbon monoxide in sheep and dogs. J. Clin. Invest. 46; 812, 1967.

118. HILL, E.P., POWER, G.G., and LONGO, L.D.: A mathematical model of placental O_2 transfer with consideration of hemoglobin reaction rates. Amer. J. Physiol. 222; 721, 1972.

119. LONGO, L.D., HILL, E.P. and POWER, G.G.: Theoretical analysis of factors affecting placental O_2 transfer. Amer. J. Physiol. 222; 730, 1972.

120. VOSBURGH, G.J., FLEXNER, L.B., COWIE, D.B., HELLMAN, L.M., PROCTOR, N.K. and WILDE, W.S.: The rate of renewal in women of the water and sodium of the amniotic fluid as determined by tracer techniques. Amer. J. Obstet. Gynec. 56; 1156, 1948.

121. PLENTL, A.A. and HUTCHINSON, D.L.: Determination of deutrium exchange rates between maternal circulation and amniotic fluid. Proc. Soc. Exper. Biol. Med. 82; 681, 1953.

122. PLENTL, A.A. and GRAY, M.J.: Hydrodynamic model of a 3-compartment catenary system with exchanging end compartments. Proc. Soc. Exper. Biol. Med. 87; 595, 1954.

123. PLENTL, A.A.: Transfer of water across the perfused umbilical cord. Proc. Soc. Exper. Biol. Med. 107; 622, 1961.

124. GRAY, M.J., NESLEN, E.D. and PLENTL, A.A.: Estimation of water transfer from amniotic fluid to fetus. Proc. Soc. Exper. Biol. Med. 92; 463, 1956.

125. HUTCHINSON, D.L., HUNTER, C.B., NESLEN, E.D. and PLENTL, A.A.: The exchange of water and electrolytes in the mechanism of amniotic fluid formation and the retlationship to hydramnios. Surg. Gynec. Obstet. 100; 391, 1955.

126. PRITCHARD, J.A.: Deglutition by normal and anencephalic fetuses. Obstet. Gynec. 25; 289, 1965.

127. CHEZ, R.A., SMITH, R.G. and HUTCHINSON, D.L.: Renal function in the intrauterine primate fetus. Amer. J. Obstet. Gynec. 90; 128, 1964.

128. SEEDS, A.E.: Amniotic fluid and fetal water metabolism. In: Intra-Uterine Development. Barnes, A.C. (ed.) Lea & Febiger, Philadelphia, 1968.

129. WILDE, W.S., COWIE, D.B. and FLEXNER, L.B.: Permeability of the placenta of the guinea pig to inorganic phosphate and its relation to fetal growth. Amer. J. Physiol. 147; 360, 1946.

130. FUCHS, A. R. and FUCHS, F.: Studies on the transfer of phosphate from mother to foetus in the rabbit. Acta Physiol. Scand. 52; 65, 1961.

131. VOSBURGH, G. J. and FLEXNER, L. B.: Maternal plasma as a source of iron for the fetal guinea pig. Amer. J. Physiol. 161; 202, 1950.

132. TWARDOCK, A. R. and AUSTIN, M. K.: Calcium transfer in perfused guinea pig placenta. Amer. J. Physiol. 219; 540, 1970.

133. WIDDAS, W. F.: Inability of diffusion to account for placenta glucose transfer in the sheep and consideration of the kinetics of a possible carrier transfer. J. Physiol. **118**; 23, 1952.

134. KARVONEN, M. J. and RÄIHÄ, N.: Permeability of placenta of the guinea pig to glucose and fructose. Acta. Physiol. Scand. **31**; 194, 1954.

135. HOLENBERG, N. G., KAPLAN, B., KARVONEN, M. J., LIND, J. and MALM, M.: Permeability of human placenta to glucose, fructose and xylose. Acta Physiol. Scand. **36**; 291, 1956.

136. DANCIS, J.: Permeability of the rabbit placenta to glucose and fructose. Amer. J. Physiol. **181**; 532, 1955.

137. DAVIES, J.: Differential permeability of the rabbit placenta to various sugars. Amer. J. Physiol. **188**; 21, 1957.

138. CHINARD, F. P., DANESINO, V., HARTMANN, W. L., HUGGETT, A. ST. G., PAUL, W. and REYNOLDS, S. R. M.: The transmission of hexoses across the placenta in the human and Rhesus monkey (macaca mulatta). J. Physiol. **132**; 289, 1956.

139. COLBERT, R. M., CALTON, F. M., DINDA, R. E. and DAVIES, J.: Competitive transfer of sorbose and glucose in placenta of rabbit. Proc. Soc. Exper. Biol. Med. **97**; 867, 1958.

140. PATERSON, P., PHILLIPS, L. and WOOD, C.: Relationship between maternal and fetal glucose during labor. Amer. J. Obstet. Gynec. **98**; 938, 1967.

141. ZUSPAN, F. P., WHALEY, W. H., NELSON, G. H. and AHLQUIST, R. P.: Placental transfer of epinephrine. I. Maternal-fetal metabolic alterations of glucose and nonesterified fatty acids. Amer. J. Obstet. Gynec. **95**; 284, 1966.

142. BATTAGLIA, F. C., HELLEGERS, A. E., HELLER, Jr., C. J. and BEHRMAN, R.: Glucose concentration gradients across the maternal surface, the placenta, and the amnion of the Rhesus monkey (macaca mulatta). Amer. J. Obstet. Gynec. **88**; 32, 1964.

143. VILLEE, C. A.: Regulation of blood glucose in the human fetus. J. Appl. Physiol. **5**; 437, 1953.

144. HUGGETT, A. ST. G.: The transport of lipins and carbohydrates across the placenta. Cold Spring Harbor Symp. Quant. Biol. **19**; 82, 1954.

145. HAGERMAN, D. D. and VILLEE, C. A.: The transport of fructose by human placenta. J. Clin. Invest. **31**; 911, 1952.

146. CAMPLING, J. D. and NIXON, D. A.: The inositol content of foetal blood and foetal fluids. J. Physiol. **126**; 71, 1954.

147. CHRISTENSEN, H.N. and STREICHER, J.A.: Association between rapid growth and elevated cell concentrations of amino acids. I. In fetal tissues. J. Biol. Chem. **175**; 95, 1948.

148. CRUMPLER, H.R., DENT, C.E. and LINDAN, O.: The Amino-acid pattern in human foetal and maternal plasma at delivery. Biochem. J. **47**; 223, 1950.

149. CLEMETSON, C.A.B., and CHURCHMAN, J.: The placental transfer of amino-acids in normal and toxaemic pregnancy. J. Obstet. Gynaec. Brit. Emp. **61**; 364, 1954.

150. GLENDENING, M.B., MARGOLIS, A.J. and PAGE, E.W.: Amino acid concentration in fetal and maternal plasma. Amer. J. Obstet. Gynec. **81**; 591, 1961.

151. GHADIMI, H. and PECORA, P.: Tree amino acids of cord plasma as compared with maternal plasma during pregnancy. Pediatrics **33**; 500, 1964.

152. DANCIS, J., MONEY, W.L., SPRINGER, D. and LEVITZ, M.: Transport of amino acids by placenta. Amer. J. Obstet. Gynec. **101**; 820, 1968.

153. JOSIMOVICH, J.B. and KNOBIL, E.: Placental transfer of I[131] insulin in the rhesus monkey. Amer. J. Physiol. **200**; 471, 1961.

154. JOST, A.: Action du propylthiouracile sur la throide de foetus de rat intacts ou decapités. C.R. Soc. Biol. **151**; 1295, 1957.

155. KNOBIL, E., and JOSIMOVICH, J.B.: Placental transfer of thyrotropic hormone, thyroxine, triiodothyroxine, and insulin in the rat. Ann. N.Y. Acad. Sci. **75**; 895, 1959.

156. GITLIN, D. and BIASUCCI, A.: Development of γG, γA, γM, βic/βia, C'l esterase inhibitor, ceruloplasmin, transferrin, hemopexin, haptoglobin, fibrinogen, plasminogen, a_1-antitrypsin, orosomucoid, β-lipoprotein, a_2-macroglobulin, and preablumin in the human conceptus. J. Clin. Invest. **48**; 1433, 1969.

157. GOLDWATER, W.H. and STETTEN, Jr., D.W.: Studies in fetal metabolism. J. Biol. Chem. **169**; 723, 1947.

158. PAPJÁK, G.: The origon of fetal lipids. Cold Spring Harbor Symp. Quant. Biol. **19**; 200, 1954.

159. KAYDEN, H.J., DANCIS, J. and MONEY, W.L.: Transfer of lipids across the guinea pig placenta. Amer. J. Obstet. Gynec. **104**; 564, 1969.

160. PORTMAN, O.W., BEHRMAN, R.E. and SOLTYS, P.: Transfer of free fatty acids across the primate placenta. Amer. J. Physiol. **216**; 143, 1969.

161. VAN DUYNE, C.M., HAVEL, R.J. and FELTS, J.M.: Placental transfer of palmitic acid-1-C^{14} in rabbits. Amer. J. Obstet. Gynec. **84**; 1069, 1962.

162. BIEZENSKI, J.J.: Role of placenta in fetal lipid metabolism. I. Injection of phospholipids, double labeled with C^{14}-glycerol and P^{32} into pregnant rabbits. Amer. J. Obstet. Gynec. **104**; 1177, 1969.

163. MIGEON, C.J., BERTRAND, J. and WALL, P.E.: Physiological disposition of 4-C^{14}-cortisol during late pregnancy. J. Clin. Invest. **36**; 1350, 1957.

164. LANMAN, J.P.: Adrenal function in premature infants. II, ACTH-treated infants and infants born of toxemic mothers. Pediatrics **12**; 62, 1953.

165. LUST, J.E., HAGERMAN, D.D. and VILLEE, C.A.: The transport of riboflavin by human placenta. J. Clin. Invest. **33**; 38, 1953.

166. RÄIHÄ, N.: On the placental transfer of vitamin C. An experimental study on guinea pigs and human subjects. Acta Physiol. Scand. **45** (Suppl. 155); 1, 1959.

167. BARNES, A.C.: The placental metabolism of vitamin A. Amer. J. Obstet. Gynec. **61**; 368, 1951.

168. SUZUKI, K., ADAMSONS, K. and FRIEDMAN, E.A.: Placental transfer of nicotine and its effect upon uterine blood flow rate in the pregnant Rhesus monkey. Presented at Twentieth Annual Meeting of Society for Gynecologic Investigation, March, 1973, Atlanta, Georgia.

169. WIGGLESWORTH, J.S.: Experimental growth retardation in the foetal rat. J. Path. Bact. **88**; 1, 1964.

170. NAEYE, R.L.: The fetal and neonatal development of twins. Pediatrics **33**; 546, 1964.

171. NAEYE, R.L.: Organ abnormalities in a human parabiotic syndrome. Amer. J. Path. **46**; 829, 1965.

172. GLUCK, L., KULOVICH, M.V., BORER, Jr., R.C., BRENNER, P.H., ANDERSON, G.G. and SPELLACY, W.N.: Diagnosis of the respiratory distress syndrome by amniocentesis. Amer. J. Obstet. Gynec. **109**; 440, 1971.

173. FREEMAN, R. K.: The use of the oxytocin challenge test for antepartum clinical evaluation of uteroplacental respiratory function. Amer. J. Obstet. Gynec. **121**; 481, 1975.

174. LUBCHENCO, L.O., HANSMAN, C. and BÄCKSTRÖM, L.: Factors influencing fetal growth. In: Nutricia Symposium—Aspects of Praematurity and Dysmaturity. Jonxis, J.H.P., Visser, H.K.A. and Troelstra, J.A. (eds.) H.E. Stenfert Kroese N.V., Leiden, 1968.

175. MEHRIZI, A. and DRASH, A.: Birth weight of infants with cyanotic and acyanotic congenital malformations of the heart. J. Pediatr. **59**; 715, 1961.

176. NAEYE, R.L., BENIRSCHKE, K., HAGSTROM, J.W.C. and MARCUS, C.C.: Intrauterine growth of twins as estimated from liveborn birth-weight data. Pediatrics. **37**; 409, 1966.

177. LICHTY, J.A., TING, R.Y., BRUNS, P.D. and DYAR, E.: Studies of babies born at high altitude. A.M.A. J. Dis. Child. **93**; 666, 1957.

178. MANN, L.I., TEJANI, N.A. and WEISS, R.R.: Antenatal diagnosis and management of the small-for-gestational age fetus. Amer. J. Obstet. Gynec. **120**; 995, 1974.

The dynamic relationship of the morphologic changes of the placenta to the feto-placental function

Hiroaki SOMA, M.D.

Department of Obstetrics and Gynecology, Tokyo Medical College, Tokyo

INTRODUCTION

The role of the placenta in fetal physiology and pathology has recently been emphasized. For example, it is considered that the placenta serves as lung, kidneys, liver and even endocrine organ for the fetus during his intrauterine life. Accordingly, if the adequate transfer mechanism across the placenta between maternal and fetal circulations be impaired, the fetal life will be in danger. Even though various morphologic changes of the placenta are seen during gestation, these alteration may be secondary to maternal factors as sees in the basal plate, placental factors as seen in terminal villi, and fetal factors as seen in the umbilical cord.

In addition, an attempt was made to detect possible relationships between abnormalities in the placenta and subsequent aberrant growth in the infant [1]. The abnormality of the placenta increased the probability of nutritional disturbances in the first six months of postnatal life.

This chapter deals with the functional significance of the morphology of the human placenta to the feto-placental-maternal relationship.

RELATION OF PLACENTAL WEIGHT TO FETAL WEIGHT

1. THE VARIATION IN SIZE AND SHAPE OF THE HUMAN PLACENTA

Whether the placental size and its form may be influenced by a hypoxic environment is yet to be evaluated. A comparative morphometric evaluation of the placenta at high altitude and at sea level was undertaken. In general, the oval shaped placenta represents the most stable form. However, a significant preponderance of placental shapes other than the round or oval form was found at high altitude compared to that at sea level [2]. As the infant born at high altitude appears to be protected from the effects of low oxygen tension in the environment, at high altitude the newborn infants weighed significantly less than those born at sea level, while the placentas at high altitude weighed more than the placentas at sea level and the number of cotyledons in high altitude placentas was half that of sea levels placentas [3]. The relative increase of other forms of placental shape should be interpreted as an adaptation or a compensation for environmental stress and oxygenation of the fetus at high altitude.

2. GROWTH RELATIONSHIP BETWEEN THE PLACENTA AND THE FETUS

Linear growth relationships between placental and fetal weights have been reported [4]. During the early stages of gestation the placental weight increases more rapidly than the fetal weight. Furthermore, the growth rate of the placenta steadily decreases, whereas that of the fetus increases. It is, however, concluded that the whole weight of the placenta is a poor indicator of its functional capacity [5], because nearly half this weight is contributed by tissues which are not part of the placenta proper. Therefore, blood-free placental weight is a rather better measure of functional capacity, but probably a still better measure would be the amount of metabolically active protein [6]. Accordingly, the placenta should be weighed after removal of blood clots and trimming the membranes and cord within 1 cm of the placenta [7].

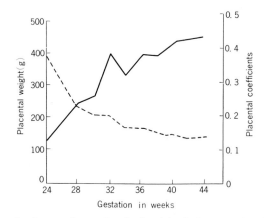

Fig. 1 The ratio of mean placental to fetal weight during gestational weeks.
——The mean placental weight.
······The mean placental coefficient.

Data on the weight ratio of placenta and fetus (Placental coefficients) are presented (Fig. 1). The ratio of normal placental to fetal weights gradually diminishes as pregrancy advances. The mean ratio decreases from 0.39 at 24 weeks to 0.15 at term. TREMBLAY [8] noted that the placental-fetal weight ratio in cases of fetal malnutrition was consistently lower than that in normal cases, but never reached the critical level. It was reported that the placental coefficient gives a mean value of 0.144 for cases at high altitude and 0.192 for cases at sea level [3]. This finding indicates that a relatively greater placenta, in comparison with the fetus, exists at high altitudes. As previously presented here, a relatively greater placental weight could be interpreted as a compensatory mechanism to favor a better irrigation and oxygenation of the fetus at high altitude [3]. On the other hand, YOUNOSZAI [9] suggested that placental decidual area may be an important determinant of infant birth weight, because infant birth weight was related to placental decidual area in all groups of the normal preterm, term, and intrauterine growth-retarded infants, but to placental weight only in the normal preterm and term infants.

In intrauterine growth-retarded infants (IUGR), placental weight does not increase significantly after the thity-sixth week, since a relation between placental weight and gestational age was not found. However, in these infants, there is an inverse relation between infant weight and placental thickness. YOUNOSZAI [9] postulated that thin placentas with a bigger area of attachment to the uterus have a circulation better distributed to the surface area available for diffusion, whereas placentas with IUGR which have smaller decidual areas and are thicker, may have a circulatory pattern which results in less efficient nutrition of the fetus.

3.   CHANGES IN VILLOUS SURFACE AREA OF THE PLACENTA RELATED TO FETAL GROWTH

It has been pointed out that it is impossible to correlate all pathological changes in the placenta with characteristic changes in the infant. WILKIN [10] developed a method of employing an integration stage in the histometric study of the placenta, by which it may be possible to obtain the quantitative variation of the placental components. AHERNE [11] demonstrated that there is a close positive correlation between the area of the chorionic villous surface and the weight of the fetus at all gestational ages. He uses point counting and mean linear intercept determination. The mean value obtained for the area of the chorionic villous surface in normal term placenta was considerably greater than that associated with hypertension or abnormally small infants. This means that the chorionic villous surface area is directly related to infant weight and to placental weight. Furthermore, in infants with low birth weight, there was a proportional reduction in weight of the placenta and in its DNA and protein contents [12].

ABNORMALITIES OF THE UMBILICAL CORD

Excessive length of the cord is found often and then it may be associated with true knots, excessive entangling in extremities or loops around the neck. Pressure or tension during delivery may then lead to obstruction of the umbilical circulation and fetal death. On occasion, coarctation of the cord may be present in association with unexplained fetal death.

KRONE [13] has attempted to correlate a variety of congenital abnormalities with the cord's insertion. He found a rather significantly higher frequency of abnormal insertion of the cord, that is velamentous and marginal, in abnormal infants when compared with normal infants. On the other hand, the most frequent umbilical abnormality described by BENIRSCHKE [14] is the absence of one umbilical artery. Incidence figures of 0.4–1.2 per cent have been found, and there is a positive correlation between single umbilical artery and fetal developmental defects. The frequency of detected anomalies varies greatly in the reports, from 16 to 65 per cent.

We found that marginal and velamentous insertions of the cord are more common in abnormal infants with lacking one umbilical artery compared to those associated with fetal abnormalities with normal cord vessels (Fig. 2, 3). Recently, out of 150 placentas of IUGR, absence of one cord artery was observed in 5 per cent [15]. In addition, it is noted that the frequency of this anomaly is much higher in low birth weight infants and in maternal diabetes.

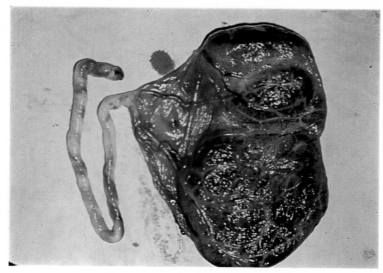

Fig. 2   Velamentous insertion of cord.

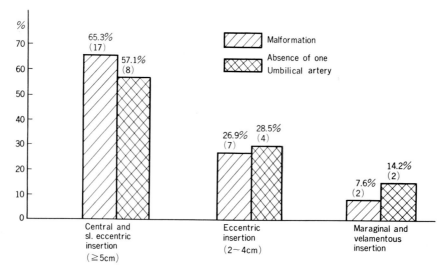

Fig. 3   Incidence of the point of insertion of cord in malformed infants and in those who had had absence of one umbilical artery.

MORPHOLOGIC AND FUNCTIONAL CHANGES OF THE PLACENTAL VILLI

1.   CHANGES OF CHORIONIC VILLI SECONDARY TO PLACENTAL CIRCULATION

The main villus below the chorionic plate divides into many branches and these again divide into third branches which go to the basal plate and anchor themselves there partly as anchoring villi. The cotyledon can be subdivided into many subcotyledons.

The placental circulation can be divided into two parts: 1) The maternal side circulation as intervillous flow through the basal plate; the maternal blood enters into the intervillous space (IVS) from the basal plate to the chorionic plate and circulates the intracotyledonary cavity. 2) The fetal side circulation through intravillous capillaries; the vessels of the main villi are terminal vessels and the terminal villi always suspend in the intervillous blood. Accordingly, it is assumed that a relative hypoxia stimulates the trophoblast of the chorionic villi and its growth depends upon the PO_2 of the IVS blood.

1) VILLOUS CHANGES RESULTING FROM PLACENTAL HYPOXIA

About 75 per cent of the total uterine blood flow perfuses the IVS and, at term, it may be as high as 90 per cent [16]. The pressure in the IVS is equal at all times to that of the amniotic fluid, and the amount of blood in the IVS is probably greater during uterine contraction which facilitates transfer of gaseous substances across the placenta.

In general, the aggressiveness of the proliferating and invading trophoblast is related to the surrounding PO_2 [17]. Thus, the viability and invasiveness of trophoblast may be influenced by placental hypoxia.

Villi from mature human placentas maintained in 26 per cent oxygen in organ culture showed little morphologic changes over a period of 10 days, while others grown under hypoxic conditions showed variable syncytial degeneration and a marked increase in tne number of cytotrophoblastic cells [18]. Furthermore, diminished concentration of oxygen content in placental tissue cultures increased the number of syncytial knots [19]. In well oxygenated conditions the fine structural integrity of the trophoblast is maintained up to 96 hours in organ culture and the tissue appears to function normally, whereas hypoxia quickly damages the syncytiotrophoblast and marked changes occur throughout the trophoblast, including apparent attempts at regeneration [20]. On electron microscopy, the hypoxic specimens showed considerable and progressive vacuolation and thinning of the syncytium, multiplication of the syncytial nuclei with frequent syncytial knot formation and clumping of the nuclear chromation, increase in the subtrophoblastic space and marked thickening and lamination of the basal lamina.

However, the syncytiotrophoblast of human chorionic villi *in vivo* is continuously regenerated by the cytotrophoblast. The function of the syncytium is unimpaired, if its regeneration is sufficient. If the cytotrophoblast regeneration is insufficient to repair the damaged syncytium, less reaction product of glycolytic enzymes is demonstrable. This fact is compensated by the activation of G6-PDH and a-GPDH. At this point polypous syncytioplasma protusions are formed and pinched off into the IVS [21]. In addition, the functional damaging effect of hypoxia on trophoblast has been confirmed by SHARP [22] who has shown a significant decrease in hydroxysteroid dehydrogenase enzyme activity in hypoxic conditions at as early as 24 hours.

The cytotrophoblastic cells can be considered as "stem cells" that undergo division and subsequent maturation, or differentiation, to form the syncytiotrophoblast. Although the cytotrophoblast cells become progressively smaller and fewer as pregnancy advances, they are present in the villi of the mature placenta. If the syncytiotrophoblast suffers ischemic damage, the cytotrophoblast proliferates in an attempt to replace the damaged tissue. Therefore, cytotrophoblastic hyperplasia is a repair phenomenon which is related to the extent of syncytial damage [23].

It has been postulated that syncytial knot formation is an ischemic change resulting from decreased maternal blood supply to the placenta, or from a functional inactivity of the syncytium [24, 25], and these epithelial plates are concerned with the passive transfer of substance of low molecular weight across the syncytium (Fig. 4) [26].

On the other hand, there is no relationship between proliferation of cytotrophoblast

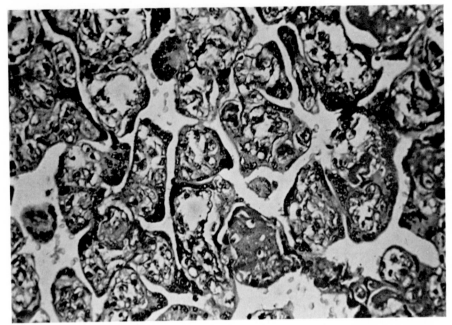

Fig. 4   Many of the villi have syncytial knots (H & E, × 200).

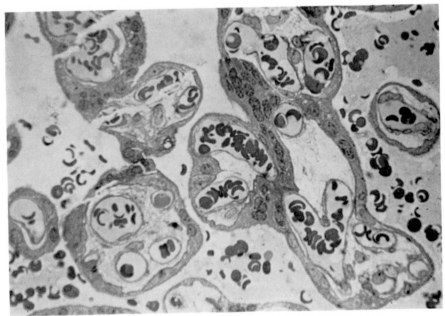

Fig. 5   The villi showing vasculo-syncytial membranes (H & E, × 400).

cells and the incidence of syncytial knot formation. It is likely that the basic change determining a high level of syncytial knot formation is a reduced fetal villous blood flow [27]. However, the significant syncytial proliferation at the periphery of placental infarctions would be the result of the hypoxic blood that bathes them [17].

2) RELATIONSHIP BETWEEN SYNCYTIAL KNOTS AND VASCULO-SYNCYTIAL MEMBRANE UNDER HYPOXIC CONDITION

To observe the number of syncytial knots, 400 terminal villi in each placenta were counted. The number of syncytial knots per field unit was counted in 30–40 per cent of the villi in 163 premature, mature and postmature placentae, whereas this knot count was found in 55 per cent of villi in 100 small term placentas (below 350 g) (Table 1), even though it has been reported that no relationship exists between variations in placental weight and variations in the incidence of syncytial knots [27].

Table 1 Relationship between placental VSM counts and Syncytial knots.

Number of Syncytial knots	Small term placenta		Premature placenta		Postmature placenta		Term placenta	
0–20	6	3	8	10	15	1	18	0
21–40	10	15	4	7	17	3	18	2
41–60	1	29	1	3	8	3	4	4
61–80	0	28	1	7	1	1	1	4
over 80	0	8	1	8	0	1	0	12
VSM	(+)	(−)	(+)	(−)	(+)	(−)	(+)	(−)

In the mature placenta the villous capillaries are sinusoidal and closely approximated to the overlying trophoblast. In many villi the dilated capilllaries bulge out towards the IVS. And then the syncytium becomes thin and anuclear. Accordingly, the syncytium may appear to fuse with the vessel wall to form a vasculo-syncytial membrane (VSM) (Fig. 5) [28].

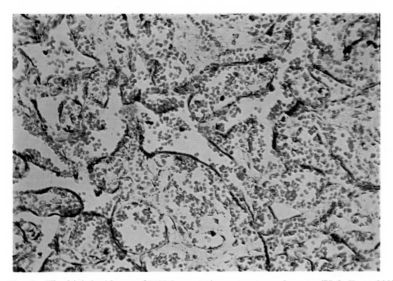

Fig. 6 The high incidence of VSM counts in postmature placenta (H & E, × 200).

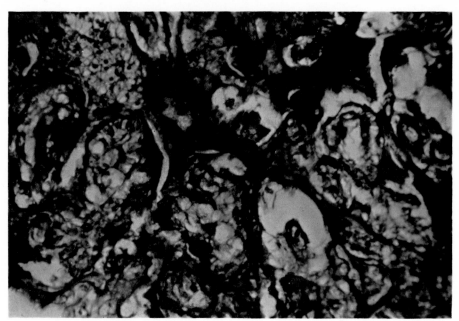

Fig. 7 The villi with a markedly thickened basement membrane in dysmature placenta (PAP, × 400).

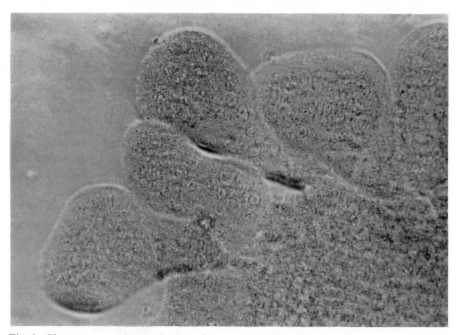

Fig. 8 Phase contrast microscopic view of many syncytial sprouts. 7 weeks pregnancy (× 200).

HORKY [29] thought that in fetal hypoxia there was an increased formation of VSM in an attempt to increase the surface available for gas transfer. However, Fox [28] suggested that a reduction of the number of VSM in prolonged pregnancies is a manifestation of villous senescence, and is accompanied by a reduction in the oxygen diffusion capacity of the placenta.

In small term and premature placentas the incidence of low VSM counts was seen, whereas there was a high incidence in mature and postmature placentas (Table 1; Fig. 6). Furthermore, the placentae with low VSM counts were characterized by high villous syncytial knot counts. It may be that such small placentas represent hypovascular villous changes responsible for low of state oxygen supply.

It has been suggested that thickening of the basement membrane can be a result of uteroplacental ischemia or the result of an immunological reaction. In fact, thickening of the villous trophoblastic basement membrane increases gradually towards term. In particular, an undue thickening of the basement membrane is also commonly seen in placentas of toxemia. Furthermore, a high incidence of placentae with thickened basement membranes was seen not only in cases of fetal hypoxia but also in those of intrauterine fetal death (Fig. 7).

3)   THE MORPHOLOGIC CHANGES OF THE CHORIONIC SURFACE
i)   **Phase contrast microscopy**

The functional importance of the morphology of the chorionic surface is well established. The work of ALVAREZ [30] and ALADJEM [31] on phase contrast microscopy of the placenta introduced a new approach to the study of the terminal villus which is considered to be the functional unit of the placenta.

In the early stage of the normal pregnancy, the syncytium of a terminal villus is strikingly active so that there are many syncytial sprouts at the apex (Fig. 8) [32]. This sprouting diminishes as the pregnancy advances and vascularization of the preterminal and terminal villi becomes more marked. The stromal edema and avascular degeneration suggesting a fetal circulatory impairment are present in the aborted villi of the mid-stage pregnancy, while lateral sprouting can often be seen at the same time. In normal terminal villi near term, syncytial sprouting is rarely observed. The syncytium becomes thinner and some parts of the terminal villi lose the syncytial covering layer. As a result, VSM is formed. After all, the ratio between stroma and capillary reduces toward term, because the capillaries become more tortuous and dilate. Thinning and hyalinization of the syncytium increase with placental age. An increasing number of syncytial sprouts appear in term placentas associated toxemia [33], these sprouts are characterized by lateral protrusion from the preterminal and terminal villi (Table 2).

Table 2   Villous change of gestational age (Phase contrast microscopic findings).

	Normal	Pathological
Early	Active sprouting Syncytial pseudopodia Vascularization	Inactive sprouts Stromal edema Sclerotic villi
Middle	Sprouting Marked vascularization Syncytial thinning	Lateral sprouts Avascular degeneration Subsyncytial edema
Term	Capllary looping and dilatation Syncytial thinning and detachment	Lateral sprouts Avascular degeneration Sclerotic villi Subsyncytial edema

By phase contrast microscopy, the main placental pathologic findings were; hypoplasia of the syncytium, ischemia, avascularity, edema and hemorrhage [34]. In particular, the hypoplasia of the syncytium is a predominant finding in cases of neonatal death, but it was never detected when the neonatal course was normal. ALADEJEM et al. [34] have done a comparison between similar diagnoses by phase contrast microscopic study and histology. It is apparent that the phase contrast microscopic study revealed a wider range of pathologic findings not usually reported by conventional histology. It also permits detection of pathology in histologic sections. However, the image of the intact terminal villus with the possibility of observing in one single specimen some 200 individual villi has a distinct advantage over fixed and stained histologic sections. Thus, it is expected that the evaluation of placental villi by phase contrast microscopy may be useful as a diagnostic tool of placental function in the future.

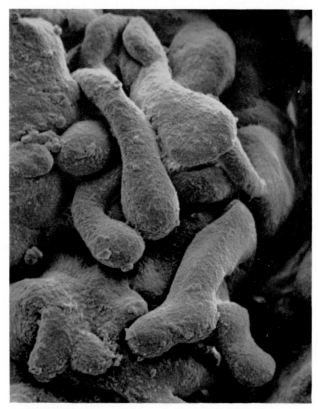

Fig. 9 Chorionic villi. Note nose-like syncytial protrusions. 2 months pregnancy (× 1,000).

ii) Scanning electon microscopy

The surface study using the phase contrast microscopy is restricted to some extent. Recently, it has been noted that the advantages of scanning electon microscopy (SEM) in the ultrastructual investigations of surfaces are evident. Thus, the surface ultrastructural study of the placenta has been further requested.

At the scanning electon microscopic levels, the placental villi in early stage of pregnancy protruded as a number of structures of various shapes and sizes from the trunk (Fig. 9), while those in late pregnancy showed an entirely different appearance in that the surface of the terminal unit was relatively smooth [35]. Besides, it has been suggested that the rounded syncytial protrusions play a role in the invasiveness of early trophoblast growth. They always seem to be undamaged and are probably not anchored in the maternal stroma to any significant extent. Their existence is easily verified in SEM [36]. The clumping of microvilli can be observed within marginal zones and with the border zones of normal placentas by SEM. It also can be seen in postmature placentas and is relatively common in placentas from toxemic pregnancies [37]. In the toxemic placenta the surface of the chorionic villi appear as narrow cylinders containing numerous prominent club-shaped syncytial protrusions, which probably correspond to the syncytial knots [38].

2. VILLOUS CHANGES RELATING TO PLACENTAL AGING

It has been pointed out that a number of metabolic processes decrease in rate as the placenta gets older untill the 25th or 30th week of gestation [39]. From then until term, the rates of most metabolic functions remain essentially constant. It is suggested that the human placenta has a modal life of approximately 38–40 weeks, after which it undergoes an aging change that results in a progressive failure to meet the nutritional demands of the fetus [40]. Furthermore, it is reported that the placental function showed a rapidly diminishing rate of oxygen in placental transfer in the end of pregnancy. Whether this functional decline can be associated with morphologic changes in the placenta of prolonged pregnancies was disputed. The cases that had senescent placentas all showed extremely low flows in the IVS and infarcts [41]. Thus, the senescent placenta showed a frank crowding of the chorionic villi with very little intervillous space. The connective tissue was strikingly dense. Therefore, the presence of numerous white infarctions was characteristic of the senescent placenta.

At the electon microscopic levels, there are no changes in the cytoplasmic organelles or endoplasmic reticulum of the syncytium of the aging placenta. In the term placenta a decreased width of the syncytium in areas between nuclear knots is noted. At these areas of decreased width there is often a decrease in the number and height of the microvilli [42].

On the other hand, though no specific histologic villous abnormalities were found in the placentae from prolonged pregnancies, the placentas from prolonged pregnancies were characterized by villous fibrosis, an excess of syncytial knots, proliferation of villous cytotrophoblast cells and thickening of the trophoblastic basement membrane [40]. Such histologic changes in the placenta in prolonged pregnancy appear to be a reflection of mild placental ischemia and may be due to a primary senescent change within the villous capillaries.

The macroscopic features of the insufficient placentas which we have observed, showed an increase of marked meconium staining, infarcts, intervillous thrombi and abnormality of the cord. WIGGLESWORTH [43] also noted that there were found intervillous thrombi in 5–10 per cent of the insufficient placentas. As regards the etiological factor in degenerative changes in the placenta which may be attributed to placental aging, one has paid attention to two main concepts; the impairment of fetal vascular supply and the circulatory impairment of villi from maternal blood.

While vascular changes appear to play no important role in the development of degenerative changes in the normal term placenta, lesions of blood vessels may develop in pathological states associated with pregnancy, in which case they may play a contributory role in intensifying these degenerative processes [44]. Furthermore, there are also reports which show a fibrillar material present in fetal endothelial cells and trophoblasts which are considered to be precursors of fibrinoid [45].

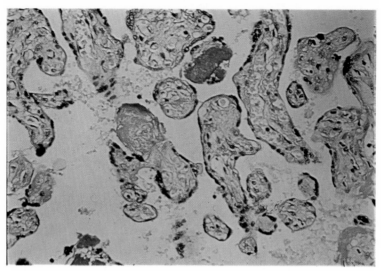

Fig. 10   Villous fibrinoid necrosia (PAS, × 200).

The villus is progressively destroyed and replaced by PAS positive material (Fig. 10). This process continues until the whole of the villus is replaced by fibrinoid material. Therefore, this lesion is termed fibrinoid necrosis [46]. It is, however, different from deposition of fibrin on the outer surface of the syncytium. In particular, there is an extremely high incidence of placentae with fibrinoid necrosis in case of rhesus incompatibility, diabetes, toxemia and hemolytic disease [46]. It has been thought that fibrinoid change is due to replacement of the villus by fibrin, this being derived either from maternal blood or fetal blood. On the other hand, the possibility has been suggested that fibrinoid necrosis may be the morphological hallmark of an immunological reaction between mother and fetus [46]. Recently, GILLE et al. [47] demonstrated by the fluorescent antibody technique that a deposit of IgG was seen on the villous epithelium of placentae from women who received

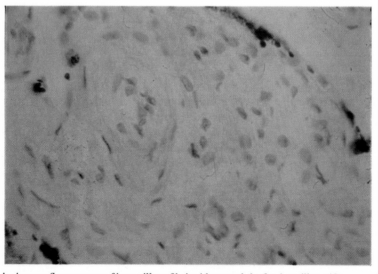

Fig. 11   An intense fluorescence of intravillous fibrinoid around the fetal capillary (Congo red, × 400).

the pepsin digested purified IgG-fragment (Fab') 2G and an immunological reation seems to take place in the villous epithelium.

Departing from the traditional view of aging of the placenta, BURSTEIN [44] proposed a new concept that the placenta undergoes senescence in a manner consistent with the misspecification—the autoimmune theory as it obtains in respect to aging of individuals generally. Then he indicates that the fibrinoid present in the placenta is comparable to amyloid, which is recognized as one of the end products of aging and immune reaction. With advancing age, the immunosurveillance system fails and neoplasms, autoimmune disorders or senile amyloidosis occur. On ultraviolet light microscopy, unstained placental sections showed some autofluorescence of intravillous fibrinoid but little if any of inter-villous or Nitabuch's fibrinoid. Sections stained with congo red showed a more intense and pink fluorescence of intravillous fibrinoid (Fig. 11). Thus, his concept is based upon the idea that intravillous fibrinoid has characteristics similar to amyloid-like substances and this substance is probably the result of an immunologic interaction between the mother and the fetus.

Although the question of the aging of the placenta as gestation proceeds has generated a great deal of discussion over years, the study of aging of the placenta is not yet clarified, and further investigation should be done from various aspects.

FETO-MATERNAL CELLULAR INTERRELATION IN THE BASAL PLATE, WITH SPECIAL REFERENCE TO THE X CELLS

The basal plate is composed of the thin layer of the maternal surface of the human placenta. This plate consists mostly of cellular elements in which fetal and maternal cells become intermixed [48]. Therefore, a dispute has arisen over the origin of such cells.

The basal plate is composed of the following layers; Rohr stria, basal trophoblast, syncy-tial giant trophoblast, X cells, fibrinoid layer of Nitabuch stria, and decidual cells. Although it has been assumed that the principal component of the basal plate is tropho-blast, being considered to be a special form, such cells have more recently been identified in the basal plate and designated X cells because of their questionable nature and origin.

1. ENZYME-HISTOCHEMICAL FEATURES OF THE X CELLS

The X cells are polygonal, almost always single-nucleated elements with unusual cytoplasmic basophilia which do not show any mitotic activity (Fig. 12). They are inter-mixed with decidual cells in the basal plate and the placental septa. Their appearance differs from the basal cytotrophoblast cells and syncytial giant cells. It is known that the X cells appear apparently from the fourth month of gestation until term.

The trophoblastic cells of the basal plate are divided into basophilic cells presenting high activity in protein synthesis and clear cells containing glycogen, whereas the decidual cells at term appear inactive [49].

Recently, on the basis of the enzyme-histochemical studies of the basal plate, three types of X cells have been delineated [50]. The primarily basal cytotrophoblast invading the basal plate during early pregnancy, mainly differentiates into homogeneous X cells. It is suggested that they have endocrine function.

In regions of intensive intermingling with decidual cells, there appear vacuolated X cells elucidated by their content of acid phosphatase. The secondarily basal cytotropho-

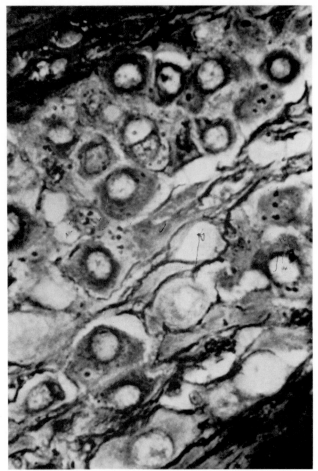

Fig. 12　X cells in the basal
plate (PAP, ×400).

blast penetrates into the basal plate during later pregnancy. It differs from the other X
cells by the transitory activity of alkaline phosphatase. After the loss of its alkaline phosphatase it develops into normal X cells.

By our enzyme-histochemical observations, the X cells were stained with lactate dehydrogenase reaction (LDH) and acid phosphatase as well as those of villous trophoblast,
and strong activity in glucose-6-phosphate dehydrogenase (G6PDH) was located in X cells
and villous trophoblast whch differ by less activity of staining of decidual cells (Table 3).

In addition, some writers have theorized that X cells have an endocrine function in
later pregnancy [49, 51]. However, the X cells contained no detectable HCG and HPL in
contrast to the hormonally active syncytial trophoblast [52, 53].

Table 3　The enzyme-histochemical localization in basal plate of the human placenta.

	Decidua cell	X cell	Villous trophoblast
LDH	—	++	+
Acid phosphatase	±	+	+
Alkali phosphatase	—	—	++
G6DH	—	+++	+++

2.   ELECTRON MICROSCOPIC FEATURES OF THE X CELLS

In ultrastructural studies of the basal plate of the human placenta, such cells in the basal plate have not always clearly been defined.

Wynn [54] pointed out that the cells of dual origin are most closely intermingled in the basal plate. Though some of the discrete cytotrophoblastic elements of the basal plate resemble mononuclear decidual cells, the two varieties can usually be distinguished. Well preserved cytotrophoblastic cells possess larger and more regular nuclei, large mitochondria and better developed endoplasmic reticulum of both the rough and smooth varieties.

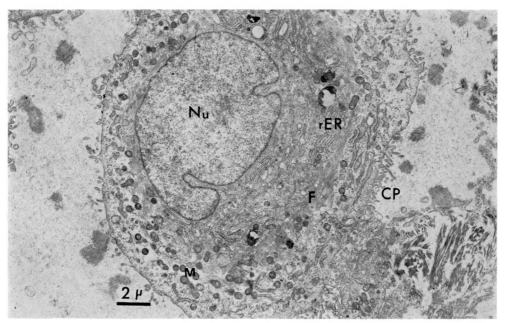

Fig. 13   Electron micrograph of X cell in basal plate of term placenta. Nucleus (Nu), rough endoplasmic (rER), fibrils (F), and mitochondria (M) are prominent ($\times$ 3,300).

On the other hand, Ruffolo et al. [55] found that X cells produce abundant amounts of glycogen and probably a mucinous material, have a well-developed endoplasmic reticulum, display microvilli, and contain abundant intracytoplasmic fine fibrils. As a result, they concluded that the ultrastructural features of X cells are more consistent with derivation from maternal tissues than from trophoblast. However, according to recent ultrastructural observations, these cells appear transitional in complexity from simple cytotrophoblast to fully developed syncytium. Our electron micrographs support the concept of the dual origin of the basal plate presented by Wynn [54]. The cytoplasm of X cells contains well-developed tubular rough endoplasmic reticulum in sheets (Fig. 13). Mitochondria are irregular with medium density and the cristae are tubular. The Golgi bodies are relatively abundant. Aggregates of fibrils are distributed in bundles within the cytoplasmic content, while giant cells contain numerous dilated vesicles of endoplasmic reticulum in the cytoplasm and the decidual cells display small nuclei and rough endoplasmic reticulum (Fig. 14) [56].

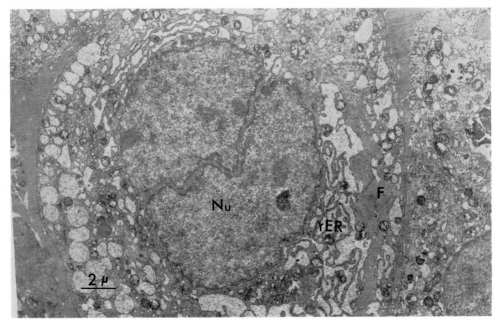

Fig. 14   Electron micrograph of giant cell in basal plate of 6 months gestation. Nucleus (Nu), rough endoplasmic (rER) and fibrils (F) are prominent (× 3,300).

3.   IDENTIFICATION OF THE X CELLS BY SEX CHROMATIN

The discovery of the Barr body in the nuclei of the intermitotic cells of many tissues led
to a new approach to the problem of the origin of the X cell. The method for identifying the
maternal or fetal nature of the X cells by the presence of sex chromatin in the nuclei of the
cells of the placental septa has been applied by several investigators [57–59]. They suggested
that the X cells are predominantly sex chromatin positive and of maternal origin. Nevertheless, dispute still exists as to whether the origin is from fetal or maternal progenitors.

BOYD and HAMILTON [60] concluded from their extensive experience that it is most
difficult to identify sex chromatin in the region where maternal and fetal tissues inter-
mingle. A fundamental difficulty in interpretation results from the structural distortion
of the tissue and degenerative changes in the area.

By means of autoradiographic technique with tritiated thymidine, KIM and BENIRSCHKE
[61] have shown that X cells in the human placenta are able to replicate, and they [62]
advanced the chromosome study of the X cells using the tissue culture techniques in order
to resolve fundamental difficulty in the identification of sex chromatin of the X cells in
the placental septa. As a result, the karyotypes of X cells in male babies had XX as female
sex chromosome complement. In this respect, they assumed that the X cells are of maternal
cell origin. However, it is suggested that X cells are poorly mitotic and that their *in vitro*
growth is affected by decidual cells that give the X cells a female karyotypic complement.

In addition, accrding to our investigation, the DNA content of nuclei of the X cells
estimated by microspectrophotometry was found to be diploid, statistically the same as that
of villous trophoblast and decidual cells.

Recently CASPERSSON et al. [63] described a band of intense fluorescence in the human Y
chromosome in metaphase and interphase nuclei. Quinacrine fluorescence microscopy is

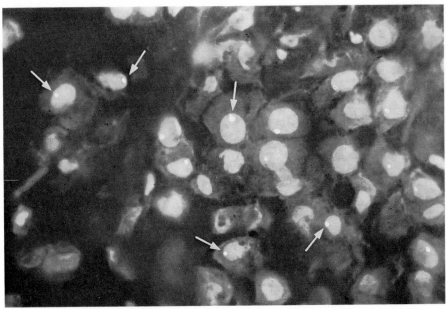

Fig. 15   F-bodies (arrows) within X cells in basal plate of the male placenta ($\times$ 1,000).

thus a valuable cytogenetic tool to determine the presence of a Y chromosome in nuclei at resting stages. Thereafter, a new application to the identification of sex chromatin of the X cells using quinacrine fluorescence of the Y chromosome (F-body) has shed further light upon studies of their origin [53, 64–66]. Khudr et al. [53] consistently demonstrated Y body fluorescence in X cells of male placentas and stated that X cells are of fetal tropho-blastic origin. However, the placental septa are composed partly of fetal and partly of maternal cells, the proportion of each changing in different septa.

Our recent data have shown that a F-body was found in the X cells of the placentas associated with male infants (Fig. 15). The incidence of F-body in each specimen was in 40.4 per cent of X cells of the male basal plate (Table 4). Although X cells are mostly of fetal origin, the question has been raised that the X cells of at least the basal plate may be derived from both sources.

From the above mentioned, it is considered that the trophoblastic cells and the X cells at the middle and end of pregnancies may have important function such as protein syn-thesis and immunological activity, in contrast to the decidual cells which appear to exert their major function at the onset of pregnancy. Thus, it is presumed that possibly the decid-ual cells are functionally replaced by the X cells.

Table 4   F-body in X cells of the basal plate.

Fetal sex	No. of specimen examined	Frequency of F-body in all specimens	Incidence of F-bodies in each specimen (%) M±SE
Male placenta			
Normal labor	44	44	12–48($\bar{X}=29.3\pm1.5$)
Cesarean section	18	18	20–54($\bar{X}=40.4\pm2.1$)
Female placenta			
Normal labor	13	2	1.0
Cesarean section	2	1	0.3

On the other hand, recently ALTSHULER et al. [67] observed that X cell proliferation was most marked in those instances where the pregnancy had progressed to term or beyond in the placentas of pre-eclamptic women. Consequently, they have speculated upon two possibilities. Either X cell proliferation represents a non-specific progression throughout pregnancy because of ultrastructural and biochemical observation or it represents an effect wherein X cell function is associated with a mechanism of delay of the onset of laber.

REFERENCES

1. HEPNER, R. and BOWEN, M.: The placenta and the fetus. J.A.M.A. **172**; 81/427, 1960.
2. CHABES, A., PEREDA, J., HYAMS, L., BARRIENTOS, N., PEREZ, J., CAMPOS, L., MONROE, A. and MAYORGA, A.: Comparative morphometry of the human placenta at high altitude and at sea level. Obstet. Gynec. **31**; 178, 1968.
3. KRÜGER, H. and ARIAS-STELLA, J.: The placenta and the newborn infant at high altitudes. Amer. J. Obstet. Gynec. **106**; 586, 1970.
4. BOYD, J.D. and HAMILTON, W.J.: Development and structure of the human placenta from the end of the third month of gestation. J. Obstet. Gynaec. Brit. Cwlth. **74**; 161, 1967.
5. THOMSON, A.M., BILLEWICZ, W.Z. and HYTTEN, F.E.: The weight of the placenta in relation to birthweight. J. Obstet. Gynaec. Brit. Cwlth. **76**; 865, 1969.
6. GARROW, J.S.: The relationship of fetal growth to size and composition of the placenta. Proc. roy. Soc. Med. **63**; 496, 1970.
7. GRUENWALD, P. and MINH, H.N.: Evaluation of body and organ weights in perinatal pathology II. Weight of body and placenta of surviving and of autopsied infants. Amer. J. Obstet. Gynec. **82**; 312, 1961.
8. TREMBLAY, P., SYBULSKI, S. and MAUGHAN, G.B.: Role of the placenta in fetal nutrition. Amer. J. Obstet. Gynec. **91**; 597, 1965.
9. YOUNOSZAI, M.K. and HAWORTH, J.G.: Placental dimensions and relations in preterm, term, and growth-retarded infants. Amer. J. Obstet. Gynec. **103**; 265, 1969.
10. WILKIN, P.: In: The Placenta and Fetal Membranes. Villee, C.A. (ed.) Williams & Wilkins, Baltimore, 1960, p. 225.
11. AHERNE, W. and DUNNIL, M.S.: Quantative aspects of placental structure. J. Path. Bact. **91**; 123, 1966.
12. WINICK, M.: Cellular growth of human placenta III. Intrauterine growth failure. J. Pediat. **71**; 390, 1967.
13. KRONE, H.A.: Pathologische Fruchtentwicklung bei Placentaanomalien. Arch. Gynäk. **198**; 224, 1963.
14. BENIRSCHKE, K. and BOURNE, G.L.: The incidence and prognostic implications of congenital absence of one umbilical artery. Amer. J. Obstet. Gynec. **79**; 251, 1960.
15. BUSCH, W.: Die Placenta bei der fetalen Mangelentwicklung. Arch. Gynäk. **212**; 333, 1972.
16. MARTIN, C.B.: The anatomy and circulation of the placenta. In: Intra-uterine Development. Barnes, A.C. (ed.) Lea & Febiger, Philadelphia, 1968, p. 35.
17. ALVAREZ, H. and BENEDETTI, W.L.: The placenta and its cord and membranes. Morphologic and functional changes of the trophoblast in relationship with oxygen pressure. In: Symposium on the Functional Physiopathology of the Fetus and Neonate. Abramson, H. (ed.) C.V. Mosby, St. Louis, 1971, p. 110.
18. FOX, H.: Effect of hypoxia on trophoblast in organ culture, A morphologic and autoradiographic study. Amer. J. Obstet. Gynec. **107**; 1058, 1970.
19. TOMINAGA, T. and PAGE, E.W.: Accommodation of the human placenta to hypoxia. Amer. J. Obstet. Gynec. **94**; 679, 1966.
20. MACLENNAN, A.H., SHARP, F. and SHAW-DUNN, J.: The ultrastructure of human trophoblast in spontaneous and induced hypoxia using a system of organ culture. J. Obstet. Gynaec. Brit. Cwlth. **79**; 113, 1972.
21. STARK, J. und KAUFMANN, P.: Trophoblastische Plasmapolypen und regressive Veränderungen am Zottentrophoblasten der menschlichen Placenta. Arch. Gynäk. **212**; 51, 1972.

22. SHARP, F., CARTY, M.J. and YOUNG, H.: The effects of hypoxia on hydroxysteroid dehydrogenase activity in placental villi maintained in organ culture. J. Obstet. Gynaec. Brit. Cwlth. **79;** 44, 1972.

23. FOX, H.: Pathological aspects of placental dysfunction. The Cong. Proc. 6th Asia. Cong. Obstet. Gynaec. 188, 1974.

24. THOMSEN, K.: Plazentarbefunde bei Spätgestosen und ihre ätiologische Zuordnung. Arch. Gynäk. **185;** 476, 1955.

25. GETZOWA, S. and SADOWSKY, A.: On the structure of the human placenta with full-term and immature foetus, living or dead. J. Obstet. Gynaec. Brit. Emp. **57;** 388, 1950.

26. HAMILTON, W.J. and BOYD, J.D.: Specialization of the syncytium of the human chorion. Brit. Med. J. **1;** 1501, 1966.

27. FOX, H.: The significance of villous syncytial knots in the human placenta. J. Obstet. Gynaec. Brit. Cwlth. **72;** 347, 1965.

28. FOX, H.: The incidence and significance of vasculo-syncytial membranes in the human placenta. J. Obstet. Gynaec. Brit. Cwlth. **74;** 28, 1967.

29. HORKY, Z.: Beitrag zur Funktionsbedeutung der Hofbauerzellen. Zbl. Gynäk. **86;** 1621, 1964.

30. ALVAREZ, H.: Morphology and physiopathology of the human placenta. Obstet. Gynec. **23;** 813, 1964.

31. ALADJEM, S.: Phase contrast microscopic observations of the human placenta from six weeks to term. An anatomic and clinical correlation. Obstet. Gynec. **32;** 28, 1968.

32. YOSHIDA, K., SOMA, H., HIRAOKA, M. and KIYOKAWA, T.: Evaluation of placental dysfunction through phase contrast microscopy. Acta Obstet. Gynaec. Jap. **22;** 37, 1975.

33. CIBILS, L.A.: The placenta and newborn infant in hypertensive conditions. Amer. J. Obstet. Gynec. **118;** 256, 1974.

34. ALADJEM, S., PERRIN, E. and FANAROFF, A.: Placental score and neonatal outcome. A clinical and pathologic study. Obstet. Gynec. **39;** 591, 1972.

35. OKUDAIRA, Y., HAYAKAWA, K., HAMANAKA, N., UEDA, G., YOSHINARE, S., SATO, Y. and KURACHI, K.: Human placental villi: Scanning electron-microscopic observations. Acta Obstet. Gynaec. Jap. **19;** 109, 1972.

36. BERGSTROM, S.: Surface ultrastructure of human amnion and chorion in early pregnancy. A scanning electron microscope study. Obstet. Gynec. **38;** 513, 1971.

37. LUDWIG, H.: Surface structure of the human placenta. In: The Placenta. Moghissi, K.S. (ed.) C.C. Thomas, Springfield, Ill. 1974, p. 40.

38. FERENCZY, A. and RICHART, R.M.: Female Reproductive System; Dynamics of scan and transmission electron microscopy. John Wiley & Sons, New York, 1974.

39. VILLEE, C.A.: The Placenta and Fetal Membranes. Williams & Wilkins, Baltimore, 1960, p.232.

40. FOX, H.: Histological features of placental senescence. In: The Foeto-placental Unit. Pecile, A. and Finzi, C. (eds.) Excerpta Medica, Amsterdam, 1969.

41. CLAVERO, J.A., ORTIZ, L., DE LOS HEROS, J.A. and NEGUERULA, J.: Blood flow in the intervillous space and fetal blood flow. II. Relation to placental histology and histometry in cases with and without high fetal risk. Amer. J. Obstet. Gynec. **116;** 1157, 1972.

42. ANDERSON, W.R. and McKAY, D.: Electron microscopic study of the trophoblast in normal and toxemic placentas. Amer. J. Obstet. Gynec. **95;** 1134, 1966.

43. WIGGLESWORTH, J.S.: Morphological variations in the insufficient placenta. J. Obstet. Gynaec. Brit. Cwlth. **71;** 871, 1964.

44. BURSTEIN, R., FRANKEL, S., SOULE, S.D. and BLUMENTHAL, H.T.: Aging of the placenta: Autoimmune theory of senescence. Amer. J. Obstet. Gynec. **116;** 271, 1973.

45. ZACKS, S.I. and BLAZAR, A.S.: Chorionic villi in normal pregnancy, pre-eclamptic toxemia, erythroblastosis, and diabetes mellitus. A light- and electron-microscope study. Obstet. Gynec. **22;** 149, 1963.

46. FOX, H.: Fibrinoid necrosis of placental villi. J. Obstet. Gynaec. Brit. Cwlth. **75;** 448, 1968.

47. GILLE, J., BÖRNER, P., REINECKE, J., KRAUSE, P-H. and DEICHER, H.: Über die Fibrinoidablagerungen in den Endzotten der menschlichen Placenta. Arch. Gynäk. **217;** 263, 1974.

48. BENIRSCHKE, K. and DRISCOLL, S.G.: The Pathology of the Human Placenta. Springer-Verlag, New York, 1967.

49. DALLENBACH-HELLWEG, G. and NETTE, G.: Morphological and histochemical observations on trophoblast and decidua of the basal plate of the human placenta at term. Amer. J. Anat. **115;** 309, 1964.

50. STARK, J. und KAUFMAN, P.: Die Basalplatte der reifen menschlichen Placenta II. Gefrier-schnitt-Histochemie. Z. Anat. Entwickl. Gesch. **135**; 185, 1971.

51. LATTA, J.S. and BEBER, C.R.: The differentiation of a special form of trophoblast in the human placenta. Amer. J. Obstet. Gynec. **74**; 105, 1957.

52. KIM, C.K., NAFTOLIN, F. and BENIRSCHKE, K.: Immunohistochemical studies of the "X cell" in the human placenta with anti-human chorionic gonadotrophin and anti-human placental lactogen. Amer. J. Obstet. Gynec. **111**; 672, 1971.

53. KHUDR, G., SOMA, H. and BENIRSCHKE, K.: Trophoblastic origin of the X cell and the pla-cental site giant cell. Amer. J. Obstet. Gynec. **115**; 530, 1973.

54. WYNN, R.M.: Fetomaternal cellular relation in the human basal plate; An ultrastructural study of the placenta. Amer. J. Obst. Gynec. **97**; 832, 1967.

55. RUFFOLO, R., BENIRSCHKE, K., CONVINGTON, H.I. and MUNRO, A.B.: Electron microscopic study of the "X-cells" in septal cysts of the human placenta. Amer. J. Obstet. Gynec. **99**; 1147, 1967.

56. ARAI, K., SOMA, H. and HOKANO, M.: Ultrastructure of the X cells in the basal plate of the human placenta. J. Clin. Electron Microscopy **7**; 284, 1974.

57. KLINGER, H.P. und LUDWIG, K.S.: Sind die Septen und die grosszelligen Inseln der Placenta aus mutterlichen oder kindlichen Gewebe aufgebaut? Z. Anat. Entwickl. Gesch. **120**; 95, 1957.

58. SERR, D.M., SADOWSKY, A. and KOHN, G.: The placental septa. J. Obstet. Gynaec. Brit. Emp. **65**; 774, 1958.

59. SOHVAL, A.R., GAINES, J.A. and STRAUSS, L.: Chromosomal sex detection in the human new-born and fetus from examination of the umbilical cord, placental tissue, and fetal membranes. Ann. N.Y. Acad. Sci. **75**; 905, 1959.

60. BOYD, J.D. and HAMILTON, W.J.: Placental septa. Z. Zellforsch. **69**; 613, 1966.

61. KIM, C.K. and BENIRSCHKE, K.: Autoradiographic study of the "X cells" in the human pla-centa. Amer. J. Obstet. Gynec. **109**; 96, 1971.

62. KIM, C.K., ALTSHULER, G.P. and BENIRSCHKE, K.: Karyotypic analysis of the X-cell in the human placenta. Obstet. Gynec. **37**; 72, 1971.

63. CASPERSSON, T., ZECH, L., JOHANSSON, C. and MODEST, E.J.: Identification of human chro-mosomes by DNA-binding fluorescent agents. Chromosoma **30**; 215, 1970.

64. MAIDMAN, J.E., THORPE, L.W., HARRIS, J.A. and WYNN, R.M.: Fetal origin of X-cells in human placental septa and basal plate. Obstet. Gynec. **41**; 547, 1973.

65. ERMOCILLA, R. and ALTSHULER, G.: The origin of "X cells" of the human placenta and their possible relationship to intrauterine growth retardation: An enigma. Amer. J. Obstet. Gynec. **117**; 1137, 1973.

66. FALLER, TH. und FERENEI, P.: Der Aufbau der Placenta-Septen Untersuchungen mit Hilfe der Quinacrinfluorescenzfärbung des Y-Chromatins. Z. Anat. Entwickl. Gesch. **142**; 207, 1973.

67. ALTSHULER, G., RUSSELL, P. and ERMOCILLA, R.: The placental pathology of small-for-gesta-tional age infants. Amer. J. Obstet. Gynec. **121**; 351, 1975.

Feto-placental unit and evaluation of estriol level

Tetsuya NAKAYAMA, M.D.

Department of Obstetrics and Gynecology, School of Medicine, Showa University, Tokyo

PURPOSE OF STUDY AND CONCEPT OF FETO-PLACENTAL UNIT

Development of a method to learn the state of a fetus in the uterine cavity of a pregnant woman, which may be termed a closed chamber, has been considered a major problem in clinical obstetrics dating back to many years, and recently, measurement of maternal urinary estriol has been calling attention. The purpose of this study is to clarify both fundamentally and clinically the significance of measurement of urinary estriol as a method of judging feto-placental functions.

Although of course a fetus in a pregnant uterus already possesses autonomy as a new life, it depends, so long as it is in the maternal body, solely on the mother for metabolism of substances through the placenta. Since the placenta assumes the various functions (such as respiration, absorption of nutriment, transfer of wastes and endocrine secretion) for sustaining life and promoting growth of the fetus so that it plays an extremely important role as the lifeline of the fetus, methods of determining the functions of the placenta as a means of elucidating fetal functions have come under study. However, as is clear from the fact that the placenta embryologically is an accessory organ of the fetus, its function is maintained normal only in harmony with the fetus and, therefore, may be considered under regulatory control by the fetus. From recent research on the endocrine mechanism of the placenta it has been disclosed that the fetus and placenta cooperate with each other as a functional unit, particularly with regard to the formation and metabolism of estrogens and progesterone, and the concept of the feto-placental unit has come vividly under the spotlight [1, 2]. Steroid hormone producing organs such as ovaries, testes and adrenals have a series of enzymes required for biosynthesis of various hormones (such as gestagens, androgens, estrogens and corticosteroids) utilizing acetate and cholesterol as materials, and possess so-called "de novo" biosynthetic functions. The distributions of enzymes involved in steroid hormone synthesis in the fetus and placenta are given in Table 1, and it has been clarified that since the enzymes possessed by each of the two are limited to only a part of the whole, they become complete as a series of steroid hormone synthesizing enzymes only when the two work together, in other words, only when the fetus and placenta work as a unit is possible the production of steroid hormones. In the following the basic researches of the author himself and his associates on the formation mechanism of estriol centering around the feto-placental unit will be introduced, and aspects of clinical application discussed.

Table 1   Distribution of steroid hormone synthesizing enzymes in fetus and placenta.

	Fetus	Placenta
Sulfokinase	+	−
Sulfatase	−	+
$\Delta_5 3\beta$-OH-steroid-dehydrogenase & isomerase	−	+
17β-OH-steroid-dehydrogenase	+	+
Aromatization enzyme	−	+
16α-hydroxylase	+	−
17-hydroxylase	+	−
11-hydroxylase	+	−
21-hydroxylase	+	−
17, 20-desmolase	+	−

ESTRIOL PRODUCTION MECHANISM IN FETO-PLACENTO-MATERNAL UNIT

1. PRODUCTION MECHANISM OF PLACENTAL ESTROGENS

1) ESTROGEN FORMATION CAPACITY OF PLACENTA

It has been known for a long time that urinary excretion of estrogens is markedly increased on conception and that estrogens exist in large quantities in the placenta. It had been assumed that estrogens increased during pregnancy were produced in the placenta from such facts as a) estrogens in the placenta exist mainly as free forms similar to those in other estrogen-producing organs (DICZFALUSY, 1953, 1955), b) increase of placental weight roughly parallels that of urinary estrogen excretion in pregnant women [3] (LEITER, 1958), c) secretion of estrogen originating from the mother's ovaries can be ignored since urinary estrogen excretion remains unchanged even when both ovaries are removed during pregnancy [4, 5] (WOLDSTEIN, 1929; GULDBERG, 1936; RIVIÈRE, 1955), and d) the adrenals of the mother cannot be considered an important source of estrogens since estrogen excretion was not changed in the case of a pregnant woman complicated by Addison's disease (SAMUELS, 1943; KNOWLTON, 1949; DE GENNES, 1959).

Previously, it was thought that the placenta, similar to ovaries, possessed a so-called de novo biosynthetic function initiating out from acetate to continue to the formation of cholesterol (C_{27} steroid) and finally to that of estrogen (C_{18} steroid). However, recent research disclosed that only a limited variant of enzymes exists in the steroid hormone producing enzyme group in the placenta (see Table 1). Parenthetically, since RYAN [6], it has widely been known that the placenta has a powerful aromatizing function with a strong action of converting the C_{19} steroid androgens into estrogens, but it was questionable whether it had the capacity of producing estrogens from cholesterol or progesterone. In perfusion experiments by the author's group using radioactive steroid precursors as substrates to verify the estrogen-producing function of the placenta (Table 2) [7, 8], androgens (C_{19} steroid) such as dehydroepiandrosterone (DHEA), Δ_4Androstenedione (Δ_4A) and testosterone (T) are readily converted into estrogens, but in cases of the C_{21} steroid progesterone and the C_{27} steroid cholesterol as substrates, estrogen production could not be recognized. This signifies that androgens are not produced from progesterone or cholesterol in the placenta, and further suggests that androgens which serve as precursors for producing estrogens are derived from some organ other than the placenta. Meanwhile, the author and his associates had reported that the majority (more than 90%) of the

Table 2 Conversion of radioactive steroids (Perfusion of human placenta).

Substrates		Conversion rate (%)		
		Estrone	Estradiol	Estriol
C_{19}	Δ_4Androstenedione-^{14}C	43.8	20.0	0.0
	Testosterone-^{14}C	47.2	15.9	0.0
	Dehydroepiandrosterone-^{14}C	42.4	7.7	0.0 16-epi 10.7
C_{21}	Progesterone-^{14}C	0.0	0.0	0.0
C_{27}	Cholesterol-^{14}C	0.0	0.0	0.0
Estrogen	Estradiol-^{14}C	60.3	5.2	0.0

urinary estrogens markedly increased during pregnancy was estriol [9]. However, in these experiments no formation of estriol (16α-hydroxyestradiol) whatsoever was disclosed in the placenta, although large quantities of estrone (E_1) and estradiol (E_2) were produced. This suggested that $\Delta_5 3\beta$-hydroxysteroid dehydrogenase ($\Delta_5 3\beta$-DHG) and 17β-hydroxysteroid dehydrogenase (17β-DHG) exist in the placenta along with aromatization enzymes, whereas 16α-hydroxylase is absent. This is indicative of the fact that for the production of estriol, which is one of 16α-hydroxysteroids, the involvement of the fetus or maternal body (livers and adrenals in particular) possessing 16α-hydroxylase is necessary, the details of which will be discussed later.

2)   ORIGINS OF PRECURSORS OF PLACENTAL ESTROGENS [10–12]

Since it is considered that the placenta has hardly any function of producing androgens which would serve as precursors of estrogens, the source of androgen production must be looked for in the maternal body or the fetus rather than the placenta. Adrenals and testes are most likely possibilities, while the mother's ovaries can be eliminated since urinary estrogens are not reduced after bilateral ovariectomies. As for the seminal glands of the fetus, they cannot be considered major sources of androgens as the quantity of urinary estrogens of the mother is unchanged regardless of the sex of the fetus. Consequently, the adrenals of the mother and fetus come under keen consideration.

i) Experiments to suppress adrenal function through administration of dexamethasone

The results of the measurement by the Brown method of urinary estrogen before and after administering 4mg of dexamethasone to a women pregnant four months (Table 3)

Table 3 Suppression of adrenal glands with dexamethasone (normal pregnancy).

	μg/day	Administration of dexamethazone	
		Before	After
Before delivery	EO	77.0	37.0
	ED	20.0	3.6
	ET	179.0	89.0
	Total	266.0	129.6
After delivery	EO	10.8	4.0
	ED	1.0	2.0
	ET	1.0	$\doteqdot 0$
	Total	12.8	6.0

showed that it was roughly halved apparently due to the suppression of adrenal cortical functions by dexamethazone given, suggesting that the adrenals of the mother and fetus were secreting precursors of estrogens. Since it was known that the principal androgen secreted from the adrenals is DHEA, subsequent investigations were centered on DEHA.

ii) Experiments of DHEA administration to fetal side of placenta

It has previously been stated (see Table 2) that as much as 50.1 per cent of radioactive substance in perfusates is converted into E_1 and E_2 when the fetal side of the placenta is perfused with DHEA-^{14}C as substrate.

In two women both at 6 months' gestation, each pregnancy was terminated by Cesarean section, then DHEA-4-^{14}C (5μC:/100μg) was injected into the umbilical cord so as to make it circulate within the feto-placental units. In mere 15 minutes the radioactivity was converted into the estrogen fraction in fairly high percentage (36.2%, 66.9%), and biosynthesis of estriol besides E_1 and E_2 was identified (Table 4). A control experiment for the case of fetus only (DHEA-^{14}C was administered to a newborn infant immediately after birth and urinary radioactive estrogens were checked) showed no production of estrogens (Table 5).

The above results indicate that $\Delta_5 3\beta$-DHG and aromatization enzymes exist in the placenta to supply it with the capability of readily converting DHEA of the fetus into estrogens.

Table 4   Conversion of radioactive steroids in feto-placental compartments (umbilical blood).

Case	Precursor	Phenolic	Estrone	Estradiol	Estriol	ET/EO ED ET
1	DHA-^{14}C	36.2	1.7	1.3	24.0	89.1
2	DHA-^{14}C	66.9	19.6	5.9	6.1	19.3

Table 5   Conversion of DHEA-4-^{14}C in vivo experiment with newborn infant (urine). (1st day of life)

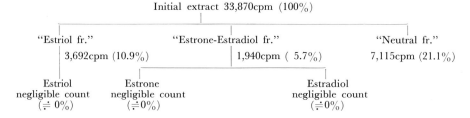

Initial extract 33,870cpm (100%)

"Estriol fr."   "Estrone-Estradiol fr."   "Neutral fr."

3,692cpm (10.9%)   1,940cpm (5.7%)   7,115cpm (21.1%)

Estriol   Estrone   Estradiol
negligible count   negligible count   negligible count
($\doteq$ 0%)   ($\doteq$0%)   ($\doteq$0%)

iii) Experiment of DHEA administration to maternal side of placenta

a) Experiment *in vitro*

A pregnant uterus removed by hysterectomy (case of cervical cancer at 4 months' pregnancy) was perfused for 3 hours from the maternal side with DHEA-4-^{14}C as substrate (apparatus the same as for the placental perfusion with a mixture of 100 ml of whole blood and 100 ml of physiological saline to which 3,000 I.U. of HCG was added), and the radioactivity was transferred to the phenolic fraction in 14.4 per cent with conversion into E_1 and E_2 recognized (Table 6).

b) Experiment *in vivo*

In two cases of analysis of 24 hour urine collections after intravenous injection of DHEA-4-^{33}C (5μC:/2.127μg) in two women pregnant 6 months' and 10 months' gestation, res-

Table 6 Perfusion of human pregnant uterus (DHA) (Perfusate).

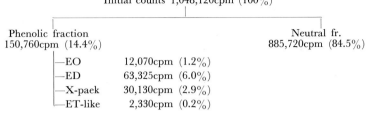

Initial counts 1,048,120cpm (100%)

Phenolic fraction 150,760cpm (14.4%)		Neutral fr. 885,720cpm (84.5%)
—EO	12,070cpm (1.2%)	
—ED	63,325cpm (6.0%)	
—X-paek	30,130cpm (2.9%)	
—ET-like	2,330cpm (0.2%)	

Table 7 Comparison of conversion rates (urine). (Conversion of dehydroepiandrosterone-^{14}C)

Maternal compartment	Delivery	Phenolic fr.	Estrone	Estradiol	Estriol
With normal fetus	before	24.1	4.2	2.0	2.7
	after	12.4	$\fallingdotseq 0$	$\fallingdotseq 0$	$\fallingdotseq 0$
With anencephalic futus	before	28.5	12.3	2.6	3.9
	after	11.2	$\fallingdotseq 0$	$\fallingdotseq 0$	$\fallingdotseq 0$

Table 8 Conversion of dehydroepiandrosterone-^{14}C (urine). (Hydatidiform mole)

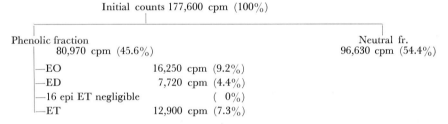

Initial counts 177,600 cpm (100%)

Phenolic fraction 80,970 cpm (45.6%)		Neutral fr. 96,630 cpm (54.4%)
—EO	16,250 cpm (9.2%)	
—ED	7,720 cpm (4.4%)	
—16 epi ET negligible	(0%)	
—ET	12,900 cpm (7.3%)	

pectively, both with anencephalic fetuses, 24 per cent and 28.5 per cent the radioactivity was converted into the phenolic fraction and production of E$_1$, E$_2$ and estriol was confirmed, while in the control tests consisting of analyses during puerperal confinement, conversion of DHEA-4-^{14}C into estrogens could not be evidenced (Table 7).

Furthermore, in case of the administration of DHEA-4-^{14}C to a woman with hydatidiform mole carrying no fetus (at 7 months' pregnancy), the radioactivity was demonstrated in the phenolic fraction in 45.6 per cent and the formation of E$_1$ (9.2%), E$_2$ (4.4%) and estriol (7.3%) was ascertained (Table 8).

The results obtained in vitro and in vivo experiments indicate that the placenta has the capability of converting DHEA on the maternal side into estrogens.

iv) Comparison between the rate of the conversion of maternal urinary DHEA of maternal side with that of fetal side

It has been ascertained through the above experiments that DHEA on the fetal as well as maternal sides is capable of assuming the role of precursors of placental estrogens, the next step of the experiment is to examine which side plays the principal part. DHEA-4-^{14}C was injected into umbilical cord at the time of the cesarean section in a woman at 6 months' gestation and made it circulate for 15 minutes within the feto-placental unit checking the amount of radioactive estrogens excreted in the maternal urine for 24 hours after injection, and this was compared with that in case of the injection into the maternal body (Table 9). On injection into the feto-placental unit (in which case metabolism at the

Table 9 Comparison of conversion rates (urine). (Conversion of dehydroepiandrosterone-^{14}C)

Administration			Phenolic fr.	Estrone	Estradiol	Estriol
Into feto-placental	exp.	1	73.9	2.7	1.5	29.9
	exp.	2	76.0	16.8	13.6	19.8
Into	normal fetus		24.1	4.2	2.0	2.7
	maternal anencephalus		28.5	12.3	2.6	3.9

maternal body also occurs) the urinary radioactive estrogen fraction is roughly twice as much as that in case of the maternal injection. This shows that the rate of the conversion of DHEA into estrogens (deducting metabolism in the maternal body) just in the feto-placental unit for 15 minutes is more or less double that in case of the maternal-placental unit. This indicates that the conversion efficiency of DHEA from the fetal side to the placenta is far higher than that from the maternal side.

v) Estrogen metabolism in case of pregnancies with anencephalic fetuses

Should the fetal adrenals be the source of placental estrogen precursors, it is conceivable that the estrogen production would be on the decrease in quantity in case of pregnancies with anencephalic fetuses whose adrenal cortical elements are known to be markedly atrophied, and as a matter of fact it has been shown that the urinary estrogens of such a gravida are only approximately one-tenth of those of a female with a normal fetus. This leads to the conclusion that the fetal adrenals are the chief source of placental estrogen precursors [13–15]. It is thought reports of marked declines in concentrations of DHEA sulfate and 16α-hydroxy-DHEA sulfate in anencephalic fetal blood (cord blood) compared with those in normal fetuses [16, 17] incidate that the androgen production from anencephalic fetus adrenals is decreased. The results of the experiments by our group are as follows:

a)   Estrogen Levels in Anencephalic Fetal Blood, Maternal Blood and Urine

The results of 9 pregnancy cases with anencephalic fetuses (Tables 10, 11) [18, 19] showed urinary estrogen of these gravidas is approximately one-tenth of or even less than that for normal cases, while the estrogen levels in maternal blood were seen conciderably lowered roughly in parallel to the urinary estrogen quantities. The estrogen levels of fetal blood also were evidenced to be considerably decreased in rough parallel with the cases of maternal urine and blood cases, and the reduction in the estriol fractions was especially prominent.

Table 10 Urinary estrogen concentrations in pregnancy with anencephalus. [19]

Case No. (weeks of gestation)	Estrone (μg/day)	Estradiol (μg/day)	Estriol (μg/day)
1 (44)	140–300	20–100	1,000–1,900
2 (39)	60	30	900
3 (33)	75	55	600
4 (40)	98	38	1,047
5 (35)	302	69	1,100
6 (40)	77	60	571
7 (39)	560	120	5,000
8 (35)	260	40	450
9 (34)	110	54	880
Normal values* near term	1,325	454	23,940

* mean values of five cases as determined in the laboratory.

Table 11   Plasma estrogen levels in pregnancy with anencephalus. [19]

Case NO. (weeks of gestation)	Cord plasma (μg/100ml)			Maternal plasma (μg/100ml)		
	Estrone	Estradiol	Estirol	Estrone	Estradiol	Estriol
1 (44)	1.7	0.9	3.9	0.7	0.2	1.0
2 (39)	1.6	—*	7.8	—*	—*	1.9
3 (33)	0.8	0.5	9.4	0.2	0.2	2.1
4 (40)	1.0	—*	3.5	0.5	0.9	0.9
5 (35)	1.2	0.5	9.0	3.4	0.9	2.1
6 (40)	0.7	0.7	1.3	0.5	0.4	0.8
7 (39)	0.3	0.8	26.7	5.7	1.1	5.9
8 (35)	0.9	0.3	0.7	0.8	0.7	0.9
9 (34)	1.5	—*	5.7	6.5	0.8	1.3
Normal values** near term	2.3	2.2	32.5	1.8	1.9	8.1

* below sensitivity of author's method.
** mean values of five cases as determined in the laboratory.

Table 12   Comparison of conversion rate in placental perfusion with dehydroepiandrosterone-[14]C.

	Phenolic fr.	Estrone	Estradiol	Estriol
Placenta with normal fetus	79.6%	42.4%	7.7%	0%
Placenta with anecephalus	95.8%	39.3%	42.8%	0%

These adrenals with the exception of one case (No. 7) were all extremely atrophied and weighed not higher than one-tenth of normal, while histologically adult zone atrophy was relatively minor but fetal zones called androgen zones were almost non-existent. In Case No. 7 of relatively large adrenal weight the estrogen value was comparatively higher than for the other cases and a parallelism between the size of fetal adrenal and the estrogen production could be surmised.

b)   Aromatization Capacity of the Placenta with Anencephalic Fetus

On checking placentae with anencephalic fetuses through perfusion experiment with DHEA-4-^{14}C as substrate (Table 12) [18], it was learned that, similar to normal placentae, they demonstrated strong capacities of conversing DHEA into estrogens. Furthermore, the aromatization capability mainly at the maternal surface of the placenta was checked by the conversion rate to urinary radioactive estrogens after administering of DHEA-4-^{14}C to the maternal side, while it had already been confirmed that placentae with anencephalic fetuses have the ability to convert maternal side DHEA into estrogens in a degree similar to those with normal fetuses (Table 7) [20].

These results lead to the presumption that although a placenta with an anencephalic fetus has the same ability as a normal placenta to convert DHEA into estrogens so long as it reaches to the placenta, its supply to the placenta is markedly reduced because of the decline in its production due to the extreme atrophy of the fetal zones of the fetal adrenals so that the estrogen production during pregnancy with anencephalic fetus is radically lowered. This is suggestive of the fact that the majority (more than 90%) of the precursors of placental estrogens is supplied by the fetal adrenals. Further, as described previously, although the ability even of a placenta belonging to a hydatidiform mole with no fetus to convert maternal DHEA into estrogen is considered fairly strong (Table 8 supra), it is suggested on the basis of previous reports that the urinary estrogen excretion of a gravida shows a subnormal value, and the DHEA secretion from the mother's adrenals is comparatively small. Consequently, it is conceivable that the precursors of placental estrogens are supplied mostly by the fetus.

3) REGULATION MECHANISM FOR PLACENTAL ESTROGEN FORMATION

Factors regulating aromatization fucntion of the placenta and DHEA production function of the fetal adrenals supplying precursors are considered principal two factors controlling the production of placental estrogens.

i) Factor regulating placental aromatization

Since the involvement of gonadotropin could be perceived in biosynthesis of steroids, placental gonadotropin (human chorionic gonadotropin: HCG) was administered to feto-placental units and the excretions of various kinds of steroids in maternal urine before and after that were checked. The cervical canals of three women pregnant 6 months authorized for termination were dilated with laminaria rods and 3,000 I.U. of HCG were injected into the umbilical cord through the vagina. Urinary estrogens were increased approximately to double the previous quantities after injections of HCG and continued to be excreted at high rates for about 36 hours, but pregnanediol, pregnanetriol, 17-KS and 17-OHCS were increased only temporarily immediately after injection (Fig. 1). When 5 ml of physiological saline was injected as controls, no change was observed. Also almost no alteration was evidenced in urinary estrogen quantity when HCG was administered to the maternal side, and in both cases the changes were only within the range of daily variations. Furthermore, as will be described below, urinary DHEA and 17-OHCS remained unchanged when HCG was administered to newborn infants immediately after delivery. From the results obtained, the increase of estrogens in the maternal urine following the administration of HCG to the fetus cannot be considered due to increase in secretion of androgens (precursors of estrogens) from the ovaries and adrenals of the mother or the

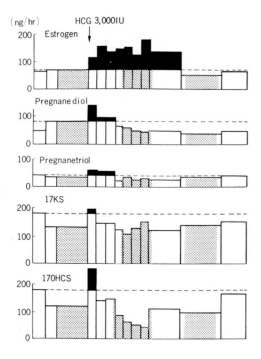

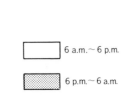

Fig. 1 HCG load on fetus in mother and maternal urinary steroids.

adrenals of the fetus, and it is suggested that the aromatization function of the placenta is activated by the administration of HCG [7].

ii) Factor regulating DHEA production of fetal adrenals

As it was considered that the chief sources of precursor production of placental estrogens were the fetal adrenals, their regulating factors were investigated [21, 22]. After confirming that the quantities of DHEA and 17-OHCS (Porter silver chromogen) in urine of newborn infants were not subject very much to time-dependent change up to the fifth day after birth, the variations in the quantities of these steroids excreted in response to the administration of ACTH, HCG and dexamethasone were checked to discern the role played by the fetal adrenal cortical function as a regulating factor (Tables 13–15). With administration of ACTH, both DHEA and 17-OCHS in urine began to increase from the first day thereafter, and on the second day prominent increases was noted approximately to 4 times and 6 times the amount prior to the administration, respectively. In case of dexamethasone, both started to decrease from the first day after the administration, and from the second day on, DHEA was reduced approximately to a quarter of the amount before the administration, while 17-OHCS declined to about 60 per cent on the second day, and in case of HCG no changes in the quantities of the two steroids could be recognized.

The results obtained are suggestive of the fact that ACTH from the fetal pituitaries regulate the secretion of DHEA by the fetal adrenal fetal zone. However, it is likely that this capacity is not existent in HCG.

Table 13 ACTH group (ACTH doses: 10 I.U./day). DHEA (μg/day)

NO.	Body weight	1st	2nd	3rd	4th	5th
1	3,560	92	209	537	1,561	
2	2,930	209	89	346	301	
3	3,200	153	431	327	1,170	
4	3,670		167	158	137	725

Note: Bold lines demarcate before and after administration. Ditto in tables following.

Table 14 Dexamethasone group (Dexamethasone doses: 500μg/day). DHEA (μg/day)

No.	Body weight	1st	2nd	3rd	4th	5th	6th
1	3,570	34	699	123	81		
2	3,440		91	80	54	13	
3	3,735		594	144	196	80	56
4	3,830		332	350	178	178	115
5	3,760		118	123	86	16	17

Table 15 HCG group (HCG doses: 5,000 I.U./day). DHEA (μg/day)

No.	Body weight	1st	2nd	3rd	4th	5th
1	3,450	79	79	65	154	
2	3,530	27	143	125	133	
3	3,580		372	146	258	340
4	3,150		140	200	126	116
5	3,050		194	242	164	233
6	3,235		249	199	240	334

2. ESTRIOL PRODUCTION AND FETO-PLACENTO-MATERNAL UNIT

In the foregoing placenta perfusion experiments, it has been disclosed that aromatization enzymes, $\Delta_5 3\beta$-DHG and 17β-DHG are contained in the placenta but not 16α-hydroxylase, and thus E_1 and E_2 are produced from DHEA, while conversion to the extent of estriol production is not to be confirmed. The involvement of the fetus and the maternal body (their livers and adrenals in particular) which do contain 16α-hydroxylase are required for the production of estriol comprising the greater part of urinary estrogens of the pregnant woman. Estriol, therefore, is produced only by the cooperative action of the fetus, mother and the placenta directly connecting them——the feto-placento-maternal unit as it is generally called.

1)   INVOLVEMENT OF FETUS OR MATERNAL BODY AND PRODUCTION OF ESTRIOL

i)   Feto-placental unit and production of estriol [11]

In order to check whether estriol is biosynthesized through the fetal involvement, DHEA-^{14}C was given to a feto-placental unit and made circulate in it, upon which in 15 minutes a fairly high rate of estriol-^{14}C production was clearly seen (Table 4, supra). Also, when estradiol-^{14}C known to be readily produced from DHEA at the placenta was administered to feto-placental compartments, the production of estriol-^{14}C was unmistakably recognized (Table 16). As a control, DHEA-^{14}C was injected into a newborn infant

Table 16   Conversion of Estradiol-^{14}C (feto-placental compartments).

Case	Conversion rate			Ratio
	EO	ED	ET	EO: ED: ET
1 (15 min)	4.4	3.8	41.5	8.8: 7.7: 83.5
2 (90 min)	2.8	3.2	10.3	16.8: 19.5: 63.7

immediately after delivery and the radioactive metabolism products in the urine were checked, but no production of estrogen-^{14}C was noted, while in case estradiol-^{14}C was given, conversion into estriol-^{14}C was recognized (Tables 17, 18).

These results indicate that a 16α-hydroxylation capacity is observed in the fetus, but not aromatization capability so that it is possible that E_1 and E_2 be produced from estriol, while 16α-hydroxy-DHEA can be formed from DHEA, although conversion further to estriol is not possible, and that the biotransformation from DHEA to estriol is feasible only by the collaboration of the fetus and the placenta.

Furthermore, on comparison between the efficiency of estradiol-^{14}C as estriol precursor and that of DHEA-^{14}C when administered to the feto-placental unit by the ratio of estriol-^{14}C production to radioactivity in cord blood, it is noticed that the trend of conversion into estriol is greater in the latter than in the former. It is suggested, therefore, that as the pathway of production of estriol from DHEA in the feto-placental unit, a neutral pathway not going through the stage of estradiol is dominant, that is to say, 16α-hydroxylation in the fetus precedes, followed by the pathway (for example, DHEA→16α-OH-DHEA→16α-Δ_4A→16α-OH-E_1→estriol) in which aromatization in the placenta takes place. Further comment will be made later in this respect.

Table 17   Conversion of DHEA-4-[14]C *in vivo* experiment with newborn infant (urine). (1st day of life)

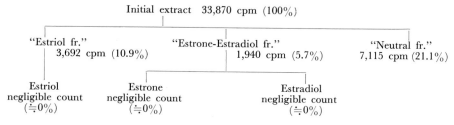

Initial extract   33,870 cpm (100%)

"Estriol fr." 3,692 cpm (10.9%)   "Estrone-Estradiol fr." 1,940 cpm (5.7%)   "Neutral fr." 7,115 cpm (21.1%)

Estriol negligible count (≒0%)   Estrone negligible count (≒0%)   Estradiol negligible count (≒0%)

Table 18   Conversion of estradiol-17β-16-[14]C *in vivo* experiment with newborn infant (1st post partum day urine).

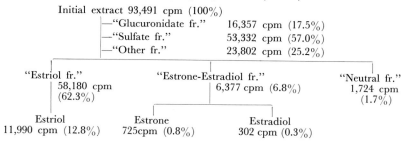

Initial extract 93,491 cpm (100%)

—"Glucuronidate fr."   16,357 cpm (17.5%)
—"Sulfate fr."   53,332 cpm (57.0%)
—"Other fr."   23,802 cpm (25.2%)

"Estriol fr." 58,180 cpm (62.3%)   "Estrone-Estradiol fr." 6,377 cpm (6.8%)   "Neutral fr." 1,724 cpm (1.7%)

Estriol 11,990 cpm (12.8%)   Estrone 725cpm (0.8%)   Estradiol 302 cpm (0.3%)

ii)   Materno-placental unit and production of estriol [11]

As mentioned previously, the production of estriol-^{14}C as a radioactive estrogen is noted when urinary metabolic substances are checked following the injection of DHEA-^{14}C in a pregnant woman, and also a considerable amount of estriol-^{14}C is formed in response to the administration of estradiol-^{14}C known to be derived from DHEA at the placenta (Table 19). When DHEA-^{14}C is given as a control to a woman in postpartal confinement, as also previously stated, the production of estrogen-^{14}C cannot be detected from the urine. Furthermore, it has been known for a long time that the urinary excretion of estriol even in a non-pregnant woman is increased when estradiol is administered.

It can be seen from the above results that the maternal body has a 16α-hydroxylation capability but not aromatization capacity worth mentioning, and, therefore, for the production of estriol from DHEA the collaboration of the placenta possessing an aromatization function and the maternal body is necessary, although the formation of estriol from estradiol may occur even at the maternal body alone.

Besides, as the efficiency of estriol synthesis at the materno-placental unit is considerably low in case of the administration of DHEA-^{14}C compared with that in case of estradiol-^{14}C, it is suggested that in the pathway of biotransformation from DHEA into estriol——

Table 19   Comparison of conversion rates (urine).

Case		Conversion rate				Ratio
		phenolic	EO	ED	ET	EO: ED: ET
ED-[14]C		90.3	8.9	7.4	34.4	17.7: 14.6: 67.7
DHA-[14]C	normal	24.1	4.2	2.0	2.7	47.2: 22.5: 30.3
	anencephalus	28.5	12.3	2.6	3.9	65.4: 13.9: 20.7

the pathway through estradiol and estrone (both being known to be mutually readily convertible by 17β-DHG)·——aromatization at the placenta is precedent, followed predominantly by a pathway (a phenolic pathway: for example, DHEA→Δ_4A→E_1→16α-OH-E_1→estriol) in which 16α-hydroxylation is formed at the maternal body. It is quite interesting to note that the principal synthesization pathway from DHEA to estriol is not the same according as the materno-placental and feto-placental units differ.

Table 20   Conversion of dehydroepiandrosterone-[14]C (urine).

Case		Conversion rate				Ratio
		Phenolic	EO	ED	ET	EO : ED : ET
Into fetoplacental	normal	73.9	2.7	1.5	29.9	7.9 : 4.4 : 87.7
	normal	76.0	16.8	13.6	19.8	33.5 : 27.1 : 39.4
Into maternal	normal	24.1	4.2	2.0	2.7	47.2 : 22.5 : 30.3
	anencephalus	28.5	12.3	2.6	3.9	65.4 : 13.9 : 20.7

Table 21   Comparison of estriol-^{14}C formation rates from DHA-^{14}C, Δ_4A-^{14}C and ED-[14]C (at feto-placental unit).

Substrate	Time circulated in cord blood (min)	Ratio to radioactivity in cord blood (%)				Ratio of 3 estrogen fractions (%)		
		Phenolic fraction	EO	ED	ET	EO	ED	ET
DHA-[14]C	15	36.2	1.7	1.3	24.0	6.3	4.8	88.9
	15	66.9	19.6	5.9	6.1	62.0	18.7	19.3
Δ_4A-[14]C	15	32.7	16.2	7.3	0.6	67.1	30.5	2.4
	15	80.8	21.3	7.6	3.1	66.6	21.3	9.7
ED-[14]C	15	—	10.6	33.8	8.4	20.1	64.0	15.9
	90	—	18.8	35.9	21.6	24.5	47.0	28.5

iii) Comparison between the efficiency of feto-placental unit as estriol production rate and that of materno-placental unit

DHEA-^{14}C was administered to both of the feto-placental and materno-placental units and the radioactive metabolities in maternal urine were analyzed to compare the estriol-^{14}C production rate in case of the former with that in case of the latter (Table 20). The result was that in case of the former, in which the fetus was involved and the circulation time of DHEA-^{14}C given was only 15 minutes, the rate of the conversion of that radioactive agent into estriol-^{14}C was just 10 times as much as that in case of the latter, and that the production of estriol from DHEA was greatly increased through such a fetal involvement. It was demonstrated further that the conversion into the phenolic fraction (estrogen fraction) was also roughly three times in efficiency. Such a trend coupled with the fact in case of the use of estradiol-^{14}C the result is almost the same irrespective of the administration site (Table 21, in which fetal involvement is hardly suggested in the conversion from estradiol to estriol) implies that the production of estriol (excreted in maternal urine) from DHEA (secreted from fetal adrenals) during pregnancy is greatly increased through the fetal involvement, and that the action of 16α-hydroxylation on DHEA occurring in the fetus plays a major role.

2) PRODUCTION OF 16α-HYDROSTEROIDS IN FETUS
i) **Metabolism of DHEA in fetal adrenals and liver**

As in the foregoing experiment, results indicating that the process of 16α-hydroxylation of DHEA in the fetus plays an important role in the mechanism of synthesis of estriol from DHEA were obtained, the 16α-hydroxylation functions of the liver and adrenals thought to be the principal 16α-hydroxylation organs were analyzed [23]. Slices (thickness, 30μ) of the liver (1.0g) and adrenals (0.98g) of a fetus at the sixth month of gestation placed in a Krebs-Ringer bicarbonate buffer (pH 7.6) solution with DHEA-4-^{14}C (0.5μ Ci/0.3545μg) were incubated for 3 hours at air temperature of 37°C, and the free fractions extracted were separated by alumina column chromatography into DHEA, Δ5Androstenediol, 16α-OH-DHEA and Δ5Androstenetriol, and the last two were further analyzed and identified (Tables 22, 23).

Table 22 Metabolism of DHA in incubation experiment with fetal liver.

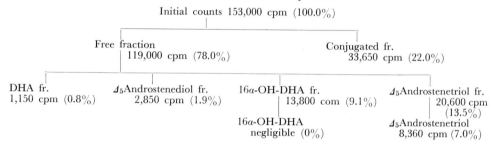

Table 23 Metabolism of DHA in incubation experiment with fetal adrenal.

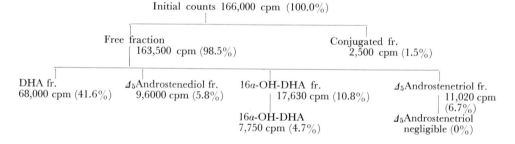

a) Adrenals

Radioactivity of 10.8 per cent was detected in the 16α-OH-DHEA fraction, and later, as specific activities were in agreement for acethylation, thin layer chromatography and recrystallization, it was possible to identify the production of 16α-OH-DHEA. At first, 6.7 per cent radioactivity was found in the Δ5Androstenetriol fraction, but in later analyses the existence of Δ5Androstenetriol could not be verified.

b) Liver

Radioactivity of 9.1 per cent was detected in the 16α-OH-DHEA fraction, but in subsequent analysis and purification, determination of 16α-OH-DHEA was not possible. In the Δ5Androstenetriol fraction 13.5 per cent radioactivity was recognized, but in the processes of subsequent analysis and purification the specific activities were in agreement and it was not possible to determine production of Δ5Androstenetriol.

The fact that 16α-OH-DHEA is formed with a fair degree of efficiency at the fetal adrenals as stated above suggests that there are secretions from the fetal adrenals in the form of 16α-OH-DHEA along with DHEA. Meanwhile, 16α-OH-DHEA was not detected at the liver, but since 16α-OH-DHEA is converted into Δ_5Androstenetriol at a fairly rapid rate, it is suggested that the 16α-OH-DHEA produced at the liver is subjected extremely quickly to 17β-hydroxylation to be converted into Δ_5Androstenetriol. It should be noted that there is a report (Solomone et al., 1965) that in perfusion experiments on a previable fetus, 16α-OH-DHEA from radioactive DHEA was found in circulating blood and Δ_5-Androstenetriol was determined in the liver, and the 16α-OH-DHEA in circulating blood in this experiment is surmised to originate from the liver, but further examination of this matter should be necessary.

ii) Metabolism of estradiol at various organs of fetus

That 16α-hydroxylation of DHEA in the fetus has much significance in conversion from DHEA into estriol in the feto-placental unit has been discussed previously. The role played by the fetus in phenolic pathways (aromatization at the fetus precedent) considered to be minor ones is studies here. In effect, the metabolic functions of fetal organs with respect to estradiol produced from DHEA at the placenta were investigated by incubation and perfusion experiments at the slice level using estradiol-^{14}C as the substrate for adrenals, liver and kidneys (Table 24) [7, 24].

Table 24 Conversion rate of estradiol-17β-16-^{14}C (fetal organs).

			Estriol(%)	16 epi Estriol (%)	Estrone(%)
Adrenal	Incubation		1.1	0	20.9
Liver	Incubation		2.2	0	30.2
	Perfusion	in Liver	12.6	0.3	8.5
		in Perfusate	4.5	0	11.1
Kindney	Incubation		0	0	29.8

It was shown that the liver and adrenals of a fetus have the capabilities of converting estradiol into estriol, that is, estriol can be produced using estradiol formed at the placenta as the material. In other words, it is possible for a pathway for production of estriol from DHEA by a phenolic pathway existing in the feto-placental unit also.

3) SUMMARY

It has been indicated that it is necessary to introduce the concepts of feto-placental and feto-placento-maternal units in regard to the estriol formation mechanism during pregnancy. In essence:

(1)   The placenta possesses a strong function to convert androgens into estrogens (aromatization), but it does not have the ability to produce the materials (androgens), and the bulk (approximately 90%) of the androgens is thought to originate in the fetal adrenals and a part is supplied from the maternal adrenals. In effect, it was shown that regarding production of placental estrogens, the co-working of fetus, placenta and maternal body as an organic functioning unit with respect to the supply of material (androgens) and processing (aromatization) of the material is necessary, and that the role played by the feto-placental unit is especially prominent. It has been suggested further that HCG acts as a regulating factor against the aromatization function of the placenta and ACTH as a regulating factor against the DHEA production function of the fetal adrenals.

(2)   Since 16α-hydroxylase required for biosynthesis of 16α-hydroxy-estrogen estriol is lacking at the placenta, it is necessary for the fetus or the maternal body having 16α-hydroxylase to become involved, and especially, the 16α-hydroxylation of the DHEA occurring in the fetus plays an important role in production of estriol from the DHEA secreted from the fetal adrenals so that there is a strong possibility that the fetal adrenals secrete 16α-OH-DHEA already subjected to 16α-hydroxylation. In other words, for the production of placental estriol, it is necessary for the cooperative action of the feto-placento-maternal unit to exist in connection with the processes of furnishing of materials, aromatization and 16α-hydroxylation, particularly that of the fetus and placenta playing the principal role as a unit. Consequently, it was clarified that the quantity of urinary estriol during pregnancy reflects the metabolism function of the feto-placental unit, and the measurement thereof could be applied to the judgment of feto-placental functions.

BIOSYNTHESIS PATHWAYS OF ESTRIOL AT FETO-PLACENTAL COMPARTMENT

1.   PHENOLIC PATHWAYS (A PATHWAYS) AND NEUTRAL PATHWAYS (B PATHWAYS)

There are a number of pathways known to exist with regard to biosynthesis of estriol from DHEA in the feto-placental compartment (Fig. 2), and a series of enzymes such as (1) $\Delta_3 3\beta$-DHG and Δ_5-Δ_4 isomerase, (2) 17β-DHG, (3) aromatization enzymes and (4) 16α-hydroxylase necessary as enzyme systems is the same for all pathways with only the order of enzymatic action being different. It has previously been described that of these enzymes (1) and (3) exist in the placenta but not in the fetus, while (4) exists only in the fetus and is lacking in the placenta. Therefore, should these pathways be broadly divided, they would be the phenolic pathways in which 16α-hydroxylation occurs in the fetus after prior aromatization in the placenta (A pathways), and in contrast, the neutral pathways in which 16α-hydroxylation in the fetus precedes and aromatization in the placenta follows (B pathways).

1)   PHENOLIC PATHWAYS (A PATHWAYS)
As the principal A pathway, the following is conceivable:

$$\text{DHEA} \xrightarrow{(1)} \overset{\text{T}}{\underset{}{\Delta_4 \text{A}}} \xrightarrow{(3)} \overset{\text{E}_2}{\underset{}{\text{E}_1}} \xrightarrow{(4)} 16\alpha\text{-hydroxy-E}_1 \xrightarrow{(2)} \text{estriol}$$

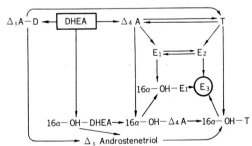

Fig. 2   Pathway to estorial (E$_3$) from DHEA in the fetoplacental compartment.

with (1) and (3) at the prior stages occurring in the placenta followed by (4) in the fetus, and the (2) at the end can be either in the fetus or the placenta (placenta perfusion experiment, Table 2; fetal organ cultivation experiment, Table 23).

i)   Pathway A-I

Using a fetal liver (6 months' gestation), a perfusion experiment (Type O whole blood 200 ml, perfusion pressure 20–30 mg Hg, perfusion rate 80 ml/min for 2 hours) with E_2-^{14}C (0.5μ Ci/80μg) as the substrate was carried out (Table 25) [25], and the quantity of estriol-

Table 25 Conversion to estriol from estradiol-^{14}C in fetal liver. (Perfusion)

		Initial counts	Conversion rate			E_3/E_1
			E_1	(E_2)	E_3	
Liver tissue	cpm	107,000	9,100	17,290	13,405	1.5
	%	100	8.5	16.3	12.6	
Perfusate	cpm	90,280	9,980	(33,000)	4,100	0.4
	%	100	11.1	(36.6)	4.5	

^{14}C detected in the perfusate was compared with the estriol-^{14}C produced in the liver tissue. This, besides indicating that the reactions of (4) and (2) occurred in the liver (Pathway A-I), also suggests that the estriol formed in the liver and released into the fetal blood is relatively small with the bulk retained in the liver constitution, and most likely it is thought this is excreted in liver bile. Furthermore, as will be described later, in an experiment of simultaneous administration of DHEA-^3H and Δ_4A-^{14}C or DHEA-^3H and E_1-^{14}C to the feto-placental compartment, it has been shown that estriol is produced by this pathway in the fetal liver (Tables 30, 31, infra). In other words, it is conceivable that estriol is formed mainly in the fetal liver in case of the A pathways although its release into the fetal blood is comparatively small, and that excretion mainly into the bile can be surmised, similar to the metabolic pathway of degradation of E_1 and E_2 secreted from the ovaries at times of non-pregnancy, converted into estriol in the liver.

From this fact, it is suggested that estriol produced in the fetal liver is a metabolic excretion type of E_1 and E_2 produced in the placenta which will be expelled from the fetal circulatory system and passing the biliary duct later will be excreted into the intestinal tract.

ii)   Pathway A-II

$$E_2 \rightleftharpoons E_1 \xrightarrow{(4)} 16a\text{-OH-}E_1 \xrightarrow{(2)} \text{estriol}$$

That the above reactions take place in the fetal liver is certain from the foregoing results. It is also possible for a pathway to exist in which $16a$-OH-E_1 produced by the reaction of (4) is carried to the placenta where the reaction of (2) occurs (Pathway A-II). As will be described later (Tables 30, 31, infra), the facts that the administration of DHEA-^3H, Δ_4A-^{14}C and E_1-^{14}C to the feto-placental compartment will result in the production of a fairly large quantity of $16a$-OH-E_1 in the cord blood, and that when $16a$-OH-E_1-^3H is given to the feto-placental unit it is readily converted into estriol in the placenta (Table 27, infra) indicate the existence of this Pathway A-II. The estriol produced by this pathway, unlike that formed at the fetal liver, moves in part immediately to the maternal side and is thought to cause some kind of physiological action.

2)   NEUTRAL PATHWAYS (B PATHWAYS)

In case of these pathways, the first question is with respect to the type of $16a$-hydroxylated

C_{19} steroid into which DHEA would be converted. In the incubation experiment previously described, the production of Δ_5Androstenetriol in the fetal liver and 16α-OH-DHEA in the adrenals have been determined and there is a possibility that these two reach the placenta through the fetal blood. According to DICZFALUSY's group, only Δ_5Androstenetriol was detected in the liver and only 16α-OH-DHEA in the fetal blood [26], as a result of the administration of radioactive DHEA to previable fetuses. Furtheron, in placenta perfusion experiments in situ using various radioactive 16α-hydroxy C_{19} steroids, 16α-OH-DHEA was converted into estriol through the pathway 16α-OH-Δ_4A→16α-OH-E_1, but a pathway through 16α-OH-T could not be proven, while, on the other hand, Δ_5Androstenetriol was converted into estriol through the stage of 16α-OH-T [27, 28]. In effect, the B pathways could be subdivided into a pathway going through the state of 16α-OH-E_1 or DHEA→16α-OH-DHEA→16α-OH-Δ_4A→16α-OH-E_1→estriol (Pathway B-I) and a Pathway B-II which ultimately goes through the stage of 16α-OH-T. The latter was said to have only the pathway of DHEA→16α-OH-DHEA→16α-OH-Δ_4A→16α-OH-T (Pathway B-IIa) with no pathway such as DHEA→16α-OH-DHEA→16α-OH-Δ_4A→16α-OH-T→estriol (Pathway B-IIb) existing so that Pathway B-I is the principal neutral pathway.

In order to study the above, radioactive 16α-hydroxysteroids were synthesized microbiologically (using RUSE and SOLOMON [29]; Streptomyces roseochromogenus), administered to the feto-placental unit and their metabolism images were investigated.

i) Experiments administering DHEA-4-^{14}C and 16α-OH-DHEA-^{3}H

Trace doses of DHEA-4-^{14}C and 16α-OH-DHEA-^{3}H were administered to cord blood at the time of termination by cesarean section, and after circulation in the feto-placental compartments for 15 minutes, the radioactive metabolites in the placentae, cord bloods, fetal livers and maternal urines were checked (Table 26) [30]. Fairly large amounts of

Table 26 Distribution of estrogenic and 16α-hydroxylated compounds isolated.*

	Placenta		Cord blood		Fetal liver	
Radioactivity Recovered (DPM)	^{3}H 249,6000	^{14}C 693,5000	^{3}H 27,300	^{14}C 40,250	^{3}H 11,800	^{14}C 19,200
Estradiol-17β	0	6.4%	0	1.2%	0	3.9%
Estrone	0	8.4%	0	7.4%	0	0
16α-OH-estrone	2.9%**	0	0	1.8%	0	0
Estriol	1.7%	0	1.0%	0	5.5%	6.3%
16α-OH-testoster.	5.5%	0	0	0	0	0
16α-OH-DHEA	3.0%	0	11.8%	2.4%	0	0
Δ_5Androstenetriol	0	0	0	0	0	0

* Steroids administered $\begin{cases} 16\alpha\text{-OH-DHEA-}^3\text{H} \ (6.9\times10^6\text{DPM}) \\ \text{DHEA-}^{14}\text{C} \ (13.2\times10^6\text{DPM}) \end{cases}$

** Figures expressed as percent of total radioactivity recovered in each source.

16α-OH-T (5.5%) and 16α-OH-E_1 (2.9%) were identified along with estriol originating from 16α-OH-DHEA-^{3}H (estriol originating from DHEA-^{14}C was not identified) in the placentae, and while only 16α-hydroxysteriod originating from 16α-OH-DHEA-^{3}H determined in cord blood was estriol, 16α-OH-DHEA (2.4%) and 16α-OH-E_1 (1.8%) originating from DHEA-^{14}C were detected. Estriol from both DHEA-^{14}C and 16α-OH-DHEA-^{3}H was further identified in the fetal liver. The fact that production of 16α-OH-T originating from 16α-OH-DHEA-^{3}H was identified in the placenta differs from the reports by the DICZFALUSY school beforementioned. This is indicative of a possibility of 16a-OH-T being converted from 16a-OH-DHEA and becoming a precursor of estriol. This suggests that in the production of estriol from 16a-OH-DHEA a Pathway B-IIb through 16a-OH-T besides a Pathway B-I through 16a-OH-E_1 (formation of which also was seen in the placenta) is existing. The fact that the production of 16a-OH-DHEA originating from DHEA-^{14}C was recognized in the cord blood, together with the above results, strongly suggests a possibility of the existence of a biosynthetic pathway (Pathway B-IIb) of DHEA →16a-OH-DHEA→16a-OH-T.

ii) Experiments administering 16α-OH-DHEA-^{14}C and 16α-OH-E_1-^{3}H

Trace doses of 16a-OH-DHEA-^{14}C and 16a-OH-E_1-^{3}H were used and similar tests were carried out for a circulation time of 15 minutes (Table 27) [25]. In these experiments,

Table 27 Conversion of $\begin{cases} 16a\text{-OH-estrone-}^3\text{H} \\ 16a\text{-OH-DHEA-}^{14}\text{C} \end{cases}$ in feto-placental compartment (Administered ^{3}H/^{14}C=2.0).

	Placenta					Umbilical blood				
	^{3}H		^{14}C		^{3}H/^{14}C	H^3		^{14}C		^{3}H/^{14}C
	cpm	(%)	cpm	(%)		cpm	(%)	cpm	(%)	
Initial counts	244,000	100,0	76,000	100.0	3.2	171,730	100.0	95,730	100.0	1.8
Estriol	37,000	19.0	11,000	14.5	3.2	1,860	1.0	660	0.7	2.8
(16a-OH-estrone)	0	0	0	0	/	(27,770)	(16.1)	750	0.8	37.0
(16a-OH-DHEA)	0	0	0	0	/	0	0	(1,725)	(1.8)	0
16a-OH-T	/	/	0	/	/	0	0	0	0	/

since the 16a-OH-T fraction was missed at the stage of gradient elation partition chromatography by celite column for the placenta, conversion to 16a-OH-T could not be verified, but production of large quantities of estriol from both 16a-OH-DHEA-^{14}C and 16a-OH-E_1-^{3}H was confirmed (19.0% and 14.5%, respectively). It was indicated further that these 16a-hydroxysteroids when reaching the placenta were very quickly subjected to metabolism and converted into estriol. Moreover, that even a small quantity of 16a-OH-E_1 originating from 16a-OH-DHEA-^{14}C was recognized in the cord blood (this is thought to have been produced in the placenta) suggests there exists a B-I pathway of 16a-OH-DHEA→16a-OH-E_1→estriol, and that the formation of estriol originating from 16a-OH-E_1-^{3}H was recognized in the liver indicates that in part of Pathway B-I there is a possibility of a mechanism of 16a-OH-E_1 made from 16a-OH-DHEA at the placenta passing through the cord blood to the fetal liver where it is converted into estriol.

On the basis of the two experiments described above, it has been confirmed that 16a-OH-DHEA is converted into estriol in the placenta, and parenthetically a neutral pathway (a B pathway) exists. It has further been indicated that besides the B-I pathway through 16a-OH-E_1, there is a possibility of a B-II pathway going through 16a-OH-T.

In case of the B pathways, the feature is that estriol is produced in the placenta (excluding Pathway B-Ib), and unlike in case of the estriol thought to be a metabolic or excretion type produced in the fetal liver in the previously mentioned A pathways (excluding Pathway A-b), it is estimated that there is a nature of what may be called a physiological pregnancy estrogen which can exert a positive influence to some extent by moving immediately from the placenta to the maternal body (and on to the fetus).

2. PRINCIPAL PATHWAYS OF PRODUCTION OF PLACENTAL ESTROGENS

As described in the preceding section, the place of estriol production differs according to the pathway (Table 28), although there are various production pathways for estriol in the feto-placental unit.

In other words, A-II and B (excluding B-Ib) are conceivable as pathways for the formation of placental estriol, while fetal estriol (mainly from liver) is produced through the pathways of A-I and B-Ib. The following describes the result of investigations mainly focused on the production pathways of placental estriol.

1) EXPERIMENT I

Radioactive DHEA, $\mathit{\Delta}_4$A and E_2 were injected into the feto-placental unit separately, made to circulate and the rates of production of radioactive estriol in cord blood were checked (Table 21, supra) [11]. A trend was seen that the quantity of E_3 formed from DHEA was clearly greater than in case of $\mathit{\Delta}_4$A administration, and also than in case of E_2 administration. This means that estriol is mainly produced from DHEA by a pathway not going through $\mathit{\Delta}_4$A or E_2, that is to say, a B pathway.

2) EXPERIMENT II

In order to confirm the above, DHEA-^{3}H and $\mathit{\Delta}_4$A-^{14}C were simultaneously administered to cord blood of the same case, made to circulate for 15 minutes in the feto-placental compartment and the ^{3}H/^{14}C ratios of radioactive estrogens produced in the cord blood were investigated (Table 29) [31]. Whereas the ^{3}H/^{14}C ratios of E_1 and E_2 were almost equal (Case 1) or slightly low as compared with the amount of steroids injected (Case 2), the ^{3}H/^{14}C ratio of estriol was roughly four times the ratios of E_1, E_2 and the injected steroids. This is indicative of the fact that the production of estriol from DHEA in the feto-placental compartment takes place mainly in a B pathway not going through the stage of $\mathit{\Delta}_4$A, in other words, a pathway in which aromatization in the placenta occurs following 16α-hydroxylation in the fetus.

Table 28   Estriol formation pathways in feto-placental unit.

		Metabolism pathway	E_3 formation organ
A Pathways	A-I	DHEA→$\mathit{\Delta}_4$A→E_1→16α-OH-E_1→E_3	Fetus
	A-II	DHEA→$\mathit{\Delta}_4$A→E_1→16α-OH-E_1→E_3	Placenta
B Pathways	B-I-a	DHEA→16α-OH-DHEA→16α-OH-$\mathit{\Delta}_4$A→16α-OH-E_1→E_3	Placenta
	B-I-b	DHEA→16α-OH-DHEA→16α-OH-$\mathit{\Delta}_4$A→16α-OH-E_1→E_3	Fetus
	B-II-a	DHEA→16α-OH-DHEA→$\mathit{\Delta}_5$Androstenetriol→16α-T→E_3	Placenta
	B-II-b	DHEA→16α-OH-DHEA→16α-OH-$\mathit{\Delta}_4$A→16α-OH-T→E_3	Placenta

Table 29 ^{3}H/^{14}C ratios of isolated estrogens following administration of $\begin{cases} \text{DHEA-}^3\text{H} \\ \mathit{\Delta}_4\text{A-}^{14}\text{C} \end{cases}$ in feto-placental compartment (umbilical blood).

	^{3}H/^{14}C ratio administered	E_1	E_2	E_3
No. 1	2.2	2.55	2.57	9.86
No. 2	2.5	0.96	1.58	9.53

Table 30 Conversion of $\begin{cases} \text{DHEA-}^3\text{H} \\ \varDelta_4\text{A-}^{14}\text{C} \end{cases}$ in feto-placental compartment (Administered $^3\text{H}/^{14}\text{C}=2.5$).

	Conversion counts (cpm)								
	Placenta			Umbilical blood			Fetal liver		
	^3H	^{14}C	$^1\text{H}/^{14}\text{C}$	^3H	^{14}C	$^3\text{H}/^{14}\text{C}$	^3H	^{14}C	$^3\text{H}/^{14}\text{C}$
Initial counts	276,605	193,310	3.0	386,680	173,230	2.2	699,830	1,175,350	0.6
Estradiol	36,400	10,520	3.5	2,090	1,370	1.7	10,430	8,420	1.2
Estrone	34,400	11,190	3.0	12,120	12,600	1.0	,360	,420	0.9
16a-OH-E$_1$	3,780	2,310	1.6	23,120	23,340	1.0	,700	,730	1.0
Estriol	39,900	7,310	5.5	35,300	3,590	9.5	37,790	21,330	1.7
16a-OH-T	14,710	770	19.8	1,330	0	∞	0	0	/
E$_3$/E$_1$+E$_2$+E$_3$	35	25	/	71	20	/	78	71	/

3) **EXPERIMENT III**

In the above experiments, it has been disclosed that estriol is produced from DHEA at the feto-placental compartment mainly by a B pathway, and in order to study this pathway in details, DHEA-^{3}H and $\varDelta_4$A-^{14}C were given simultaneously as in Experiment II. After circulation for 15 minutes in the feto-placental compartment, the radioactive metabolites in the fetus, cord blood, fetal liver and maternal urine were examined, and the converted amounts and the ^{3}H/^{14}C ratios for estriol and the intermediate metabolic steroids in the process to the estriol were investigated (Table 30) [25, 32].

i) **Estriol**

Whereas estriol originating from DHEA-^{3}H is seen to the same degree in the placenta, cord blood and fetal liver, estriol originating from $\varDelta_4$A-^{14}C is produced in largest amount in the fetal liver and is relatively small in quantity in the placenta and fetal blood. On examination of the ^{3}H/^{14}C ratios, the ratio in the placenta (5.5) is distinctly higher than that (2.5) of the steroids given, while in the fetal liver (1.7) it is clearly lower. This leads to the conclusion that placental estriol is produced from DHEA chiefly by B pathway, while fetal liver estriol mainly by A pathway.

Further, that the ^{3}H/^{14}C ratio (9.5) of estriol in cord blood is extremely higher than that (1.7) in the liver and is close to that (5.5) in the placenta suggests that this is principally estriol produced at the placenta, and that its production by B pathway occurs sooner than that by A pathway, and therefore the ^{3}H/^{14}C ratio of estriol produced in the placenta at the early stage of perfusion is extremely high, and due to its transfer to the cord blood it may be interpreted that it is higher than the ^{3}H/^{14}C ratio of estriol in the placenta at 15 minutes of perfusion.

The ^{3}H/^{14}C ratios of the various estrogens in maternal urine are roughly equal to those of estrogens in the placenta, and ^{3}H/^{14}C ratio (4.4) of estriol higher than those (1.0) of E$_1$ and E$_2$ means that estriol produced in the placenta is transferred extremely quickly to the maternal side.

ii) **16a-Hydroxysteroids**

As it was evidenced that the precursors immediately prior to the formation of estriol are the two of 16a-OH-E$_1$ (A pathway and Pathway B-I) and 16a-OH-T (Pathway B-II), these were focused on and investigated.

a) 16a-OH-E$_1$

16a-OH-E$_1$ originating from both DHEA-^{3}H and $\varDelta_4$A-^{14}C was shown in a largest amount in umbilical cord blood, while that in the placenta was relatively small in quantity and that determined in the fetal liver was even less. That 16a-OH-E$_1$ detected in the cord blood was the one formed (by A pathway) mainly in the fetal liver from E_1 and trans-ferred there should be understandable from the facts that the $^3H/^{14}C$ ratio is equal to that of the $16a$-OH-E_1 steroid in the fetal liver (both 1), and that the ratios (1.0 and 0.9 respectively) are roughly equal to those of El in the same liver and El in the cord blood (this originates from the placenta). On the other hand, that the $^3H/^{14}C$ ratio (1.6) of $16a$-OH-E_1 in the placenta is slightly higher than the ratio in the cord blood (1.0) is considered due to partial inclusion of $16a$-OH-E_1 produced through aromatization of $16a$-OH-DHEA and $16a$-OH-$\varDelta_4$A in the placenta (in effect, through B pathway) besides the transfer of $16a$-OH-E_1 from the cord blood.

b) $16a$-OH-T

$16a$-OH-T originating from DHEA-^3H was identified in a fairly large quantity in the placenta. A small amount was also noted in cord blood, while $16a$-OH-T originating from $\varDelta_4$A-^{14}C was determined in an extremely small amount in the placenta alone. That the $^3H/^{14}C$ ratio is exceedingly high at 19.8 indicates that $16a$-OH-T is produced mainly by a pathway not going through $\varDelta_4$A from DHEA-^3H, that is, B pathway. In the results ob-tained by the author's group mentioned previously (Table 25), it was pronounced that $16a$-OH-T is derived from $16a$-OH-DHEA in the placenta, and it is thought that besides $16a$-OH-T converted from $\varDelta_5$Androstenetriol reported by DICZFALUSY's group (Pathway B-IIa), there is another $16a$-OH-T converted from $16a$-OH-DHEA (Pathway B-IIb).

c)   Respective Weight of Two $16a$-Hydroxysteroids as Estriol Precursors

(a)   Placental Estriol : From the fact that the $^3H/^{14}C$ ratio of estriol in the placenta is 5.5, the ratio of $16a$-OH-E_1 is 1.7 and that of $16a$-OH-T is 19.8, the calculation that approx-imately two-thirds of the estriol in the placenta are converted from $16a$-OH-T and rough-ly one-third from $16a$-OH-E_1 is valid. And considering the previously mentioned result that a portion of the latter is produced in Pathway B-I, it is calculated roughly 70 per cent of placental estriol is produced in B pathways (the majority at Pathway B-II) and only about 30 per cent in A pathway.

(b)   Liver Estriol : Based on the facts that estriol from both DHEA-^3H and $\varDelta_4$A identified in the liver is fairly large in quantity, and moreover, that $^3H/^{14}C$ ratio (1.7) is slightly higher than the $^3H/^{14}C$ ratio (1.0) of $16a$-OH-E_1 in the same liver, the calculation that the greater part (approximately 93%) of the estriol is converted in the liver from $16a$-OH-E_1 and that part (approximately 7%) of the estriol in the cord blood (estriol originating from DHEA-^3H is far greater in quantity than that from $\varDelta_4$A-^{14}C and thus the $^3H/^{14}C$ ratio is high at 9.8) is transferred is well-founded. Since it may be considered that $16a$-OH-E_1 in the liver is converted from E_1 and transferred there from the cord blood (as beforementioned), it is thought the greater part, more than 90 per cent, of the liver estriol is produced in A pathways.

Based on the result stated above, it is to be suggested that the production pathway of placental estriol differs from that of estriol in the liver, in other words, it is produced chiefly through B pathway, especially through Pathway B-II (a pathway not going through $16a$-OH-E_1 but through $16a$-OH-T)——a matter which in the past reports had tended to be refuted.

4)   EXPERIMENT IV

In order to examine further the results of Experiment III, E_1-^{14}C already subjected to aromatization was administered (in lieu of $\varDelta_4$A-^{14}C) simultaneously with DHEA-^3H to the feto-placental compartment and made to circular for 5 minutes and similar searches as in Experiment III were made (Table 31) [30].

Table 31 Conversion of DHEA-^{3}H and E1-^{14}C in feto-placental compartment
(Administered ^{3}H/^{14}C=0.9).

| | Converction counts (cpm) | | | | | | | | |
| | Placenta | | | Umbilical blood | | | Fetal liver | | |
	^{3}H	^{14}C	^{3}H/^{14}C	^{3}H	^{14}C	^{3}H/^{14}C	^{3}H	^{14}C	^{3}H/^{14}C
Initial counts	235,350	200,930	1.2	278,980	345,690	0.8	62,860	289,730	0.22
Estradiol	13,900	13,300	1.1	0	6,040	0	0	15,220	0
Estrone	45,000	41,100	1.1	0	90,200	0	0	43,360	0
16α-OH-estrone	0	0	/	0	13,050	0	0	890	0
Estriol	10,600	8,700	1.2	5,100	5,250	0.97	9,290	15,750	0.59
16α-OH-T	5,900	0	∞	1,150	0	∞	0	0	/

i) Estriol

Estriol originating from both DHEA-^{3}H and E$_1$-^{14}C was identified in the placenta, cord blood and fetal liver. The ^{3}H/^{14}C ratios were 1.2 at the placenta and clearly higher than the 0.9 of the steroids administered, while they were low in the fetal liver at 0.59.

ii) Estriol precursors

E$_1$ and E$_2$ originating from DHEA-^{3}H were demonstrated in the placenta only and were not detected in the cord blood and the fetal liver. Regarding 16α-OH-E$_1$, only that originating from E$_1$-^{14}C was evidenced in the cord blood and fetal liver, while 16α-OH-T only from DHEA-^{3}H was noted in the placenta and umbilical cord blood.

As described above, E$_1$ and E$_2$ originating from DHEA-^{3}H, and 16α-OH-E$_1$ could not be verified in the umbilical blood and liver, and the ^{3}H/^{14}C ratio of estriol in the placenta was higher than that of the steroids administered. This is enough to lead to the assumption that placental estriol produced follows a pathway from DHEA-^{3}H that does not go through E$_1$ but mainly through 16α-OH-T, or Pathway B-II, while fetal liver estriol is produced following A pathway from DHEA-^{3}H mainly through E$_1$ and 16α-OH-E$_1$ ——all substantiating the presumption of the author's group previously mentioned.

3. SUMMARY

Pathways for the production in the feto-placental compartment of estriol from DHEA were examined and the following results were obtained:

(1)   This estriol formation contains phenolic pathways (A pathways) and neutral pathways (B pathways), but in the placenta and fetal liver considered the prinicipal estriol producing organs, the respective production pathway differs. While estriol in the former is chiefly produced by B pathway in which 16α-hydroxylation in the fetus precedes followed by aromatization in the placenta, estriol in the latter is mainly formed by A pathway in which aromatization occurs first.

(2)   In regard to the details of the production pathways of placental estriol, it has been noted that of the three pathway including Pathway A-II (DHEA→Δ_4A→E$_1$→16α-OH-E$_1$→estriol) and Pathway B-I (DHEA→16α-OH-DHEA→16α-OH-Δ_4A→16α-OH-E$_1$→estriol) the principal pathway (approximately 70%) is Pathway B-II going through 16α-OH-T. It has further been implied that the placental estriol is quickly transferred from fetus to mother and is capable of influencing physiological processes so that from the biosynthesis mechanism aspects estriol is considered to possess the physiological character of a pregnancy estrogen.

FETO-PLACENTAL FUNCTION AND ESTRIOL LEVEL IN MATERNAL URINE

1. FACTORS INFLUENCING ESTRIOL QUANTITY IN MATERNAL URINE

As is clear from the formation mechanisms of estriol in the feto-placento-maternal unit previously described, the three factors given in Table 32 are conceivable as those influencing estriol quantities in maternal urine. Actual cases are cited below.

Table 32   Principal factors influencing maternal urinary estriol.

---

1) Condition of production of material (DHEA) from fetal adrenal tissue
2) Conversion capacity of DHEA to estriol in feto-placental unit
    1. 16α-hydroxylation capacity of fetus (adrenal or liver)
    2. Aromatization capacity of placenta
    3. $\Delta_5 3\beta$-OH-Steroid-DHG activity of placenta
    4. 17β-OH-Steroid-DHG activity of placenta anf fetus
3) Blood circulation condition of feto-placento-maternal unit

---

1)   DHEA FORMATION CAPACITY OF FETAL ADRENALS

Of the maternal urinary estrogens of anencephalic pregnancy cases in which fetal adrenals showed extreme atrophy (Table 10, supra), estriol quantities were shown to be markedly reduced to approximately one-tenth of those of normal fetuses, in which as in Case No. 7 with relatively slight atrophy of the adrenals the reduction in estriol quantity was smaller, and the growth of the fetal adrenals was thus roughly parallel to the quantity of estriol in maternal urine. Since it is thought that the fetal adrenal growth and DHEA production capability run roughly parallel, the lowering of DHEA production capability can be considered the cause of reduction in the quantity of estriol in maternal urine. It is also known that concentrations of DHEA and 16α-OH-DHEA in anenecephalic fetus blood are greatly lowered.

2)   METABOLIC FUNCTION OF DHEA TO ESTRIOL IN FETO-PLACENTAL COMPARTMENT

The aromatization function of the placenta and the 16α-hydroxylation function of the fetus are problems of particular attention. In cases of anencephalic fetuses in which the estriol levels in maternal urine are low, the estrogens in umbilical blood are likewise low (Table 12, supra), and the lowering of 16α-hydroxylation function of the fetus is implied by the prominent decline in the estriol fraction compared with the reductions in the E_1 and E_2 fractions. The following is the result of the investigation to this effect. Injecting trace doses of ^{3}H-DHEA into umbilical cord blood in case of an anencephalic fetus at the time of the termination by cesarean section and allowing circulation for 15 minutes in the feto-placental compartment, the radioactive estrogens (E_1 and E_2) biosynthesized in the placenta and umbilical blood and 16α-hydroxyestrogens (E_3 and 16α-OH-E_1) were examined, and comparisons were made with cases of normal fetuses (Table 33) [34, 35].

Although there were no great differences in quantity of formation of total estrogen, the production rate of 16α-hydroxyestrogen in the case of an anencephalic fetus was prominent-

Table 33 ^{3}H-DHEA metabolic capability in anencephalic fetus cases (16α-hydroxylation capability and aromatization capacity).

		Placenta		Cord blood	
		Anencephalic fetus	(Control)	Anencephalic fetus	(Control)
	Initial counts	148,560 dpm	276,605 dpm	163,530 dpm	380,680 dpm
Conversion rate (%)	E_1	9.5	12.5	2.3	3.2
	E_2	11.0	13.2	0.7	0.5
	16α-OH-E_1	0.2	1.4	0.5	6.0
	E_3	3.3	14.5	0.4	9.1
	(total E)	23.3	41.4	3.9	18.8
	(total 16α-OH-E)	3.5	15.9	0.9	15.1
totl 16α-OH-E/total E (%)		13.0	38.0	23	80
$E_3/(E_1+E_2)$		0.15	0.56	0.12	2.48

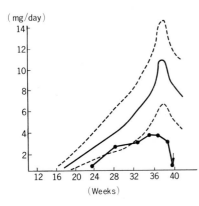

Fig. 3 Transition in urinary estorial in case of intra-uterine fetal death. Progress good in final stages of pregnancy. Apearance of hypertention, albuminuria (slight) from 38W. Labor initiated at 39W 2D and fetal heart rate extinct, stillbirth, excessive torsion of umbilical cord recognized. Abnormally low estriol level in urine was noticed by chance the previous day. Infant 3,280 g, placenta 500 g, placental infarct (—).

ly decreased, suggesting the lowering of 16α-hydroxylation functions in amencephalic fetuses. It is believed that the reason for the small amount of estriol production in case of anencephalic pregnancy is closely related to, in addition to the small amount of formation of DHEA as a material, the lowering of 16α-hydroxylation functions in anencephalic fetuses.

3) STATE OF BLOOD CIRCULATION AT FETO-PLACENTO-MATERNAL COMPARTMENT

Fig. 3 is a case in which torsion of the umbilical cord was marked, and the circulatory obstruction of the feto-placental compartment was estimated to have been a major cause of fetal death. In this case the transitions of estriol into the maternal urine was observed as pregnancy progressed. From midterm of pregnancy on the estriol quantity was close to the lower limit of the normal range and continued at a relatively low level until immediately before death of the fetus the estriol quantity showed a sudden abnormal decline.

4) SUMMARY

The above results indicate that the fetus plays the main role in biosynthesis of estriol and that the condition of feto-placental circulation is of extreme importance, and it is seen that an impediment in any of the above 3 factors will cause the lowering of the estriol quantity in maternal urine. Each of these 3 factors is an important aspect of the fetal metabolic function, and furthermore, the three are functionally interrelated and it may be comprehended that by measurement of estriol the metabolic function of the fetus as a composite of the 3 factors can be ascertained.

2. SIMPLE METHODS OF QUANTITATIVE MEASUREMENT OF URINARY ESTRIOL OF PREGNANT WOMAN

The basis for the great significance that measurement of urinary estriol of a pregnant woman has on monitoring the fetus in the mother by way of checking the function of the feto-placental compartment has been described in the foregoing. For application to actual clinical aspects, development of a simple yet highly accurate method of quantitative measurement is required. The methods used by the author's group are briefly introduced below.

1) METHOD A [36, 37]
i) Procedure
A quantity of 5 ml of a pregnant woman's urine (0.5 to 1 ml in the third trimester) is taken and diluted with 10 ml of distilled water. Adding 0.6 ml of conc H_2SO_4, this is hydrolyzed at 100°C for 90 minutes. Extracts are taken twice using 10 ml of ether and washed once with 10 ml of 5 per cent $NaHCO_3$ and twice with 10 ml of distilled water. Then vacuum distillation and drying are performed, followed by column chromatography using 1 g of alumina, and first estrone, estradiol, 17-KS, pregnanediol and corticosteroid are removed beforehand by eluting with 5 per cent methanol-benzene (M-B), and further estriol fraction is eluted with 30 per cent M-B. The latter is vacuum-distilled and dried, then caused to be colored by Kober chromogen using 2 per cent hydroquinone sulfuric acid (65%), and the absorption at 513 mμ is measured with a spectrophotometer with the reading corrected by ALLEN's formula using the absorptions at 480 mμ and 546 mμ.
ii) Accuracy of method
Alumina column chromatography is applied for separating estriol in this method, and it has been confirmed that almost all of the various steroids in the urine of a pregnant woman are eluted by 5 per cent M-B. The rate of recovery by this method in case 10 μg of pure estriol are added is 58 per cent, while scatter is not more than about 10 per cent.
iii) Transitions of estriol level in normal pregnancy
In Fig. 4 the estriol levels in urine by week of gestation are given for 324 instances (381 samples) of normal preganacies whereby healthy infants weighing 2,801 to 3,800 g were later delivered at full terms. This shows estriol increases rapidly from around the fifth month of pregnancy when the placenta has become completely formed, reaching a peak at around the thirty-eighth week, after which a gradual decline is noted until delivery.

2) METHOD B [38, 39]
Although there is no problem in reproduceability with Method A, a shortcoming is that the rate of recovery is slightly low. Therefore, at present, Method B which is a simplification of the method of BROWN (1957) is being used and this method will now be introduced. Still further, the X-AD method (a simplified method of extracting steroids in urine in combined form using the absorbent X-AD and extracting as well as measuring only the Kober chromogen coloring substances of estrogens following ITTRICH's Method) recently coming into practical use is being examined and its report will be published soon.
i) Procedure
A quantity of 0.2 ml (0.5 ml at the second and third trimesters, 1 to 3 ml at the first trimester of pregnancy) of a pregnant woman's urine is taken and diluted with 10 ml of distilled water. Adding 1.5 ml of conc HCl, this is hydrolyzed at 100°C for one hour.

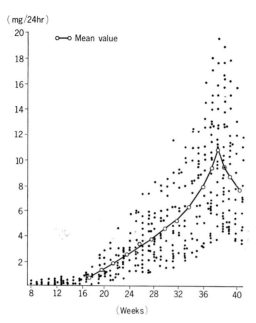

Fig. 4 Urinary ET in normal pregnancy (Method A).

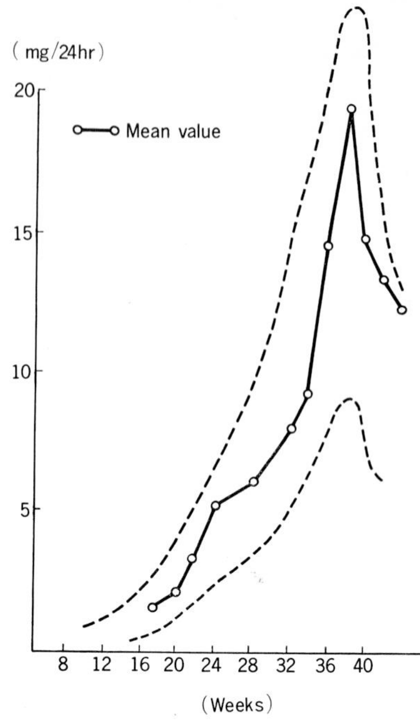

Fig. 5 Urinary estriol in normal pregnancy (Method B).

Extracting twice with 20 ml of ether, the extract is washed once with 10 ml of carbonate solution (pH 10.4), once with 3 ml of 8 per cent $NaHCO_3$ and once with 1.5 ml of distilled water. Following this, the ether portion is vacuum-distilled and dried, then redesolved in 20 ml of a mixed solution (1 : 1) of benzene and petroleum ether. From this the estriol portion is extracted twice with 10 ml of distilled water, and is further estriol back-extracted from the distilled water twice with 20 ml of ether. Quinol sulfuric acid reagent (2% hydroquinone solution of 70% v/v H_2SO_4) is added in the amount of 3 ml and hydrolyzation is performed for 20 minutes at 100 °C, followed by cooling. Adding 1 ml of H_2O, this is heated again for 10 minutes at 100 °C to cause Kober chromogen coloration. Within one hour of coloration, following Method A beforementioned, the absorption at 513 mμ is measured by spectrophotometer and corrections are made by ALLEN's formula.

ii) Accuracy and Normal Levels of Method

The rate of recovery with this method in case 6 μg of pure estriol is added is approximately 80 per cent, while scatter is not more than about 10 per cent. The transitions into estriol values by weeks of gestation in cases of normal pregnancies are shown in Fig. 5. Sharp increases are seen after 6th month of pregnancy.

3. FETO-PLACENTAL DYSFUNCTION AND ESTRIOL LEVEL

1) ESTRIOL LEVELS IN CASES OF TOXEMIAS OF PREGNANCY

It is known from researches in the past that in cases of toxemias of pregnancy the rates of underdeveloped and infarcted placentae are high and placental dysfunctions are frequently seen, coupled with a rate of delivery of premature infants 2.5 times (4.5 times for serious cases) that of normal pregnancies and a high rate of intrauterine fetal deaths

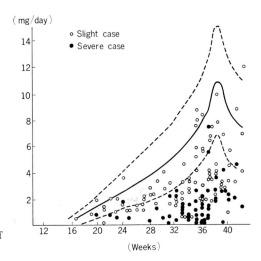

Fig. 6 Urinary estriol levels in case of pregnancy toxemias.

amounting to 10 times (20 times for serious cases) normal [40]. Fig. 6 gives urinary estriol values measured for 120 instances (141 samples) of toxemias of pregnancy showing that more than 90 per cent of the cases had distributions under the average level, with 90 per cent of the 60 serious cases especially indicating abnormally low values below the normal range. This suggests that there exists a distinct parallel relation between clinical statistics on prognoses of infants and abnormalities of placentae in toxemic pregnancy and urinary estriol levels, or inversely there is a dysfunction from the aspect of estriol formation capability in feto-placental units in toxemia cases of pregnancy indicating a close relationship between that pregnancy and prematureness of fetuses.

2) ESTRIOL LEVELS IN OVERTERM PREGNANCY

In overterm pregnancies so-called difficult deliveries are known to be relatively high in frequency with the rates of perinatal fetal death and of infant asphyxy two to three times those of normal term deliveries. It is thought that in some of these cases is playing what can be considered a dysfunction in the labor initiating mechanism, parenthetically, an abnormal symptom in which there is no onset of labor, although a condition of latent feto-placental disproportion has developed resulting in the endangerment of fetal life (NAKAYAMA, 1968).

In order to cut down the relatively high rate of perinatal fetal mortality incident to such a pathological condition, it is essential that deliveries be completed while the feto-placental units are still normally functioning, and it is necessary, therefore, to continuously measure the estriol levels in order to check the function of feto-placental unit and provide an indication of labor at an appropriate time.

In the following, cases in which it is thought the lives of infants were made survived through the continuous measurements of estriol are briefly described (Table 34) [41].

i) Case 1

A 28-year-old primigravida experiencing no labor pains even at 42W 0D was hospitalized. The oxytocin test at 0.02 unit positive, no meconium staining of amniotic fluid checked by hysteroscope, the cervix dilated for one finger, the uterine muscles sensitive to oxytocin so that with the expectation that onset of natural labor could be looked forward a watch was initiated. Since labor was not started even after waiting for 3 days, oxytocin drips (3 units) were administered for 5 hours to 42W 3D without, however, any effect. On the

Table 34   Estriol levels in overterm cases.

	Weeks and days of gestation	Estriol level	Delivery induction method	Observations on infant	Observations on placenta
Case 1	42W-3D	5.9mg	Oxytocin drip	3,410g ♂ Asphyxy (−)	Placental dysfunction syndrome (Clifford)
	42W-0D	3.8mg			
	43W-1D	2.2mg	Cesarean section		
Case 2	42W-4D	28.9mg	Oxytocin drip	2,980g ♂ Apgar score 4 recovery	Placental dysfunction syndrome (Clifford)
	42W-6D	16.7mg			
	43W-1D	13.6mg	Forceps delivery		
Case 3	42W-3D	20.6mg		3,290g ♀ Apgar score 7 2min later 10	Prominent white infarcts
	42W-4D	15.8mg	Cesarean section		
	42W-6D	8.6mg			

other hand, as the urinary estriol count (Method A: NAKAYAMA, 1961) showed a gradual drop of 5.9 mg→3.8 mg→2.2 mg, induction of labor was carried out again by oxytocin drip at 42W 1D upon which the fetal heart sounds got impaired, and as it was diagonosed as fetal distress, emergency delivery by cesarean section was performed. The infant was a male weighing 3,410 g indicating a placental dysfunction syndrome (CLIFFORD) together with placenta, yellowish-green color, while there were marked indications of peeling of the fetal tissues, but the prognosis was good.

ii) Case 2

A 20-year-old woman in her first pregnancy was hospitalized past the estimated date of confinement at 42W 3D. The oxytocin test positive at 0.04 unit, and the amniotic fluid checked by hysteroscope indicated no meconium staining, but the cervix was more or less closed. Since a trend of gradual decline in estriol levels (Method B : NAKAYAMA, 1967) of 28.9 mg→16.7 mg→13.6 mg was recognized, oxytocin drip (2 units) was performed at 42W 2D, upon which labor was initiated and the cervix was fully dilated without trouble, but from around this time the fetal heart beats became alarmingly impaired so that forceps delivery was performed.

The infant was a male weighing 2,980 g with the Apgar score immediately after delivery 4, but it recovered through resuscitation and the subsequent progress was favorable. The fetus and the placenta showed a placental dysfunction syndrome (CLIFFORD) when delivered.

iii) Case 3

A 23-year-old woman (primigravida) was hospitalized past the estimated date of confinement at 42W 3D. The oxytocin test was positive at 0.02 unit and meconium staining of the amniotic fluid checked by hysteroscope was not recognized, while the cervix was dilated for one finger. The estriol level (Method B) dropped rapidly (20.6 mg→15.8 mg→ 8.6 mg), in addition to which a slight staining of the amniotic fluid was recognized by the hysteroscope so that delivery was made by cesarean section. The infant was a female weighing 3,290 g with the Apgar score at delivery 7, but this was recovered to 10 two minutes later. Staining of the amniotic fluid at delivery was prominent while numerous white infarcts were demonstrated in the placenta.

3)   CASE OF PREMATURITY AND MORTALITY OF INFANTS AND ESTRIOL LEVEL [7]

i)   Weight of infant and estriol level

The correlation between the urinary estriol levels during the 4 weeks before delivery and

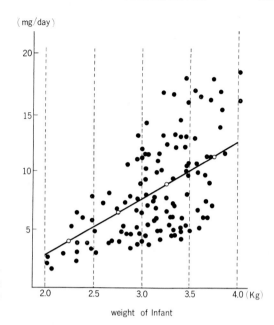

Fig. 7 Weight of infant and urinary estriol: Measurements with in 4 weeks prior to deliverry without complications of pregnancy toxemias.

weight of Infant

the weight of the infants at birth is given in Fig. 7. Although there is a fair amount of scatter, the line connecting the average values of every 500 g of infant weights is perfectly straight and a parallel relation between the two can be surmised. This result is significant in that the estriol levels are reflecting quite well the feto-placental unit's functions in accordance with the degree of fetal growth.

ii) Rate of birth of premature infants, rate of perinatal fetal mortality and estriol levels

Two hundred fifteen cases of single pregnancy including those with toxemias of pregnancy and those past maturity were divided into 4 groups according to the estriol levels measured during the 4 weeks prior to delivery and the rates of birth of premature infants and those of perinatal fetal deaths for the various groups were compared (Table 35). In the group of low estriol levels under 2 mg/day the birth rate of premature infants reached 75.8 per cent while the perinatal fetal mortality rate also showed an abnormally high value of 7.9 per cent. In the group of 2 to 5 mg/day also still high rates of 30 per cent premature infants and 8.3 per cent mortality were noted, but as the estriol level became higher the rates of both premature infant deliveries and perinatal mortality were decreased, and in the group of more than 8 mg/day there was not a single case of premature birth or infant mortality. This result indicates that the estriol level will serve as a fairly effective supple-

Table 35 Premature infant birht rate, perinatal fetal mortality rate and urinary ET.

ET (mg/24hr)	Premature infant birth rate (%)		Perinatal fetal mortality rate (%)	
0–2	25/33	75.8	19/33	57.6
2–4	18/60	30.0	5/60	8.3
4–8	5/71	7.0	1/71	1.4
8–	0/51	0	0/51	0

Note: Urinary ET measured with in 4 weeks prior to delivery (by Method A).

mentary diagnostic method in predicting the prematureness and the prognosis of an infant. If the estriol value is higher than 8 mg/day no danger is feared, while in case it is under 4 mg/day it is necessary to be on the alert anticipating that premature infants and perinatal deaths are liable to occur. Especially, in case estriol is less than 2 mg/day, dysfunction of the feto-placental unit is certain and the continuation of pregnancy would be dangerous to the child so that it is necessary to resort to emergency delivery or cesarean section, particularly when the estriol levels are consistently low or a trend of decline is prominent by continuous estriol measurements.

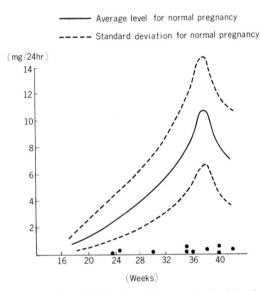

Fig. 8 Urinary ET in cases of intrauterine fetal death.

iii)   Estriol level in case of intrauterine fetal death

The estriol values of urine in cases of cessation of the fetal heart sounds during the process of pregnancy and subsequent confirmation of intrauterine fetal death (Fig. 8) show extemely low figures of less than 1 mg/day regardless of the number of weeks of gestation indicating that this can be utilized for diagnosing intrauterine fetal death at the late stages of pregnancy.

4)   SUMMARY

The results of clinical studies relating to the methods of measuring estriol in maternal urine as a means of checking feto-placental functions have been described.

(1)   Citing actual examples, the principal factors influencing estriol quantity in maternal urine have been described as i) DHEA formation capacity in the fetal adrenals, ii) metabolism (aromatization and 16α-hydroxylation) from DHEA to estriol in the feto-placental compartment, and iii) blood circulation of the feto-placento-maternal unit.

(2)   In order to supply the feto-placental function checking methods through estriol level measurement in actual clinical aspects, simple and accurate procedures of quantitative measurement have been developed.

(3)   Relations between prognoses of infants in cases of dysfunctions of feto-placental units and the transitions of urinary estriol have been described giving cases of pregnancy toxemias, prolonged pregnancy and intrauterine fetal death. From the fact that there

exist close parallel relationships between prognoses of premature infant birth, perinatal fetal mortality rate and the estriol levels, respectively, the significance of estriol measurement as a method of checking feto-placental functions has been established.

CONCLUSIONS

This research was carried out with the purpose of clarifying both basically and clinically the great significance of the measurement of estriol during pregnancy in care of the fetus in the maternal body. The results obtained are summarized as follows :

(1)   In regard to estriol formation during pregnancy, there is an ingeneous confunctioning of the fetus, placenta and maternal body as an organic unit involving supply of material (androgens), the processing thereof (aromatization and 16α-hydroxylation) and transport, and it has been indicated that the role played by the feto-placental unit is extremely important.

(2)   As for the formation mechanisms leading to estriol (formed in the placenta) from DHEA (secreted from fetal adrenals) in the feto-placental unit, the so-called neutral pathways (B pathways) account for the greater part, while it has been shown that DHEA first is subjected to 16α-hydroxylation at the fetus, which on reaching the placenta is converted into estriol. In particular, it has been indicated that this is dependent on Pathway B-II going through 16α-OH-T. It should be noted additionally that there exists a great possibility of the fetal adrenals secreting 16α-OH-DHEA already subjected to 16α-hydroxylation.

(3)   The major factors influencing estriol quantity in maternal urine have been identified as the three of i) furnishing material (DHEA from fetal adrenals), ii) processing in the feto-placental unit (aromatization and 16α-hydroxylation), and iii) transport thereof (blood circulation condition of feto-placento-maternal unit).

(4)   Simple estriol measurement methods of high accuracies have been developed for application to actual clinical cases.

(5)   The existence of a parallel relationship between the transition in estriol level and prognosis of the infant has been clarified for cases of toxemic pregnancy and overterm pregnancy regarded as the dysfunction of the feto-placental unit.

The urinary estriol level of a pregnant woman is believed to reflect the metabolic function of the feto-placental unit, and a basic view has been indicated that measurement of the estriol is extremely of usefulness in monitoring the fetus in the mother.

This research was conducted in part by the support of a U.S. National Institute of Health Grant.

REFERENCES

1.   DICZFALUSY, E.: Endocrine function of the human feto-placental unit. Fed. Proc. **23;** 791, 1964.
2.   ZANDER, J.: Progesterone and its metabolites in the placental-foetal unit. Proceedings of the Second International Congress of Endocrinology, Part 2, 715, 1965.
3.   BROWN, J.B.: The relationship between urinary oestrogens and oestrogens produced in the body. J. Endocrinol. **16;** 202, 1957.
4.   SZARKA, S.: Hormonale Verhältnisse während der Schvangerschaft bei Fehlen der Eierströcke. Zentrabatt. f. Gynäk. **54;** 2211, 1930.

5. DICZFALUSY, E. and LAUTRIZER, CHR.: Oestrogene beim Menschen. Springer-Verlag, Berlin, 1961.

6. RYAN, K.J.: Conversion of androstenedione to estrone by placental microsomes. Biochim. Biophys. Acta 27; 658, 1958.

7. NAKAYAMA, T.: Estrogen metabolism and its significance in the field of obstetrics. Abstracts of Compulsory Theme Reports for the Seventeenth Congress of the Japanese Obstetrical and Gynecological Society, 1965. (in Japanese)

8. NAKAYAMA, T., ARAI, K., TABEI, T., YANAIHARA, T., SATOH, K., NAGATOMI, K. and FUJITA, Y.: Oestrogen metabolism in anencephalus. Endocrinol. Japon. 14; 251, 1967.

9. NAKAYAMA, T., KINOSHITA, K., NAKAZAWA, H., TSUKADA, I., SHIRAISHI, H., HARA, F. and OKINAGA, S.: ESTROGENS originating from placenta. Folia Endocrinol. Japon. 39; 1919, 1964. (in Japanese)

10. NAKAYAMA, T., ARAI, K., SATOH, K., YANAIHARA, T., NAGATOMI, K. and TAKANEZAWA, Y.: Origin of precursors of placental estrogens. Sanfujinka no Sekai 19; 1048, 1967. (in Japanese)

11. NAKAYAMA, T.: Transitions in estrogen metabolism at the placenta—Feto-placento-maternal relationship. Proceedings of the Seventeenth Japan Medical Congress, III, 710, 1967. (in Japanese)

12. NAKAYAMA, T., ARAI, K., SATOH, K., YANAIHARA, T., NAGATOMI, K. and FUJITA, K.: The placenta and hormones—Particularly the background for method of judging placental function by measurement of estriol in maternal urine. Sanfujinka Chiryo 14; 392, 1967. (in Japanese)

13. TEN BERGE, B.S.: Oestriol excretion in intrauterine foetal death. Gynaecologia 149; 40, 1960.

14. FRANDSEN, V.A. and STAKEMAN, G.: The site of production of oestrogenic hormones in human pregnancy. Acta Endocrinol. 38; 383, 1961.

15. FRANDSEN, V.A. and STAKEMAN, G.: The site of production of oestrogenic hormones in human pregnancy, II. Acta Endocrinol. 43; 184, 1963.

16. COLÁS, A. and HEINRICHS, W.L.: Pattenkofer chromogens in the maternal and fetal circulations: Anencephalic pregnancy, caesarean section and tentative identification of 3β, 17β-dehydroxyandrost-5-en-16-one in umbilical cord blood. Steroids 5; 753, 1965.

17. EASTERLING, W.E., JR., SIMMER, H.H., DIGNAM, W.J., FRANKLAND, M.V. and NAFTOLIN, F.: Neutral C_{19}-steroids and steroid sulfates in human pregnancy. II. DHEA sulfate, 16α-OH-DHEA, 16α-OH-DHEA sulfate in maternal and fetal blood of pregnancies with anencephalic and normal fetuses. Steroids 8; 157, 1966.

18. NAKAYAMA, T., ARAI, K., YANAIHARA, T., TABEI, T., SATOH, K. and NAGATOMI, K.: Oestrogen metabolism in anencephalus. Acta Endocrinol. 55; 369, 1967.

19. YANAIHARA, T.: Origin of estrogen in woman during pregnancy. Acta Obstet. Gynaecol. Japon. 15; 279, 1968.

20. KOBAYASHI, T., NAKAYAMA, T., YANAIHARA, T., ARAI, K., FUJITA, K., SATOH, K. and NAGATOMI, K.: Estrogen metabolism in anencephalic pregnancy. Proceedings of the Third Asia & Oceania Congress of Endocrinology, p. 718, 1967.

21. NAKAYAMA, T., ARAI, K., FUJITA, K., SATOH, K., NAGATOMI, K. and YANAIHARA, T.: Metabolism of urinary dehydroepiandrosterone in newborn infant: 17-ketosteroids in female urine. Shindan to Chiryo 60, 1969. (in Japanese)

22. FUJITA, K.: Considerations of regulatory factors in secretion of dehydroepiandrosterone from newborn infant adrenals. Nippon Sanka-Fujinka Gakkai Zasshi 21; 1377, 1969. (in Japanese)

23. NAKAYAMA, T., ARAI, K., SATOH, K., YANAIHARA, T., NAGATOMI, K. and FUJITA, Y.: 16α-hydroxylation of dehydroepiandrosterone by human fetal tissues. Endocrinol. Japon. 14; 269, 1967.

24. NAKAYAMA, T., ARAI, K., SATOH, K., NAGATOMI, K., TABEI, T. and YANAIHARA, T.: The formation of estriol from estradiol-17β by human fetal adrenal tissues. Endocrinol. Japon. 13; 153, 1966.

25. NAKAYAMA, T.: Estriol biosynthesis pathways in human feto-placental unit. Folia Endocrinol. Japon. 46; 758, 1970. (in Japanese)

26. BOLTÉ, E., WIQVIST, N. and DICZFALUSY, E.: Metabolism of dehydroepiandrosterone and dehydroepiandrosterone sulfate by the human foetus at midpregnancy. Acta Endocrinol. 52; 583, 1966.

27. DELL'ACQUA, S., MANCUSO, S., WIQVIST, N., RUSE, J.L., SOLOMON, S. and DICZFALUSY, E.: Studies on the aromatization of neutral steroids in pregnant women. 5. Metabolism of androst-

5-ene-3β, 16β, 17β-triol in the intact foeto-placental unit at midpregnancy. Acta Endocrinol. **55**; 389, 1967.

28. DELL'ACQUA, S., MANCUSO, S., ERIKSSON, G., RUSE, J.L., SOLOMON, S. and DICZFALUSY, E.: Studies on the aromatization of neutral steroids in pregnant women. 6. Aromatization of 16α-hydroxylated C-19 steroids by midtern placentas perfused in situ. Acta Endocrinol. **55**; 401, 1967.

29. RUSE, J.L. and SOLOMON, S.: The in vivo metabolism of 16α-hydroxyprogesterone. Biochemistry **5**; 1065, 1966.

30. NAKAYAMA, T. et al.: Metabolism of DHEA-^{14}C and 16α-OH-DHEA-^{3}H in the feto-placental unit. Proceedings of the Forty-Fourth Annual Meeting of the Japan Endocrinological Society, 1971. (in Japanese)

31. NAKAYAMA, T., ARAI, K., YANAIHARA, T., SATOH, K., NAGATOMI, K., TABEI, T. and FUJITA, Y.: Formation of estrogens in the feto-placental compartments. Endocrinol. Japon. **15**; 135, 1968.

32. NAKAYAMA, T. et al.: The pathway to estriol from dehydroepiandrosterone in the feto-placental unit at midpregnancy. Excerpta Medica, International Congress Series, No. 157, p. 171, 1968.

33. NAKAYAMA, T. and KANAGAWA, S.: Study on estriol formation mechanism at feto-placental unit. II. Metabolism of DHEA-^{3}H and estriol-^{14}C at feto-placental unit. Proceedings of the Twenty-Third Congress of the Japanese Obstetrical and Gynecological Society, p. 230, 1971. (in Japanese)

34. NAKAYAMA, T., ARAI, K. and SATOH, K.: Estriol metabolism in anencephalic pregnancy. Proceedings of the Sixth World Congress of Gynecology and Obstetrics, p. 270, 1970.

35. NAKAYAMA, T., ARAI, K. and SATOH, K.: Estriol metabolism in anencephalic pregnancy. Proceedings of the Twenty-Second Congress of the Japanese Obstetrical and Gynecological Society, p. 33, 1970. (in Japanese)

36. NAKAYAMA, T.: Simple method of measuring urinary estriol during pregnancy. Folia Endocrinol. Japon. **37**; 845, 1961. (in Japanese)

37. NAKAYAMA, Y., ARAI, K., TSUKADA, I., YANAIHARA, T., TABEI, T., NAGATOMI, K. and SHIRAISHI, H.: Hormones and the fetus. Sanka to Fujinka **41**; 1163, 1967. (in Japanese)

38. NAKAYAMA, T. and NIIZUMA, K.: Daily variation in urinary estrogens of pregnant women. Folia Endocrinol. Japon. **42**; 379, 1966. (in Japanese)

39. NAKAYAMA, T., ARAI, K. and NIIZUMA, K.: Method of measuring urinary estriol during pregnancy. Sanka to Fujinka **38**; 505, 1971. (in Japanese)

40. KOBAYASHI, T., TANAKA, T. and TSUKADA, I.: Prematurity and placental function in pregnancy toxemias. Sanka to Fujinka **31**; 1578, 1964. (in Japanese)

41. NAKAYAMA, T.: Measurement of estriol of maternal urine as method of monitoring fetus. Sanfujinka no Sekai **23**; 125, 1971. (in Japanese)

An investigation of the materno-fetal hormonal milieu with special emphasis on the maternal influence

Shigeo TAKAGI, M.D., Takao YOSHIDA, M.D.
and Katsuo TSUBATA, M.D.

Department of Obstetrics and Gyneclogy, School of Medicine, Nihon University, Tokyo

INTRODUCTION

In pregrancy, mother, placenta and fetus comprise a functional system in which each of the three compartments, while maintaining specificity within its own system, interacts for the purpose of the development of the fetus, and alters the maternal metabolism to comply with the gravid state and prepares for the termination of pregnancy by parturition.

The maternal steroids or their precursors which can pass to the fetus and affect the fetal target organs attain a state of equilibrium to maintain a homeostatic balance between the maternal steroids and the native fetal steroids. The fetus, then, progresses through an interdependant endocrine status to an independant endocrine status, free from maternal influence.

This report intends to investigate the maternal as well as the fetal endocrine milieu from early pregnancy to parturition, thereby clarifying the controlling mechanism involved in the maintenance of balance in the materno-fetal relationship.

The procedures which are employed in this report are shown in Table 1.

THE DYNAMICS OF MATERNO-FETAL HORMONES IN PREGNANCY

1. STEROIDS

1) CORTICOIDS
i) **Unconjugated cortisol** (Fig. 1)

In normal pregnancy, the dynamics of cortisol concentration in the peripheral blood are as in Fig. 1. As pregnancy proceeds, cortisol levels increase and at 29–32 weeks show an accelerated increase. At the onset of labor, the stress of labor causes a more marked increase which peaks immediately post partum at 532 ng/ml or 6 times non-gravid levels. In the puerperium, cortisol levels decrease rapidly and return to non-gravid levels by the 4th post partum day.

Table 1

RADIOIMMUNOASSAY		
steroid	antigen	sensitivity
estrone	estrone-6-oxime-BSA	10 pg
estradiol	estradiol-6-oxime-BSA	10
estriol	estriol-6-oxime-BSA	10
DHA	DHA-7-oxime-BSA	50
DHA-S	DHA-3-succinate-BSA	50
Δ^4-androstenedione	Δ^4-androstenedione-3-oxime-BSA	20
testosterone	testosterone-3-oxime-BSA	5
16α-OH-DHA	16α-OH-DHA-3-succinate-BSA	500
16α-OH-DHA-S	16α-OH-DHA-3-succinate-BSA	1,000
progesterone	progesterone-3-oxime-BSA	10
17α-OH-progesterone	17α-OH-progesterone-3-oxime-BSA	10
20α-OH-progesterone	20α-OH-progesterone-3-oxime-BSA	10
cortisol	cortisol-21-succinate-BSA	5
cortisone	cortisone-21-succinate-BSA	10
DOC	DOC-3-oxime-BSA	10
aldosterone	aldosterone-3-oxime-BSA	10
hFSH	double antibody	0.21 mIU
hLH	double antibody	5 mIU
ACTH	dextran coated charcole	10 pg
hPL	double antibody	10 ng
hCG	double antibody	13.2 mIU
hCG-β-subunit	double anitibody	1 ng
GASCHROMATOGRAPHY		
steroid	column	sensitivity
pregnenolone	1.5 %SE	20 ng
pregnenolone-s	1.5 %SE	20 ng

Fetal levels of unconjugated cortisol at term are 53.0 ng/ml compared to maternal levels of 312 ng/ml, a remarkable contrast between the two levels.

Cortisol levels in umbilical blood are 114 ng/ml in the umbilical arteries and 82 ng/ml in the umbilical vein. The slightly higher concentration of cortisol in the umbilical arteries than in the umbilical vein suggests the probability of fetal production of cortisol.

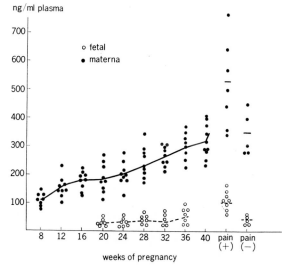

Fig. 1 Plasma cortisol.

According to MURPHY [1], the umbilical blood cortisol increases with the advance of pregnancy, and in cases of spontaneous onset of labor pains, the umbilical cortisol levels are higher than in cases where labor is artificially induced, suggesting that the fetal adrenals may play a role in the induction of labor.

ii) Unconjugated cortisone (Fig. 2)

In normal pregnancy, cortisone increases gradually until the 28th week, then rapidly to 42.5 ng/ml at term. With the onset of labor, a slight increase is observed, then decreases rapidly to non-gravid levels by the 4th post partum day. At term the peripheral cortisone levels are 4 times non-gravid levels.

The fetal cortisone concentrations are remarkably higher than the maternal peripheral blood, and immediately post partum the umbilical arterial concentration is 110 ng/ml and the venous is 151.8 ng/ml.

iii) Unconjugated desoxycorticosterone (DOC) (Fig. 3)

In the maternal peripheral circulation, DOC gradually increased until the 20th week of pregnancy, thereafter it increased to peak levels at 40 weeks of 2.53 ng/ml or 5 times the levels of the non-gravid state.

The fetal DOC pattern was similar to that of the maternal DOC, however, the fetal levels were slightly higher than maternal levels.

Umbilical levels sampled immediately post partum revealed a ratio where the venous blood (3.82 ng/ml) was slightly higher than the arterial blood (2.94 ng/ml).

iv) Aldosterone (Fig. 4)

Aldosterone in the maternal blood showed a gradual increase throughout pregnancy with the concentration at term 0.52 ng/ml, roughly 5 times that of the non-gravid levels of 0.10 ng/ml.

The fetal pattern was highly correspondent with the maternal pattern.

The umbilical blood sampled immediately post partum showed a slightly higher concentration in the umbilical veins (0.52 ng/ml) than in the umbilical artery (0.36 ng/ml).

Our findings on corticoids at the time of parturition and their distribution in the materno-fetal system reveal a complex pattern dependant on the steroids measured. This may be attributed to the differences between the corticoid binding proteins in the maternal circulation and those in the newborn circulation. Other factors involved may include differences in the rate of placental transfer of the various corticoids, rates or degrees of metabolism by placental enzymes, and hepatic metabolism in the fetal system. However, all the mechanism mentioned above are yet to be elucidated.

2)   PROGESTERONE AND RELATED STEROIDS

i) Progesterone (Fig. 5)

In normal pregnancy, progesterone levels in the peripheral blood show an increase up to the 9th week, when there is a slight decrease coinciding in time with the luteo-placental shift as reported by CSAPO [2] and YOSHIMI [3]. Thereafter, there is a rapid increase up to about the 24th week followed by an increase starting from about the 28th week, and peaks at 168.7 ng/ml at 37–40 weeks. Prolonged pregnancies show a slight decrease from 40 week levels.

The onset of labor coincides with a decrease in progesterone levels, and just prior to parturition progesterone concentrations show a slight elevation, then decreases rapidly, and following the expulsion of the placenta decrease still further.

The fetal levels show a 6 times as high as that of the maternal circulation during the second trimester of pregnancy, and thereafter shows a gradual increase, and at term fetal levels are roughly twice that of the maternal circulation.

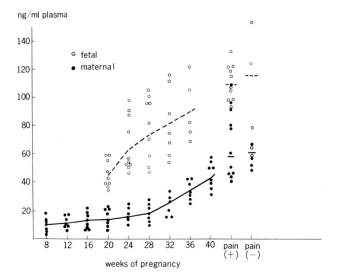

Fig. 2 Plasma cortisone.

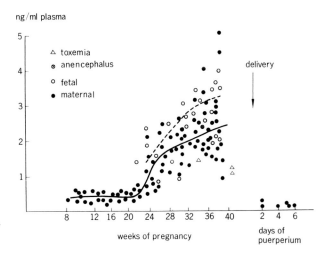

Fig. 3 Plasma desoxycorticosterone.

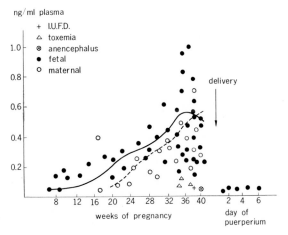

Fig. 4 Plasma aldosterone.

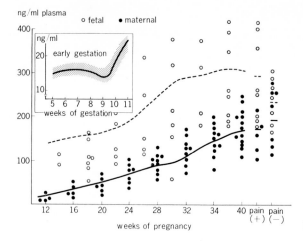

Fig. 5   Plasma progesterone.

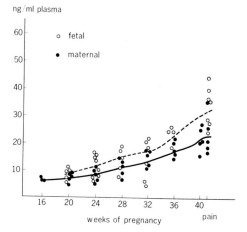

Fig. 6   Plasma 20α-OH-progesterone.

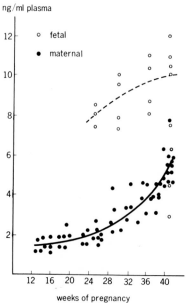

Fig. 7   Plasma 17α-OH-progesterone.

Feto-maternally, the highest concentrations are found in the retroplacental blood at 652.2 ng/ml, followed by the umbilical vein at 466.3 ng/ml, umbilical arteries at 231.4 ng/ml, and the maternal peripheral blood at 168 ng/ml in decreasing order of concentration. The ratio of umbilical venous to umbilical arterial progesterone is roughly 2 : 1. This difference between the umbilical venous and arterial progesterone levels of 234.0 ng/ml may be explained as a result either of fetal metabolism or its being metabolized as a substrate for other steroids. Further, the high concentrations of progesterone in the retroplacental blood suggests that the placenta is most likely the major site of progesterone production.

ii) 20α-hydroxy-progesterone (20α-OH-progesterone) (Fig. 6)

20a-OH-progesterone is a reduced product of progesterone that has only minimal progestational effect, and in the peripheral circulation at term is found in concentrations of roughly 20 ng/ml or one-eighth that of progesterone levels. 20a-OH-progesterone shows a gradual increase throughout pregnancy and at term is 22.1 ng/ml or roughly 7 times the 3.4 ng/ml of the luteal phase.

In contrast, fetal levels of 20a-OH-progesterone were consistently slightly higher than that of the maternal circulation.

iii) 17α-hydroxy-progesterone (17α-OH-progesterone) (Fig. 7)

In the maternal circulation 17a-OH-progesterone increases rapidly from the 28th week of pregnancy and at term is 5.2 ng/ml, a 7 fold increase over the non-gravid levels of 0.76 ng/ml.

The fetal levels are at roughly 3 times that of maternal levels.

iv) Pregnenolone (Figs. 8, 9)

Pregnenolone is found in the conjugated and free form, of which the sulfo-conjugated form predominated in the human circulation.

The peripheral pregnenolone sulfate concentrations gradually increase up to the 24th week, rapidly increase after the 36th week and peaks at the 40th week with an average of 313.8 ng/ml or roughly 11 times that of non-gravid levels of 28.0 ng/ml (Fig. 8).

At parturition, the feto-maternal relationship of pregnenolone sulfate shows 1,863.6

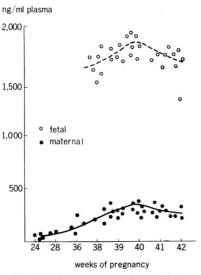

Fig. 8 Plasma pregnenolone sulfate.

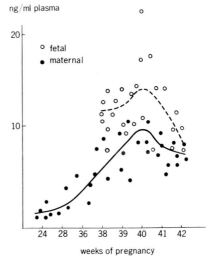

Fig. 9 Plasma unconjugated pregnenolone.

ng/ml in the umbilical arteries, 1,372.9 ng/ml in the umbilical vein and 369 ng/ml in the retroplacental blood, suggesting that pregnenolone sulfate is produced in the fetus and a portion of it is metabolized in the placenta.

The placenta is abundant in sulfatase and Δ^5-3β-hydroxysteroid-dehydrogenase. Pregnenolone which is produced in the fetus and cleared in the placenta may be therefore postulated as metabolized into progesterone.

Unconjugated pregnenolone is very low in concentration in the human circulation compared with pregnenolone sulfate. In normal pregnancy, unconjugated pregnenolone increases after the 28th week of gestation and in the 40th week peaks at 97.7 ng/ml or roughly 8 times that of non-gravid levels (Fig. 9). The feto-maternal distribution of unconjugated pregnenolone at the time of parturition shows the highest concentration of 146.0 ng/ml in the umbilical vein, 115.0 ng/ml in the umbilical arteries, and 118.0 ng/ml in retroplacental blood.

Although unconjugated pregnenolone is found in slightly higher concentrations in the umbilical vein than in the umbilical arteries, the differences are not of statistical significance, suggesting that unconjugated pregnenolone of fetal origin is not likely a major source of progesterone precursors.

On the other hand, maternal pregnenolone secreted from the adrenal cortex may have little significance as a progesterone precursor, because both conjugated and unconjugated pregnenolone are found in higher concentrations in the retroplacental blood than in the maternal peripheral circulation.

3)   ANDROGENS (Fig. 10)

Testosterone levels increase throughout pregnancy and at term is 2.08 ng/ml or 4 times that of 0.5 ng/ml in non-gravid females, but the rate of increase is low in comparison with estrogens and progesterone. Following parturition, testosterone levels return to non-gravid levels 3–4 days post partum.

Fetal levels are lower than maternal levels, and during the second trimester of pregnancy a sex difference was observed. Male fetuses at 16 weeks showed 0.99 ng/ml, a concentration significantly higher than the 0.36 ng/ml measured in female fetuses. However, following the 24th week of pregnancy the female levels increased and by 26 weeks, the female levels approximate male levels making the identification of sex differences inconclusive after the 26th week of pregnancy.

Immediately post partum the average testosterone levels are 0.89 ng/ml in the umbilical arteries, and 0.82 ng/ml in the umbilical vein. Testosterone concentration is slightly higher in the umbilical arteries than in the umbilical vein, though statistically not significant.

On the other hand, the retroplacental blood shows an extremely high concentration of 5.0 ng/ml, suggesting that testosterone may be also produced in the placenta and secreted toward the maternal compartment.

The maternal serum testosterone binding globulin increases with the advance of pregnancy, in late pregnancy is roughly 4 times that of the non-gravid state, and may explain the decreased rate of testosterone elimination via the renal system resulting in elevated serum levels.

4)   ESTROGENS AND THEIR PRECURSORS
i)   **Estrone** (Figs. 11, 12)

In the normal pregnancy at 5–6 weeks unconjugated estrone levels are slightly lower than in the luteal phase of non-gravid females. However, with advance of pregnancy a tendancy for a gradual increase is noted and at term is 12.5 ng/ml or 300 times that of the luteal phase.

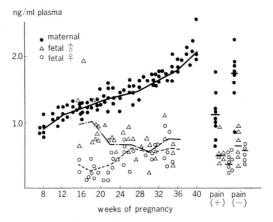

Fig. 10 Plasma testosterone.

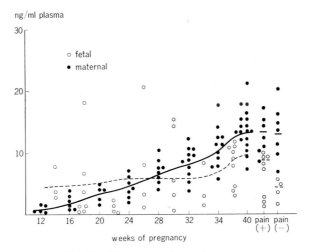

Fig. 11 Plasma unconjugated estrone.

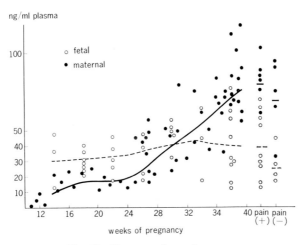

Fig. 12 Plasma conjugated estrone.

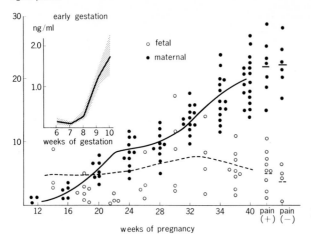

Fig. 13 Plasma unconjugated estradiol.

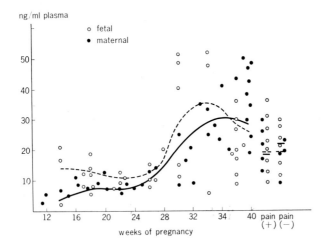

Fig. 14 Plasma conjugated estradiol.

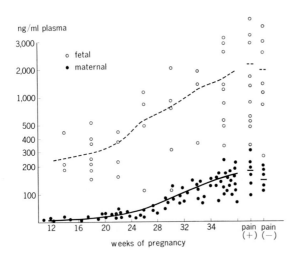

Fig. 15 Plasma conjugated estriol.

In early pregnancy, the fetal levels are higher than those of the maternal peripheral circulation. In the second trimester the fetal and maternal levels are roughly equivalent, and at term, the fetal levels are roughly two-thirds that of the maternal circulation.

The materno-fetal distribution of unconjugated estrone shows the highest concentration of 26 ng/ml in the retroplacental blood, followed by 17 ng/ml in the umbilical vein and 3.0 ng/ml in the umbilical arteries in decreasing order. This suggests that the placenta is the source of unconjugated estrone production and that estrone is secreted toward both the fetus and the mother. Further, because of the difference of concentration between the umbilical vein and arteries, it may be inferred that the greater portion of unconjugated estrone secreted toward the fetus is metabolized by the fetal organs.

Conjugated estrone which is obtained by HCl hydrolysis gradually increases throughout pregnancy, and is found in concentrations 5–10 times that of the unconjugated form.

ii) Estradiol-17β (Figs. 13, 14)

Unconjugated estradiol compared to the luteal phase, decreases slightly at 7 weeks, increases gradually to the 8th week, after which it increases rapidly to 21.05 ng/ml at 40 weeks of gestation, an increase of 100 times that of roughly 0.2 ng/ml at ovulation. With the onset of labor the concentration decreases and following the expulsion of the placenta decreases rapidly to return non-gravid levels at 6 hours post partum.

Unconjugated estradiol in fetal blood gradually increases throughout pregnancy. However, in the first trimester it is higher than in the maternal circulation, in the second trimester almost equal to, and at term is 6.0 ng/ml, roughly 1/4 that of 21.1 ng/ml in the maternal circulation.

Conjugated estradiol in the maternal circulation showed a pattern of increase similar to that of unconjugated estradiol in that until mid-pregnancy it gradually increases, and after the 28th week, shows a rapid increase in concentration. The fetal conjugated estradiol pattern of increase closely follows that of the maternal pattern, but is found in slightly higher concentrations.

A comparison of feto-maternal unconjugated estradiol at the time of parturition shows the highest concentration in the retroplacental blood at 64.9 ng/ml followed by 21.05 ng/ml in the maternal peripheral blood. The concentration in the umbilical vessels is at very low levels. The distribution of feto-maternal estradiol at parturition is similar to that of progesterone, and opposite to unconjugated estriol, which allows the assumption that unconjugated estradiol is produced in the placenta and is secreted much more readily into the maternal circulation.

iii) Estriol (Figs. 15, 16)

Peripheral unconjugated estriol increases very gradually until the 14th week of pregnancy and thereafter increases rapidly. After the 28th week the rate of increase further accelerates and at term reaches 16.39 ng/ml or roughly 1,000 times that of 0.015 ng/ml in the non-gravid state.

The fetal peripheral unconjugated estriol levels are twice that of the maternal peripheral circulation levels of 16.4 ng/ml, increase throughout pregnancy and at term is 32 ng/ml in the umbilical blood.

The maternal peripheral conjugated estriol (152.1 ng/ml) is roughly 10 times that of unconjugated estriol, and as with the unconjugated form increases throughout pregnancy. The fetal conjugated estriol levels are more than 10 times that of maternal conjugated estriol, and were 1,723 ng/ml in umbilical plasma at term.

As estriol, whether conjugated or free, is found in dramatically highter concentrations in the fetus, it is possible to assume that the majority of the estriol is produced in the fetal compartment.

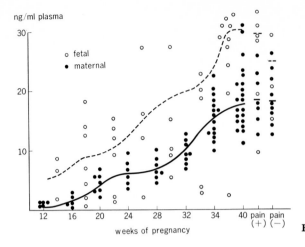

Fig. 16 Plasma unconjugated estriol.

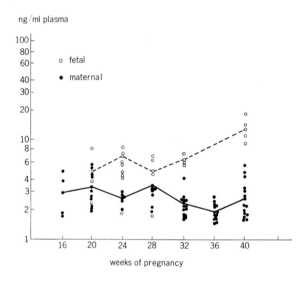

Fig. 17 Plasma DHA.

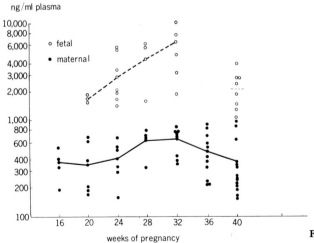

Fig. 18 Plasma DHA-S.

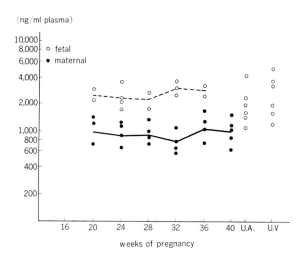

Fig. 19 Plasma 16α-OH-DHA.

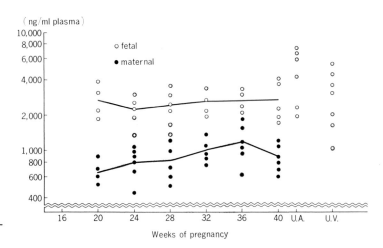

Fig. 20 Plasma 16α-OH-
DHA sulfate.

iv) Dehydroepiandrosterone (DHA) and dehydroepiandrostene-sulfate (DHA-S) (Figs. 17, 18)

In pregnancy, both DHA and its sulfate are transformed to estrogens and are considered to be important precursors for estrogen production. The dynamics of the materno-fetal DHA and DHA-S have been investigated with the following results. The maternal DHA decreases with the advance of pregnancy and at term is 2.27 ng/ml, whereas the fetal plasma DHA is at higher levels than the maternal and increases throughout pregnancy and at term is roughly 13.2 ng/ml or 5 times that of the maternal.

The major portion of DHA in plasma is as sulfate, and the maternal peripheral blood concentration of DHA-S is 529.7 ± 188.6 ng/ml in the non-gravid state and during pregnancy shows a fluctuating decrease to roughly 400 ng/ml. However, this fluctuation has no statistical significance.

v) 16α-hydroxy-dehydroepiandrosterone (16α-OH-DHA) and its sulfate (16α-OH-DHA-S) (Figs. 19, 20)

16α-OH-DHA is an important steroid precursor of estriol and in pregnancy may be involved in the control of the quantitative production of estriol.

The maternal peripheral plasma 16α-OH-DHA levels remain relatively constant throughout pregnancy at roughly 1 ng/ml, and fetal 16α-OH-DHA levels are roughly 3 times higher than maternal peripheral levels.

The maternal peripheral plasma 16α-OH-DHA-S levels increase in accordance with the progress of pregnancy peaking at the 36th week of gestation and at 40 weeks is roughly 900 ng/ml. The fetal peripheral plasma 16α-OH-DHA-S levels are markedly higher than the maternal levels and are maintained at levels of roughly 2,000–3,000 ng/ml.

The evidence of high levels of both 16α-OH-DHA and its sulfate in the fetal peripheral plasma seems to indicate an active participation of the fetus in the synthesis of estriol.

2. PROTEOHORMONES

1) HUMAN CHORIONIC GONADOTROPIN (hCG) AND ITS β-SUBUNIT
    (hCG-β-SUBUNIT) (Figs. 21, 22)

In normal pregnancy, hCG in the maternal peripheral circulation shows a distinctive pattern characterized by a peak in early pregnancy and another near its term.

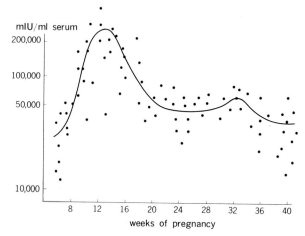

Fig. 21 Serum hCG.

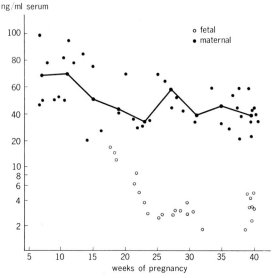

Fig. 22 Serum hCG-β-subunit.

The materno-fetal distribution in descending order is as follows: 60 mIU/ml in the maternal peripheral circulation, 20 mIU/ml in the retroplacental blood and the levels in the umbilical vessels are too low to be of significance.

On evaluation of hCG-β-subunit, the peaks observed in early pregnancy and at term with hCG were not seen (Fig. 22). In fact, with the β-subunit, levels ranging from 50–100 ng/ml were consistently observed throughout pregnancy, and only a slight tendency toward a decrease in concentration was observed with the advance of pregnancy. Further, the umbilical blood concentrations were roughly 4 ng/ml with a slightly higher concentration in the umbilical veins than in the umbilical arteries.

2) HUMAN LUTEINIZING HORMONE (hLH)

LH concentrations during pregnancy could not be adequately evaluated because of our inability to differentiate between LH and hCG either by bio- or radioimmunoassay.

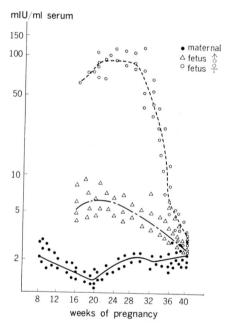

Fig. 23   Serum FSH.

3) HUMAN FOLLICLE STIMMULATING HORMONE (hFSH) (Fig. 23)

There have been reports stating that maternal serum FSH levels during pregnancy are constant, and maintained at the relatively high levels of 11.7 mIU/ml [4]. However, Jaffe et al. [5] reported that, coincident with the increasing concentrations of hCG, the hypophyseal secretion of FSH is decreased to less than 2.0 mIU/ml. Our findings indicate that at 8 weeks of pregnancy, the average FSH levels are 2.1 $\pm$0.4 mIU/ml and, thereafter, show a slight tendency toward a decrease in concentration. At 20 weeks, average levels were 1.25$\pm$0.4 mIU/ml followed by a gradual increase, and at 40 weeks, FSH levels averaged 2.3$\pm$0.5 mIU/ml. All our findings on the maternal FSH levels showed concentrations consistently lower than those observed during normal menstrual cycles.

In contrast, investigation of fetal umbilical serum levels of FSH in induced and/or spontaneous abortions, premature deliveries and term pelvic deliveries, revealed that in the first trimester of pregnancy, male fetuses showed FSH levels of 2–10 mIU/ml and female fetuses 50–130 mIU/ml, a definite indication that in early to mid-pregnancy, female fetuses have a consistently higher FSH concentration than do male fetuses. Following the 30th week of pregnancy, female fetuses show a dramatic decrease, while male fetuses show only a relative tendency toward a decrease in FSH levels. After the 35th week of preganancy, we were unable to definitely establish a sex difference between male and female fetuses based on FSH levels. However, in the post partum period a sex difference in FSH levels could be determined, with female FSH concentrations slightly higher than male FSH concentrations.

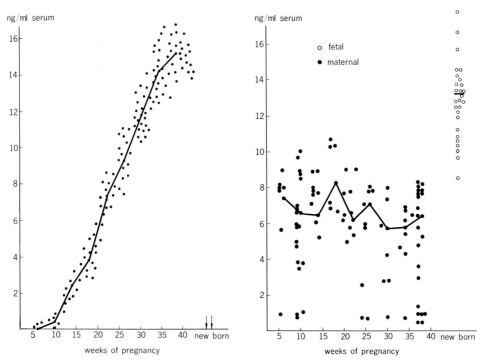

Fig. 24   Serum hPL.   Fig. 25   Serum hGH.

4)   HUMAN PLACENTAL LACTOGEN (hPL) (Fig. 24)

HPL in the maternal peripheral circulation increases during pregnancy and reaches a peak at 36 weeks, then decreases. Following parturition, a sudden decrease is seen and at 2–3 days post partum hPL is almost undetectable.

Its materno-fetal distribution shows the highest concentrations in the retroplacental blood, followed by the maternal peripheral circulation. The umbilical blood contained insignificant amounts.

5)   HUMAN GROWTH HORMONE (hGH) (Fig. 25)

Human growth hormone in normal pregnancy is in slightly higher concentrations than in the non-gravid state. Its concentration in the retroplacental blood is on the average 3 ng/ml, much less than 20 ng/ml in umbilical blood, of which the arterial concentrations are slightly higher than that of the veins.

Further, because it is difficult to demonstrate the transplacental passage of hGH and, its short half life and presence in high concentrations (10 ng/ml or more) in neonatal infants, it has been postulated that both fetal and maternal hGH is synthesized independently in the respective hypophyses.

6) ADRENOCORTICOTROPIC HORMONE (ACTH) (Fig. 26)

Maternal peripheral plasma ACTH levels in pregnancy could not be definitely established as having a fluctuation pattern during pregnancy. The range of ACTH levels in the maternal peripheral plasma was 15–140 pg/ml with an average of 52.5±25.2 pg/ml. Throughout pregnancy as in the non-gravid state, ACTH revealed a definite diurnal

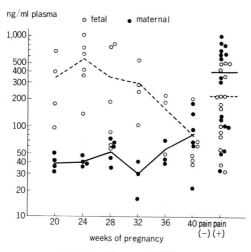

Fig. 26 Plasma ACTH.

pattern with the highest levels seen in the early morning to pre-noon hours, followed by a gradual decrease, with the lowest concentrations seen in the middle of the night.

In the fetal plasma, peak levels are noted in the second trimester, with the concentrations at 20–24 weeks of pregnancy 570.1±325 pg/ml, followed by a decrease, and at cesarean section at term, in the absence of labor pains, ACTH levels were 100 pg/ml.

MATERNAL INFLUENCE ON THE INTERACTION OF
THE MATERNO-FETAL ENDOCRINE MILIEU

1) CORTICOIDS

As seen in Figs. 1, 2, 3, and 4, the maternal corticoids are present in high concentrations and at parturition increase still further and may exceed by 2–10 times non-gravid levels. According to MEGEON [6], in humans corticoids readily pass through the placenta and, therefore, maternal corticoids can easily influence the fetal metabolism. Based on these finding, it was proposed that all corticoids in the fetal circulation are maternal in origin.

However, it has been demonstrated that the fetal adrenals differentiate into the fetal zone as early as the 6th week of gestation and are equipped with 11β, 17α and 21-hydroxylases by the 11th week of gestation [7]. Histochemically Δ^5-3β-hydroxysteroid-dehydrogenase has been demonstrated throughout the entire fetal adrenal as early as the 9 to 12th week of gestation [8].

From the above finding it is most likely that corticoids are synthesized in the fetal adrenal relatively early in fetal development. Further, from finding of a statistically significant difference of cortisol concentrations between the umbilical arteries and the umbilical vein at parturition, it may be assumed that the fetal adrenals secrete cortisol.

Administration of dexamethasone to the maternal organism results in decreases in maternal urinary estriol [9]. The mechanism involved in the inhibition of estriol excretion may be due to the direct passage of dexamethasone to the fetus via the placenta causing an inhibition of the fetal hypophysis, suppressing the release of ACTH, which in turn inhibits the fetal adrenals from secreting DHA-S [10]. Based on these hypotheses, it may be assumed that there is a hypophyseal adrenal feedback system operating during the intrauterine period. Further, it may be postulated that the corticoids from the maternal adrenals which pass through the placenta have a regulatory function on the fetal hypophysis and in turn affects the fetal adrenals. However, whether or not this takes place has yet to be elucidated.

2) PROGESTERONE AND ITS PRECURSORS

It has been accepted that progesterone plays an important role in the maintenance of pregnancy, and the alteration of its major site of secretion from the corpus luteum to the placenta, the "luteoplacental shift", occurs early in pregnancy.

Csapo et al. [2] by clinical observation reported that this shift occurs at the 8–11th week of pregnancy. Based on determinations of circulatory progesterone levels, Yoshimi et al. [3] reported the shift in the 9th week of pregnancy, and there are reports claiming that it occurs 38 days after the LH surge [11]. Our determinations of circulatory progesterone levels also indicated the shift at about the 9th week of pregnancy. Thus, the placenta takes over the responsibility for the secretion of the major portion of progesterone after the 8–9th week of gestation.

However, it has not been possible to demonstrate the de novo synthesis of progesterone in the placenta, and it has been thought that the placenta is an incomplete endocrine organ. The obstacle to de novo synthesis has been shown as existing in the pathway from acetate to cholesterol [12]. Therefore, the placental synthesis of progesterone is dependant on an adequate supply of cholesterol and/or pregnenolone as precursors or substrates.

Pregnenolone has been shown to be efficiently converted to progesterone by the placenta [13–15] and the determination of materno-fetal distributions of this progesterone precursor is shown in Figs. 8 and 9. It is noticed that in the maternal circulation there is no statistically significant difference between the peripheral circulation and retroplacental blood. Therefore, it is unlikely that maternal pregnenolone is a major precursor for the placenta synthesis of progesterone.

On the other hand, as the pregnenolone concentration in the fetal circulation is high and arterio-venous difference has been demonstrated, it is much easier to accept the fetus as the major contributor of pregnenolone to the placenta.

As shown in Figs. 8 and 9, the amount of both conjugated and un-conjugated pregnenolone secreted into the placenta from the fetal compartment is calculated to be 25 mg per diem [16]. Even if all of the pregnenolone from the fetus is converted to progesterone in the placenta, it would account for only 10 per cent of the daily requirement of progesterone precursor, when contrasted with per diem production of placental progesterone of 250 mg at term [17]. Thus, it is not likely that fetal pregnenolone is the major contributor to placental progesterone production. This leaves only cholesterol to be considered as the major precursor of placental progesterone.

Hellig's [18] investigations using tritium labeled cholesterol administered to the maternal circulation followed by measurement of specific activity of both the pregnanediol in maternal urine, and cholesterol and progesterone in the placenta revealed a close correlation of the radioactivity of these steroids. From these findings, he concluded that the major precursor for placental progesterone is cholesterol from the maternal circulation.

MATHUR et al. [19] reported active fetal de novo synthesis of cholesterol. However, he was unable to accurately determine the amount of placental progesterone converted from fetal cholesterol. Further, HELLIG et al. [18] and DAVIS et al. [20] reported that the fetus produces 80 per cent of its cholesterol, which further indicates the probability of the utilization of fetal cholesterol as a precursor for conversion. However, it is more likely that the major source of cholesterol is maternal rather than fetal, when the circulating blood volume of the fetus is considered.

The evidence that although progesterone synthesis shifts from the corpus luteum to the placenta, the major source of progesterone precursor remains maternal in origin is a point of continuing interest.

3)   ESTROGENS AND THEIR PRECURSORS

Estrogens as well as progesterone are demonstrated to be vital hormones necessary for the process of the intrauterine implantation of the zygote, and early in pregnancy the site of estrogen's secretion shifts from the maternal ovaries to the placenta.

Our investigations of estradiol levels in the peripheral blood during pregnancy suggests the ovary to syndesmal layer shift occurs at about the 8th week of gestation, which correlates closely with the luteoplacental shift of progesterone [21].

Although the major site of estrogen synthesis shifts early in pregnancy, the placenta has little capacity for the de novo synthesis of estrogens. The impaired pathway that have been clarified are the conversion from acetate to cholesterol, and the conversion from C-21 steroids such as pregnenolone and progesterone to C-19 steroids [22].

The precursors of estrogens necessary for the synthesis and maintenance of adequate estrogen levels have been postulated to be C-19-Δ^5-3β-hydroxysteroids, for example, DHA-S and 16α-hydroxy-DHA-S [23–25]. Clinical and biochemical determinations indicate that these precursors are fetal in origin, more specifically the fetal zone of the adrenal cortex.

Our investigations revealed that DHA-S and 16α-OH-DHA-S levels are high in the blood from umbilical vessels, especially the umbilical arteries. Further, there is a significant difference between the umbilical arteries and vein, suggesting that there is an active uptake of DHA-S and 16α-OH-DHA-S in the placenta from fetal sources.

In contrast, the maternal peripheral circulation and retroplacental blood contain low levels of DHA-S and 16α-OH-DHA-S, making it difficult to cite maternal DHA-S and 16α-OH-DHA-S as major sources of estrogen synthesis during pregnancy.

HARKNESS et al. [26] reported a case of woman with Cushing's syndrome who became pregnant following bilateral adrenalectomy. Analysis of her urinary steroids during pregnancy revealed a dramatic decrease in all three classic estrogens as well as pregnanediol. The decreases reported were roughly half the normal non-gravid levels. This report would seem to indicate that the maternal source of precursors be half the total. However, the patient was on a 40 mg/day cortisol regimen which passing through the placenta reached the fetus. On reaching the fetus, the hypophyseal secretion of ACTH may have been inhibited, which in turn may have inhibited the fetal adrenals DHA-S secretion. This report suggesting the importance of the maternal adrenals as a source of estrogen precursors contains information of great value.

SIITERI et al. [27] using radioactive isotope-labeled steroids administered to the maternal system to investigate estrogen synthesis during pregnancy, found that the rate of utilization of materno-fetal estrogen precursors varied with the stage of pregnancy, and that at or near the term, roughly 50 per cent of estrone and estradiol, and less than 10 per cent of estriol are from precursors that are maternal in origin.

We found the dramatic increase in estrogens during pregnancy in the materno-fetal system has limitations in that the placenta does not have adequate endocrinological function to directly convert acetates to estrogen, but must rely on specific precursors of both maternal and fetal origins in order to synthesize sufficient levels. The major portion of the precursors was found to be fetal origin, although the maternal adrenals also play an important but minor role in the synthesis and maintenance of estrogen levels.

4)   PROTEOHORMONES

The fetal hypophysis begins functioning early in pregnancy as is shown by our electron microscopic observations of human fetal hypophysis. Adrenocorticotropic hormone (ACTH) secreting granules were identified in 10 week fetuses and growth hormone (GH) secreting granules by the 12th week [28].

Fetal growth, development and maintenance by fetal endocrinological systems are thought to begin in early pregnancy. However, both maternal and fetal proteohormones are considered unable to pass through the placenta. Thus, it is difficult to present a valid argument for the materno-fetal interaction of proteohomones.

But, as some of the proteohormones act as regulating mechanisms on steroid hormones, it is possible to speculate that the proteohormones may exert influence via steroids which can pass the placental barrier.

i)   Adrenocorticotropic hormone (ACTH)

The fetal hypophysis has been demonstrated to contain ACTH as early as the 10th week of gestation [29]. Aso [30] reported that ACTH levels in the umbilical blood at parturition are 300–700 pg/ml, which are slightly lower than in the maternal peripheral blood. As mentioned previously, our investigations show that in the second trimester of pregnancy the fetal ACTH levels are extemely high, and thereafter gradually decrease.

Our finding coincide with those reported by WINTERS et al. [31], and seem to indicate

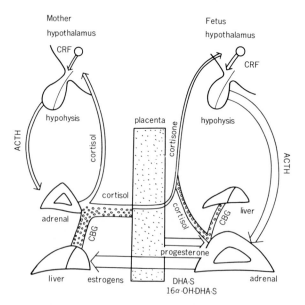

Fig. 27   The interrelation of the hypothalamo-hypophyseo-adrenal systems of both mother and fetus during pregnancy.

a high degree of activity in the fetal pituitary resulting in an accelerated release of ACTH during intrauterine fetal development and growth.

In anencephalic pregnancies, there is an associated adrenal cortical hypotrophy which can be reversed with ACTH [32] and infusion of corticoids in the maternal compartment causes a decrease in estriol concentration. These findings seem to indicate that by the second trimester of pregnancy, the fetal hypophyseo-adrenocortical functional integrity is established. Further, the increased fetal production and release of ACTH may be due to a decreased amount of cortisol released by the fetal adrenals acting as a feed back mechanism on the hypothalamo-hypophyseal tract, as seen in Fig. 27. This increased release of fetal ACTH acts on the fetal adrenals to promote growth and the increased production and release of pregnenolone, its sulfate, DHA and its sulfate, resulting in an increase in the levels of estriol.

The maternal ACTH levels are slightly higher than umbilical levels [30], and ACTH may cross the placenta readily [33]. However, it is difficult to conclude that maternal ACTH has significant direct influence on fetal development, if one considers the case of anencephaly where there is a retardation of adrenal cortical development.

We found that the maternal peripheral plasma ACTH in comparison to non-gravid levels remains relatively constant throughout pregnancy in the presence of ever increasing cortisol. This may be explained as in Fig. 27 that the greater proportion of cortisol is bound to corticoid binding globulin (CBG), and the form which more actively affects the hypophysis remains at relatively constant levels. Maternal peripheral ACTH levels are more affected by whether the fetus is delivered by cesarean section or transvaginally than the presence or absence of labor. This difference may be due to the stress inhibition effects of lumbar anesthesia [30].

ii)   Human chorionic gonadotropin (hCG)

Human chorionic gonadotropin is synthesized by the syncytial cells of the placenta and the major portion of hCG is secreted into the maternal system, and a minor portion may be said to be released toward the fetus. This is further substantiated by our investi-

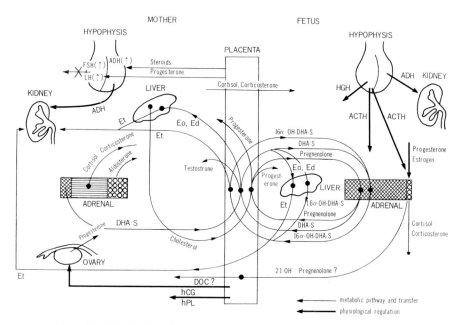

Fig. 28   Metabolic pathway and physiological regulation of hormone.

gation of the hCG-β-subunit, although the mechaism involved in the release of hCG have yet to be adequately elucidated.

At present, it is considered that the hCG secreted into the maternal system stimulates the ovaries enhancing or elevating corpus luteum activity. In vitro, hCG stimulates the secretion of progesterone by the corpus luteum and it is reasonable, therefore, to assume that in early pregnancy maternal blood progesterone levels are under the influence of hCG.

The small amount of hCG found in the fetal circulation is thought to affect the fetal adrenals by increasing the secretion of DHA-S, and in the placenta it is believed to enhance aromatization [34].

Consequently, being secreted both to the maternal and fetal systems, hCG may be considered as a regulator in the materno-fetal relationship.

The relationships between steroids and proteohormones as they affect the materno-placento-fetal system are inferred to be as shown in Fig. 28.

REFERENCES

1. MURPHY, B.E.P.: Does the fetal adrenal play a role in parturition? Amer. J. Obstet. Gynec. **115**; 521, 1973.
2. CSAPO, A.I., PULKKINEN, M.O., RUTTNER, B., SAUVAGE, J.P. and WIEST, W.G.: The significance of the human corpus luteum in pregnancy maintenance. I. Preliminary studies. Amer. J. Obstet. Gynec. **112**; 1061, 1972.
3. YOSHIMI, T., STROTT, C.A., MARSHALL, J.R. and LIPSETT, M.B.: Corpus luteum function in early pregnancy. J. Clin. Endocr. **29**; 225, 1969.
4. FAIMAN, C., RYAN, R.J., ZWIREK, S.J. and RUBIN, M.E.: Serum FSH and HCG during human pregnancy and puerperium. J. Clin. Endocrinol. Metab. **28**; 1323, 1968.
5. JAFFE, R.B., LEE, P.A. and MIDGLEY, A.R., JR.: Serum gonadotropins before, at the inception of, and following human pregnancy. J. Clin. Endocrinol. Metab. **29**; 1281, 1969.
6. MEGEON, C.T., BERTRAND, T. and GEMZELL, C.A.: The transplacental passage of various steroid hormones in mid-pregnancy. Recent Prog. Hormone Res. **17**; 207, 1961.
7. VILLEE, D.B., ENGEL, L.L. and VILLEE, C.A.: Steroid hydroxylation in human fetal adrenals. Endocrinology **65**; 465, 1959.
8. NIEMI, M. and BAILLIE, A.H.: 3β-hydroxysteroid dehydrogenase activity in the human foetal adrenal cortex. Acta Endocr. **48**; 423, 1965.
9. WRAY, P.M. and RUSSELL, C.S.: Maternal urinary oestriol levels before and after death of the foetus. J. Obstet. Gynaec. Brit. Cwlth. **71**; 97, 1964.
10. SIMMER, H.H., WILLIAM. J.D., EASTERLING, W.E., JR., FRANKLAND, M.V. and NAFTOLIN, F.: Neutral C-19 steroid and steroid sulfates in human pregnancy. III. Dehydroepiandrosterone sulfate, 16α-hydroxydehydroepiandrosterone, and 16α-hydroxydehydroepiandrosterone sulfate in cord blood and blood of pregnant women with and without treatment with corticoids. Steroids **8**; 179, 1966.
11. SOBREVILLA, L., HAGERMAN, D. and VILLEE, C.A.: Metabolism of pregnenolone and 17α-hydroxypregnenolone by homogenates of human term placentas. Biochim. Biophys. Acta **93**; 665, 1964.
12. VILLEE, C.A. and TSAI, S.: The de novo synthesis of steroids by the placenta. In: The Foeto-Placental Unit. Pecile, A. and Finzi, C. (eds.) Excerpt Medica, Amsterdam, 1969.
13. SOLOMON, S., LENZ, A.L., VANDE WIELE, R. and LIEBERMAN, S.: Pregnenolone, and intermediate in the biosynthesis of progesterone and the adrenal cortical hormones. Abstracts 126th Meeting of the American Chemical Society, New York, p. 29 C, 1954.
14. MORRISON, G., MEIGS, R.A. and RYAN, R.T.: Biosynthesis of progesterone by the human placenta. Steroids **6** (Suppl. II): 117, 1965.
15. RYAN, K.J., MEIGS, R. and PETRO, Z.: The formation of progesterone by the human placenta. Amer. J. Obstet. Gynec. **96**; 676, 1966.

16. NISHII, T.: Dynamics of plasma pregnenolone and its sulfate in pregnancy. Nippon Sanka-Fujinka Gakkai Zasshi **22**; 579, 1970. (in Japanese)

17. PEARLMAN, W.H.: (16-³H) progesterone metabolism in advanced pregnancy and in oophorectomized-hysterectomized women. Biochem. J. **67**; 1, 1957.

18. HELLIG, H., GATTEREAU, D., LEFEBVRE, Y. and BOLTÉ, E.: Steroid production from plasma cholesterol. I. Conversion of plasma cholesterol to placental progesterone in humans. J. Clin. Endocr. **30**; 624, 1970.

19. MATHUR, R.S., ARCHER, D.F., WIQVIST, N. and DICZFALUSY, E.: Quantitative assessment of the de novo sterol and steroid synthesis in the human feto-placental unit. I. Synthesis and secretion of cholesterol and cholesterol sulphate. Acta Endocr. **65**; 663, 1970.

20. DAVIS, M.E., PLOTZ, E.T., LEROY, G.V., GOULD, R.C. and WERBIN, H.: Urinary steroids after the administration of labelled cholesterol. Amer. J. Obstet. Gynec. **72**; 740, 1956.

21. YAMAJI, M.: Dynamics of plasma estrogen in non-gravid women and in early pregnancy by radioimmunoassay. Nippon Sanka-Fujinka Gakkai Zasshi **24**; 1045, 1972. (in Japanese)

22. SOBREVILLA, L., HAGERMAN, D. and VILLEE, C.A.: The metabolism of pregnenolone and 17α-hydroxyprogesterone by homogenates human term placentas. Biochim. Biophys. Acta **93**; 665, 1964.

23. MAGENDANTZ, H.G. and RYAN, K.T.: Isolation of an estriol precursor, 16α-hydroxydehydroepiandrosterone, from human umbilical sera. J. Clin. Endocr. **24**; 1155, 1964.

24. SIMMER, H.H., EASTERLING, W.E., JR., PION, R.J. and DEGNAM, W.J.: Neutral C-19 steroids and steroid sulfates in human pregnancy. I. Identification of dehydroepiandrosterone sulfate in fetal blood and quantification of this hormone in cord arterial, cord venous and maternal peripheral blood in normal pregnancies at term. Steroids **4**; 125, 1964.

25. EASTERLING, W.E., JR., SIMMER, H.H., DEGNAM, W.J., FRANKLIND, Y.W. and NAFTOLIN, F.: Neutral C-19 steroids and steroid sulfates in human pregnancy. II. Dehydroepiandrosterone sulfate, 16α-hydroxydehydroepiandrosterone and 16α-hydroxydehydroepiandrosterone sulfate in maternal and fetal blood of pregnancies with anencephalic and normal fetuses. Steroids **8**; 157, 1966.

26. HARKNESS, R.A., MENINI, E., CHARLES, D., KENNY, F.M. and ROMBAUT, R.: Studies of urinary steroid excretion by an adrenalectomized woman during and after pregnancy. Acta Endocr. **52**; 409, 1966.

27. SIITERI, P.K. and MACDONALD, P.C.: Placental estrogen biosynthesis during human pregnancy. J. Clin. Endocr. **26**; 751, 1966.

28. TAKAGI, S.: Hormone synthesis and metabolism with emphasis on materno-fetal interrelations and their clinical significance. Nippon Sanka-Fujinka Gakkai Zasshi **23**; 750, 1971. (in Japanese)

29. TAYLOR, N.R.W., LORAINE, J.A. and ROBERTSON, H.A.: Estimation of ACTH in human pituitary tissue. J. Endocr. Metab. **9**; 334, 1953.

30. ASO, T.: Studies on maternal and fetal pituitary adrenal function; Plasma corticosteroids and ACTH levels during pregnancy and those of maternal, umbilical vein and artery of full term delivered cases. Nippon Sanka-Fujinka Gakkai Zasshi **25**; 1201, 1973. (in Japanese)

31. WINTERS, A.J., OLIVER, C., COLSTON, C., MACDONALD, D.C. and PORTER, J.C.: Plasma ACTH levels in the human fetus and neonate as related to age and parturition. J. Clin. Endocrinol. Metab. **39**; 269, 1974.

32. JOHANISSON, E.: The fetal adrenal cortex in the human: Its ultrastructure at different stages of development and different functional states. Acta Endocr. (Suppl.) **130**; 1, 1968.

33. GEMZELL, C.A., HEIJENSKJÖLD, F. and STRÖM, L.: A method for demonstrating growth hormone activity in human plasma. J. Clin. Endocrinol. Metab. **15**; 537, 1955.

34. BERLE, P.: Chorionic gonadotrophin in the foeto-placental unit. In: Abstracts. International Symposium on Foeto-Placental Unit. Pecile, A. and Carruthers, G.B. (eds.) ICS 170, Excerpta Medica, Amsterdam, 1968.

Sonar as a detecting method of fetal informations

Mitsunao KOBAYASHI, M.D.

Department of Obstetrics and Gynecology, National Defense Medical College, Tokorozawa, Saitama

One of the most remarkable recent advances in obstetrics and gynecology is perhaps the diagnostic ultrasound (sonar), which has revolutionized the diagnosis in many areas of our specialty.

Attempts to properly assess and evaluate the fetal growth and the state of fetal health in utero have involved a number of investigators in obstetrics and its related specialties.

With the advent of ultrasonic compound B-scanning in obstetrics, we have witnessed many significant contributions and remarkable progresses made by sonar in the rapidly expanding area of fetal medicine.

This versatile investigative technique began with the work of IAN DONALD and his colleagues [1], who showed the potential usefulness of sonar and has subsequently published many papers on its diagnostic applications in every facet of obstetrics and gynecology [1–13], thus attracting an ever-increasing number of investigators into this field. A majority of the reports, however, have dealt with obstetrical applications, because sonar is particularly suited for pregnant patients with an enlarged uterus filled with amniotic fluid.

In this paper an attempt is made to present the current status of sonar applications in the area of fetal diagnostic informations.

1. EARLY PREGNANCY

1) DIAGNOSIS OF PREGNANCY AND NORMAL GROWTH OF THE GESTATIONAL SAC

Sonar has naturally found an important application in the diagnosis of early pregnancy and the monitoring of early fetal growth prior to the appearance of the fetal head.

An early pregnancy is characterized by a round cystic-appearing sac, gestational sac, located in the uterine fundus (Figs. 1, 2).

The gestational sac is an important structure in that it can be useful indices of monitoring fetal growth and assessing the integrity of pregnancy as to the subsequent outcome.

The gestational sac can be measured in three greatest diameters on the longitudinal and transverse scans and thus fetal growth can be monitored for the assessment of the adequancy of fetal growth in its early developmental stage. The gestational sac persists until the 10th week of pregnancy. Then the period of dissolution of the gestational sac follows

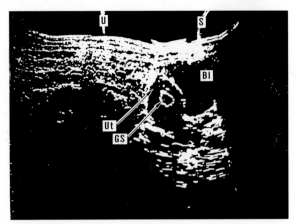

Fig. 1   Pregnancy 6 weeks. Bl, bladder; GS, gestational sac;
S, symphysis pubis; U, umbilicus; Ut, uterus.

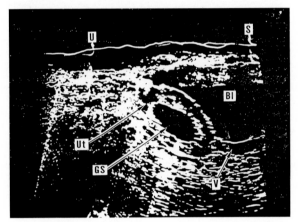

Fig. 2   Pregnancy 8 weeks. Bl, bladder; GS, gestational sac;
S, symphysis pubis; U, umbilicus; Ut, uterus; V, vagina.

between the 11th and 13th week of pregnancy, coinciding with the time of fusion of the decidua capsularis and parietalis. This is the period of neither a gestational sac nor a demonstrable fetal head. Only the placenta can be clearly seen at this sonographically somewhat confusing period, and the placenta at this stage is a reliable structure in the diagnosis of pregnancy.

The fetal head begins to become demonstrable sometime between the 12th and 15th week of pregnancy with a clearly linear midline echo.

Extending their original work [1], DONALD and MACVICAR explored the diagnostic potential of sonar in early pregnancy and its complications [14]. They examined a total of 135 cases of pregnancy ranging from 9 to 20 weeks with various complications, and could detect fetal echoes as early as 8 1/2 weeks of pregnancy, proving sonar in early pregnancy to be a valuable adjunct to our clinical judgment.

DONALD is to be credited with the invention of the invaluable "full bladder technique" for the purpose of clearly visualizing the pelvic vicera in early pregnancy [3, 4].

DONALD [5, 8, 9] described the "ring appearance" of the early gestation sac, discussing the significance of measuring this structure in relation to the maturity of the embryo.

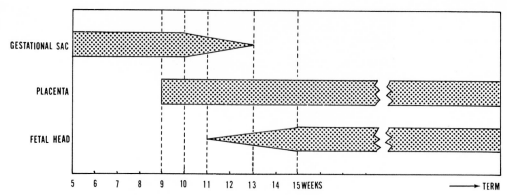

Fig. 3   Three important intrauterine structures in pregnancy (From KOBAYASHI, M.: Illustrated Manual of Ultrasonography in Obstetrics and Gynecology. Igaku Shoin, Tokyo, 1974).

He noted the very rapid growth between the sixth and tenth week of pregnancy. After 11 weeks this characteristic "ring appearance" of the gestation sac began to fragment, then followed by a difficult period of the 11th through the 14th week until the appearance of the fetal head.

The chronological sequence of these findings was later confirmed by HELLMAN and his colleagues [15], who, in a series of 103 gravidas from the 5th to the 20th week with precisely known last menstrual periods, measured 3 separate structures, namely, the gestational sac, the uterine size (uterine length and AP diameter) and the fetal head. The size of the gestational sac was measured in three diameters, the antero-posterior and longitudinal diameters on the longitudinal scan and a transverse diameter on the transverse scan. These three measurements were averaged. The biparietal diameter of the fetal head was measured from the 12th through the 20th week of pregnancy. They described the three phases of early gestation, namely, that of the gestational sac which persists from the 5th to the 10th

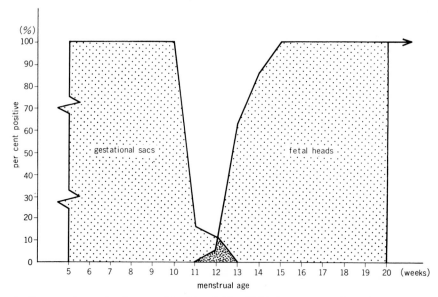

Fig. 4   Per cent of gestational sacs and fetal heads identifiable in sonograms from the fifth to the 20th week of pregnancy (From HELLMAN, L.M. et al.: Amer. J. Obstet. Gynec. **103**; 789, 1969).

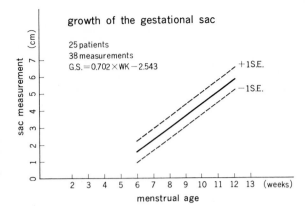

Fig. 5 Least squares regression line and standard error of the estimate of the relation between the diameter of the gestational sac and the duration of pregnancy (From HELLMAN, L.M. et al.: Amer. J. Obstet. Gynec. **103;** 789, 1969).

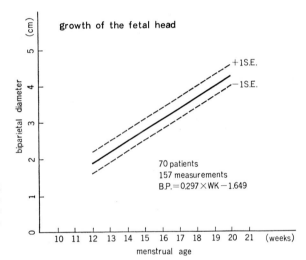

Fig. 6 Least squares regression line and standard error of the estimate of the relation of the fetal biparietal diameter to the duration of pregnancy (From HELLMAN, L.M. et al.: Amer. J. Obstet. Gynec. **103:** 789, 1969).

week, that of dissolution of the sac from the 11th to the 13th week, and that of the fetal head from sometime between the 12th and the 15th week. These periods merged into one another as shown in Figs. 3 and 4. The growth of the gestational sac and that of the fetal head are shown in Figs. 5 and 6. A summary of sonographic features of pregnancy is presented in Fig. 7.

Regression equations and standard errors for the growth of the gestational sac, and the fetal head were as follows:

Gestational sac (cm) $=0.70 \times$ wks -2.54 (Standard error 0.64)
Biparietal diameter (cm) (prior to the 20th week) $=0.30 \times$ wks -1.65 (Standard error 0.29)

Whereas the slope of the least squares regression line showing the relation between the biparietal diameter of the fetal head and the duration of pregnancy in normal gravidas from the 24th to the 40th week was 0.21[16], that of the least squares regression line from the 12th to the 20th week of pregnancy was 0.30 [15]. This difference in the slopes indicated a slightly faster growth rate of the biparietal diameter in early pregnancy (0.30 vs. 0.21 cm/week). Significant deviations from these normal rates may indicate abnormal fetal development. These early growth curves of pregnancy will contribute greatly to our knowledge of early fetal development and the sonographic study of normal and

M. KOBAYASHI

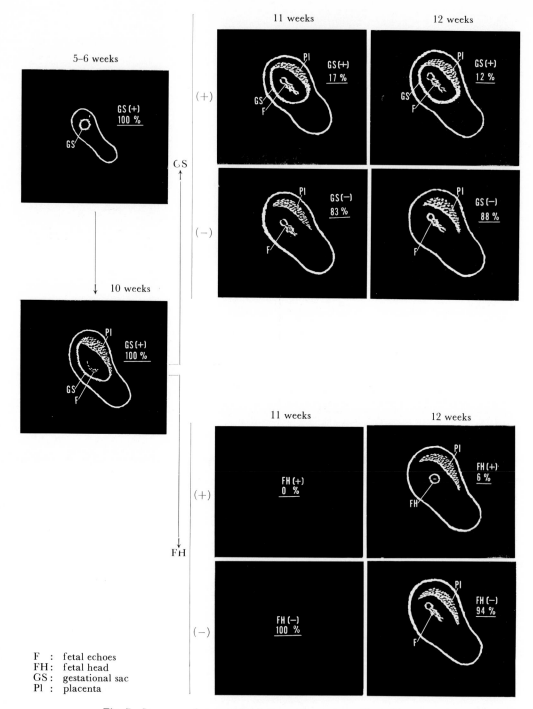

F : fetal echoes
FH: fetal head
GS : gestational sac
Pl : placenta

Fig. 7 Summary of sonographic features of pregnancy (From KOBAYASHI .M.: Illustrated

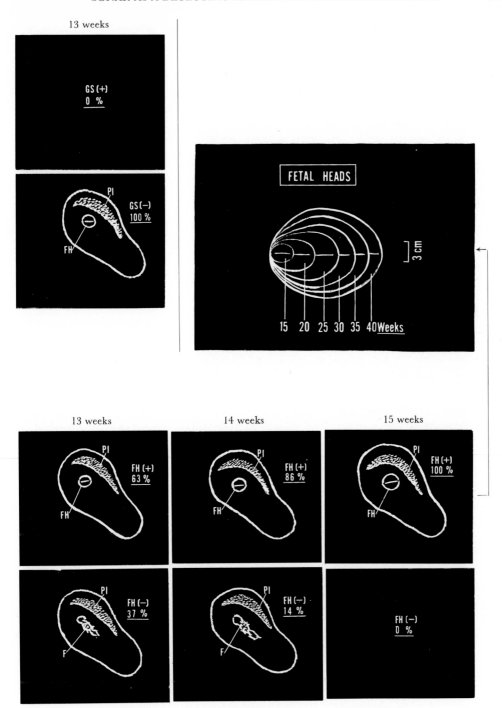

Manual of Ultrasonography in Obstetrics and Gynecology. Igaku Shoin, Tokyo, 1974).

abnormal early fetal growth has great impact on the future of the fetal medicine. With refinement and sophistication of the sonar equipment, more and more important informations will be obtained.

2) ABNORMAL EARLY PREGNANCY

In 1969, DONALD [9] recognized two sonographic signs that suggested failure of the normal intrauterine rate of growth: (1) the presence of a poorly shaped incomplete ring that failed to enlarge, and (2) a ring that was replaced by a blotchy mass of speckles. In addition, he described an increased likelihood of subsequent abortion in the case of low implantation of the gestation sac just over the internal os.

In an extension of his earlier work, DONALD [13] presented 5 ultrasonographic features of blighted ovum. They were as follows:

1. *Loss of definition of the gestation sac:* Poor definition or actual fragmentation of the gestation sac.
2. *Absence of fetal echoes:* In normal pregnancy, from 8 weeks onward, fetal echoes should be seen within the gestation sac.
3. *Small-for-dates gestation sac:* The gestation sac two weeks smaller is suspect. Examination should be repeated a week later.
4. *Failure of growth:* Growth failure over 1 to 2 weeks' period is significant. Shrinkage of the gestation sac may be seen.
5. *Low position of the sac:* This usually occurs as the sac is about to be expelled. This is significant when associated with an open cervix.

The demonstration of one isolated ultrasonographic abnormality, however, is not usually diagnostic of a blighted ovum: in many cases several of the signs above described were present.

He recommended that in case of any doubt serial examinations should be performed at weekly intervals to confirm the developmental failure. In his series, 23 of the 29 patients (79%) with a "poor ring" subsequently aborted. Abortion occurred in 24 of the 27 cases (89%) in which the pregnancy was at least two weeks smaller than dates, and in all patients in whom the gestation sac failed to grow in the serial examinations. Five of the 6 patients with a low gestation sac aborted soon after examination, this sign being most significant when associated with a dilating cervix.

The clinical usefulness of sonar in the management of bleeding complications in early pregnancy was also confirmed by others [17, 18].

HELLMAN and his colleagues [19] analyzed their sonographic data based on 140 gravidas with histories of previous obstetrical difficulties and described 6 different types of embryonic or fetal malformations. Of their series, 114 patients aborted. The sonographic prediction of abortion showed an over-all accuracy of 78 per cent. The six types of embryonic malformations they described were as follows:

1. *Poorly defined gestational sac:* 71 of 140 gravidas (50.7%) showed poorly defined gestational sacs, appearing as fragmented non-round structures with thin walls (Fig. 8). Of the patients showing the poorly defined gestational sac, 83 per cent aborted.
2. *Small gestational sac:* Of 63 cases (45%) showing the gestational sac smaller than dates, 94 per cent aborted.
3. *Abnormal intrauterine echoes:* Of 54 cases (38.5%) showing abnormal intrauterine echoes (Fig. 9), 90.7 per cent aborted.
4. *Growth failure:* Of 38 cases (27.1%) showing growth failure on successive sonograms, 92.2 per cent aborted.

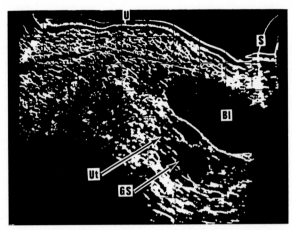

Fig. 8   A longitudinal sonogram of early pregnancy with a poorly defined thin-walled gestational sac within the uterine cavity. Abbreviations used in Figs. 8, 9 and 10 are as follows: Bl, bladder; GS, gestational sac; S, symphysis pubis; U, umbilicus; Ut, uterus.

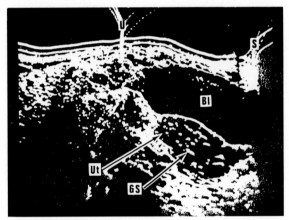

Fig. 9   A longitudinal sonogram of early pregnancy with intrauterine echoes showing no form. Abortion is usually inveitable.

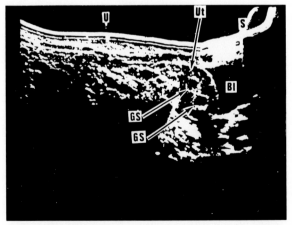

Fig. 10   A fundally implanted double gestational sac which subsequently aborted.

5. *Double gestational sac:* An apparent double-appearing sac (Fig. 10) may signal the presence of abnormal pregnancy. Of 22 cases (15.7%) shwoing double gestational sac, 9 had received artificial ovulants. All of the remaining 13 patients with spontaneously occurring double sacs aborted, whereas the 9 patients later gave birth to only 5 sets of twins and 3 singletons.

6. *Low implanted gestational sac:* Since ovum nidation normally occurs near the fundus, low implantation is an unfavorable prognostic sign. Of the 6 patients (4.3%) showing low implantation, 5 (83.3%) aborted. However, in one patient, the sac appeared to rise in the uterine cavity and the patient had spontaneous vaginal delivery.

In this study there were 114 patients who eventually aborted; in 12 of these abortion was not predicted by sonar. Thus the percentage of false negative error was 10.5 per cent. In 132 patients, abortion was predicted in 18 who did not abort, thus the false-posive error was 13.6 per cent. There were, therefore, 30 errors in the entire series (140 cases), with a total error in the sonar prediction of abortion of 21.2 per cent.

It is generally agreed that serial examinations are necessary to predict abortion in suspected growth retardation or abnormality [13, 19, 20].

Obviously, a large number of cases will have to be accumulated for more definitive analysis of data on embryonic and early fetal abnormalities and malformations.

2. BIPARIETAL CEPHALOMETRY AND FETAL GROWTH

One of the most important contributions of sonar in the fetal medicine is the fetal cephalometry as a means of assessing fetal growth and maturity.

Fetal cephalometry using sonar was first described by DONALD and BROWN [2] and this has naturally led to the numerous subsequent publications on this matter [15, 16, 21–52].

WILLOCKS [50], after making more than 300 measurements of fetal biparietal diameter, confirmed its great value in studying the growth of the fetal head in utero from the 30th week of 7.5 cm to term of 9 cm or more and described an average rate of growth of 1.5 mm a week, the growth being more rapid between the 30th and 36th week than between the 36th week and term. He was the first to call attention to an interesting finding: the growth of the fetal biparietal diameter was significantly retarded in some cases of preeclampsia and placental insufficiency.

WILLOCKS and his colleagues [51] found a correlation between birth weight and ultrasonic measurement of the biparietal diameter. Their simple rule was as follows : if the biparietal diameter is 8.5 cm or more, the baby is unlikely to weight less than 4 pounds, and if the diameter is 9.0 cm or more, the fetal weight will be 5 pounds or more with the expectation of being right in over 80 per cent of cases.

They noticed that in the last quarter of pregnancy the biparietal diameter was found to increase linearly. In 2 of the 25 cases growth faltered, one being a case of hypertension and the other a case of albuminuric preeclampsia. Their observation indicated that the average growth rate of the biparietal diameter in the last 10 weeks of pregnancy was 1.6 mm per week and the diameter correlated with maternal height.

In the serial biparietal diameter determinations in 108 cases in which dysmaturity seemed likely, a comparison made between the biparietal growth rate and gestational age and birth weight of the infant revealed the following results [52]:

1. 70.4 per cent of the dysmature babies had a growth rate of less than 1.7 mm a week.
2. 69.1 per cent of the non-dysmature babies had a growth rate of 1.7 mm a week or more.

3. When the growth rate exceeded 1.7 mm a week, 87.5 per cent of the babies were not dysmature.

It was further suggested that the measurements should be started as early in pregnancy as possible.

THOMPSON and his colleagues [47] showed that the growth of the biparietal diameter was 1.8 mm per week during the last trimester of pregnancy. Using the formula (Weight (g) = 1,060 × Biparietal diameter − 6,575) for estimating fetal weight, they could predict, in 68 per cent of patients, the fetal weight within ±484 g of the actual weight by using A-scan measurement of the biparietal diameter. In 91 per cent, when the fetal biparietal diameter was 8.5 cm or more, the fetal weight was in excess of 2,500 g. In attempting to estimate the fetal weight by measuring the fetal chest circumference in utero by B-scan, they used the following formula:

$$W = 1,000 \sqrt{\frac{Max^2 + Min^2}{2}} - 7,000$$

Where W: Weight, Max: maximum diameter of the fetal thorax, Min: minimum diameter of the fetal thorax.

With this formula, there was an error of about 500 g in 20 per cent. By the combined use of biparietal diameter and fetal chest circumference, it was possible to estimate within 400 g of the actual weight except in large babies where the tendency is to underestimate the weight.

HELLMAN and his colleagues [16] presented the correlations between the biparietal diameters and duration of pregnancy and made from normal and abnormal gravidas the least squares regression lines to the means of the observations (Figs. 11, 12). The formulas for the least squares regression lines made between the biparietal diameter and the duration of pregnancy for normal and abnormal gravidas are shown below:

Normal pregnancy	BP (cm) =	1.14 + 0.21 wk
Diabetes mellitus	BP (cm) =	0.88 + 0.22 wk
Chronic hypertension	BP (cm) =	1.95 + 0.18 wk
Pyelonephritis	BP (cm) =	−0.94 + 0.27 wk

These growth rates, however, were based on too few observations to represent more than

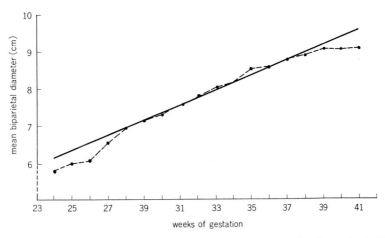

Fig. 11   Least squares line fitted to the mean biparietal diameter by weeks of gestation in 91 normal gravidas (From HELLMAN, L.M. et al.: Amer. J. Obstet. Gynec. **99**; 662, 1967).

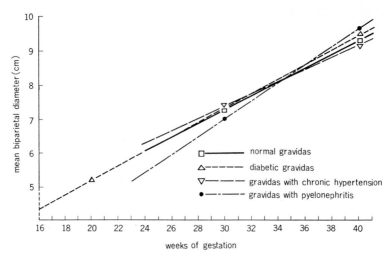

Fig. 12   Comparison of least squares lines fitted to the mean biparietal diameters by weeks of gestation in normal and several types of abnormal pregnancies (From HELLMAN, L.M. et al.: Amer. J. Obstet. Gynec. **99**; 662, 1967).

approximations, and obviously a large number of cases are required before definitive formulas can be constructed.

KOHORN [38], discussing the limitations and the difficulties of the A-scan cephalometry, first described the importance of obtaining the midline echo in defining the biparietal diameter in order to eliminate the error of measurement.

DONALD [53] found the biparietal measurement more useful in assessing maturity. He stated that any biparietal diameter of 9.8 cm indicates maturity and a measurement of over 10 cm almost certainly indicates the postmature fetus whatever its birthweight.

CAMPBELL has made significant contributions to the fetal cephalometry and fetal medicine [22–29, 54–56]. In 1968, he described a method of fetal cephalometry known now as "Campbell technique" [22]. This was the first time that the accurate technique of cephalometry had been presented. As was described in detail in the CAMPBELL's original paper, the Campbell technique utilizes the combined A and B scan, the B-scan being done by means of two scans made at right angles to each other.

The basic steps in obtaining accurate biparietal diameter by the Campbell technique involve the following steps:

1.   In case of occipito-transverse (OT) position or slightly rotated OT:
    (1)   The longitudinal B-scan is first made to determine the angle of asynclitism of the fetal head.
    (2)   With this information concerning the angle, the transducer of the transverse scan is tilted to the angle of asynclitism.
    (3)   A-scan beam is directed along the bipariental diameter, vertically to the midline echo.

2.   In case of occipito-anterior (OA) or occipito-posterior (OP) position:
    (1)   The longitudinal scan is first made with the beam directed along the occipito-frontal diameter.
    (2)   Transverse scan is tilted to the angle of asynclitism.
    (3)   The beam is directed along the biparietal diameter, vertically to the midline echo.

There are crucial signs necessary to minimize the error in obtaining an accurate measurement [28]:

    (1)   The transverse section of the fetal head must show a strong continuous midline echo completely bisecting the head.

    (2)   Provided that the midline echo is still visualized, the largest transcoronal diameter must be obtained.

The Campbell technique, however, is not easy to perform in practice [28–30, 32] and it should be remembered that considerable experience and a good ultrasonic equipment specifically designed for cephalometry are necessary before it can be done with consistent accuracy. According to CAMPBELL, his 95% confidence limits for measuring weekly growth of the biparietal diameter are ± 0.71 mm [28].

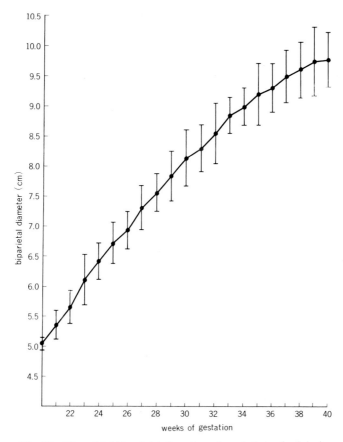

Fig. 13   Mean fetal biparietal diameter values $\pm$ 2 standard deviations for each week of gestation during the second half of normal pregnancy in 186 patients whose gestation was known (471 individual measurements) (From CAMPBELL, S.: J. Obstet. Gynaec. Brit. Cwlth. **76;** 603, 1969).

Applying his combined A and B scan method to various stages of pregnancy, CAMPBELL made a total of 471 individual observations of the fetal biparietal diameter from the 20th week of pregnancy onward (Fig. 13). He showed that up to the 30th week inclusive, the growth was more rapid (mean 2.8 mm per week) than in the last 10 weeks (mean 1.5mm per week) and that in the later weeks of pregnancy the values showed a wider scatter about the mean. It was, therfore, suggested that measurement of the fetal biparietal diameter between the 20th to the 30th week is more useful in the estimation of fetal maturity. He could also predict the true week of gestation $\pm$ 8.4 days in 95 per cent of cases from the regression line fitted to his data.

Stressing that the midline echo should be seen to be bisecting the fetal head for accurate cephalometry [24], CAMPBELL demonstrated that the fetal head could be measured with a high degree of accuracy from the 13th week of pregnancy onward, and constructed the growth curve of the biparietal diameter (Fig. 14) [25]. The important point to emerge

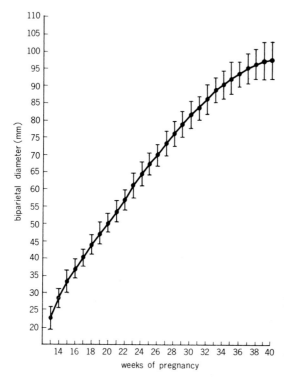

Fig. 14 Mean fetal biparietal diameter (mm) $\pm$ 2 standard deviations for each week of pregnancy from 13 weeks to term (1,029 measurements) (From CAMPBELL, S. and NEWMAN, G.B.: J. Obstet. Gynaec. Brit. Cwlth. **78**; 513, 1971).

from this study was that fetal head growth was almost linear until about 30 weeks and less rapid but more variable in growth thereafter. A measurement taken after 30 weeks correlates less accurately with the expected date of confinement, and ultrasonic cephalometry clearly is the most satisfactory method of assessing the duration of pregnancy if a measurement is taken before 30 weeks [33].

The value of serial cephalometry was assessed in the diagnosis of the small-for-dates fetus [26]. In a series of 406 patients whose fetus was considered to be at risk from placental failure, serial ultrasonic cephalometry was performed and the following results were obtained:

(1)   When the ultrasonic growth was "normal" (above the 10th percentile), 83 per cent of the babies were of normal weight, 8 per cent were borderline, and 9 per cent were small-for-dates.

(2)   When the ultrasonic growth was "borderline" (between the 5th and 10th percentile), 69 per cent of the babies were of normal weight, 15 per cent were borderline, and 15 per cent were small-for-dates.

(3) When the ultrasonic growth was "retarded" (below the 5th percentile), 18 per cent of the babies were of normal weight, 14 per cent were borderline, and 68 per cent were small-for-dates.

(4) Retarded ultrasonic growth rates were associated with a significant increase in the number of low Apgar scores, perinatal deaths, and gross fetal anomalies.

(5) Serial ultrasonic cephalometry was confirmed to be an important aid in the diagnosis of the fetus at risk from chronic placental insufficiency.

In order to assess fetal maturity and growth in monitoring high risk pregnancies, attempts have been made to use fetal cephalometry in combination with estriol [10, 27, 33, 49, 57] and other examinations [58].

WILLOCKS and his colleagues [52] made serial observations of biparietal growth and estriol excretion, proving their combination to be valuable in detecting fetal growth or its failure and showed (1) that the estriol excretion tended to be low in the group of dysmature fetus who had shown the average growth rate of 0.14 cm per week and (2) that the extriol excretion tended to be high in the group of non-dysmature infants who had shown the average growth rate of 0.20 cm per week.

Subsequent reports confirmed the clinical usefulness of serial cephalometry coupled with estriol in high risk pregnancies [10, 27, 33, 49, 57].

CAMPBELL and KURJAK [27] performed urinary estrogen assay and serial ultrasonic cephalometry on 284 patients who were at risk of having a growth-retarded fetus and found that ultrasonic cephalometry was significantly better than urinary estrogen in predicting fetal growth retardation. Of the 14 stillbirths, 3 were in the normal ultrasonic growth rate group, and 5 were in the normal estrogen exeretion group. They found that both methods were of value in diagnosing fetal growth retardation although cephalometry appeared to have some advantages, especially in distinguishing between fetal growth retardation and mistaken maturity.

In assessing the fetal growth by serial ultrasonic cephalometry and urinary estrogen assays in 150 cases of uncomplicated placenta previa, VARMA [49] found that there were 24 (16%) small-for-dates infants, more accurately predicted by serial cephalometry than by serial maternal urinary estrogen assays. Whereas serial ultrasonic cephalometry produced correct predictions in 22 of the 24 small-for-dates infants, estrogen assay was abnormal in only 17 of the 24. In the group of the 150 patients followed until delivery, 24.7 per cent were found to have abnormal estrogen levels in two or more successive determinations, and abnormal serial cephalometry below the 10th percentile was found in 22.7 per cent in two or more successive determinations. His finding indicated that the placental insufficiency and fetal growth retardation might be a common problem in placenta previa where the bleeding episodes were recurrent even in small amount.

3. PLACENTAL ULTRASONOGRAPHY

The value of ultrasonic placental localization in clinical obstetrics has been firmly established, and its scanning and interpretation have been described [6, 49, 54, 59–68].

The accuracy of this technique was reported to be 94–97 per cent, with the salient features of simplicity, rapidity and safety [69–80].

The characteristically thicker and ultrasonically more "opaque" placenta [6] with a stronger fetal surface echo [12] was described in a case of rhesus iso-immunization. It should, however, be remembered that the placenta scanned not vertically to the chorionic and basal plates but either with angles or tangentially to the plates produces a picture of an unduly thick-appearing placenta. It should also be noted that the placenta

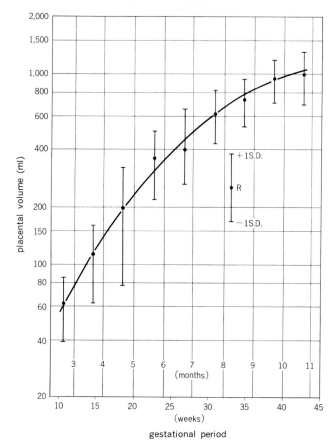

Fig. 15 Composite placental growth curve derived from 207 gravidas at
various stages of gestation (From HELLMAN, L.M. et al.: Amer. J. Obstet.
Gynec. **108**; 740, 1970).

in abruptio placentae may, depending upon its severity, appear thick along with the chorionic plate bulging into the amniotic cavity [61, 62].

With increasing use of transabdominal amniocentesis for various obstetric and genetic
indications, the ultrasonic examination has found one of its greatest indications in local-
izing the placenta [64, 65] because of its capability of clearly delineating the exact location of the placenta even at its thinnest periphery.

There has been some innovation attached to the transducer to facilitate the procedure of
amniocentesis [65, 81].

We used to perform amniocentesis after careful scanning of the placenta with the patient's
bladder full as in the examination for placenta previa. However, we no longer think it
necessary. We simply perform amniocentesis on the examining table of the ultrasonic
equipment immediately after having confirmed the exact location of the placenta. This
will eliminate the time lag between the ultrasonic examination and scheduled amniocentesis. This time lag may occasionally alter the positional relationship between the lower
uterine segment and the bladder which may be progressively distending with urine.

In an attempt to study placental volumetric growth in vivo and construct a placental
growth curve, HELLMAN and his colleagues [82] measured the placental thickness, and

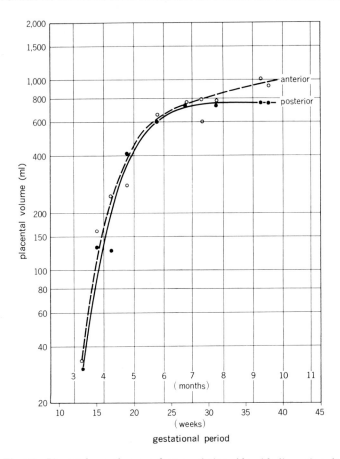

Fig. 16   Placental growth curves from a primigravida with dizygotic twins
(From HELLMAN, L.M. et al.: Amer. J. Obstet. Gynec. **108**; 740, 1970).

the length of the chorionic plate and the basal plate from 207 gravidas at various stages of pregnancy.

The measurements were applied to a formula based on a theoretical planoconvex model to derive the placental volume. Relations between the calculated ultrasonic placental volumes and post-cesarean section immerson volumes as well as comparisons between the preoperative and postoperative placental measurements were used to check the accuracy of the ultrasonic intrauterine measurements. Ultrasonic placental volumes thus calculated were found to be compatible with the measurements of placentas delivered by cesarean sections. A logarithmic plot of placental volume versus pregnancy duration illustrated that the growth rate of the human placenta showed the dramatic change between the 3rd and the 11th month. Fig. 15 shows a curve of the placental volume as a function of a gestational age. Fig. 16 illustrates placental growth curves constructed from a primigravida with Clomid-induced twins. This patient developed mild preeclampsia between the 35th and 36th week of pregnancy, and cesarean section was done one week later. Whereas the larger twin nourished by the anterior placenta weighed 2,250 g, the smaller twin with the posterior placenta which had ceased to grow after 28 weeks, weighed 1,680 g. This might be interpreted to suggest that the placental growth may be a determinant of fetal growth.

4. MULTIPLE PREGNANCY

Since the fetal head is the most reliable, unmistakable structure to identify in the uterine cavity, the confirmation of multiple pregnancy is made by identifying more than one fetal head. Becuase the timing of appearnce of the fetal head in the sonogram is sometime between the 12th and the 15th week, the definitive diagnosis cannot usually be made before this time. However, there is another ultrasonic finding suggestive of multiple pregnancy before the appearance of fetal heads: the presence of plural gestational sacs.

It is agreed that before the 10th week of gestation the number of gestational sacs should be identified, and after the 13th or 14th week, that of fetal heads is to be counted [55, 61, 62, 83].

In cases of more than twin pregnancy of early gestation, the diagnosis becomes more difficult with increasing number of gestational sacs, the reason for this being considerable difficulty of ultrasonic examination to demonstrate all the gestational sacs in one plane of scan.

In scanning plural heads, a skillful external manipulation over plural heads will show the accurate number of heads in one ultrasonogram. Often, a composite picture may have to be made of two or more ultrasonograms [55].

Twin gestations of 5 weeks [61] and 7 weeks [7, 8, 61] and a triplet pregnancy [61] have been described.

Campbell [55] diagnosed a quintuplet pregnancy at 9 weeks menstrual age and assessed the fetal maturity and size. Although it was unlikely that a quintuplet fetus would show a similar growth rate, the two fetal biparietal diameters that could be accurately measured at 30 weeks were only slightly smaller than the expected size of a single fetus and the three other heads seemed to be of similar size.

In general, the serial cephalometry for assessing the individual growth rate of fetuses of multiple pregnancy is not possible because of inability to identify the individual heads in the subsequent examinations.

5. FETAL ANATOMY AND MALFORMATIONS

At the earlier developmental stage of ultrasonic examination, only gross deformities of either the fetal head (hydrocephalus and anencephalus) or the fetal abdomen (ascites) were considered to be the subject of ultrasonic examination. With the refinement and sophistication of the ultrasonic equipment and experience, more and more infrafetal structures and their abnormal changes will be clarified with the development of the promissing "grey-scale" ultrasonography.

Anencephaly can be diagnozed by total inability to detect a clearly defined fetal head [61]. In presenting a case of anencephaly, a scan along the long axis of the fetal body is necessary so that the absence of a fetal head can be confirmed next to the fetal neck and body.

Hydrocephalus is suspected when an obviously large fetal head is seen to occupy either the upper half or the lower half of the uterine cavity [61]. There is a marked discrepancy between the size of the head and the cross-section of the fetal body. The biparietal diameter commonly exceeds 11 cm, sometimes 13 cm or more [12].

Hydramnios associated with or without fetal head deformities can be readily identified by the sonographic finding of a disproportionately large amniotic cavity in relation to the fetal volume.

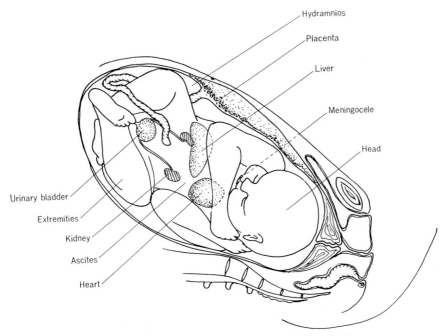

Fig. 17 Fetal parts and organs for ultrasonic investigation.

Cross and longitudinal sections of the fetal body and extremities as well as the gross deformities previously described have been identified and presented [61, 66, 84, 85].

Sonar has been applied to various parts and organs of the fetus to aid in the understanding of fetal physiology and development. The fetal parts and organs that have thus far been investigated by ultrasound are illustrated in Fig. 17.

Fetal heart: In the fetal trunk, the heart appears as a circle in the lower half of the thorax.

The fetal heart is distinguishable from the fetal bladder by its position in relation to the rest of the trunk and by its pulsating walls. On many occasions the interventricular septum is outlined [85]. Fig. 18 demonstrates the fetal heart by the grey scale ultrasonography.

GARRETT and ROBINSON [86] measured the fetal heart in vivo by using two-dimensional ultrasonic echoscopy and showed that the heart occupied 21% of the cross-sectional area of the chest and its widest diameter was found to be 52% of the diameter of the chest at the same level. It was also shown that the fetal heart grew at the same rate as the chest in the last 8 weeks of pregnancy.

In an attempt to test the validity of the heart size as an indicator of fetal maturity, SUZUKI and his colleagues [87] measured the fetal heart volume and biparietal diameter by B-scan. They found that the fetal heart volume correlated well with the gestational age and biparietal diameter. It was suggested that the combined use of fetal biparietal diameter and heart volume is useful for the rough estimation of whether the birthweight is above or below 2500 g. When the biparietal diameter was less than 9 cm but the heart volume was more than 30 cu cm, birthweight was most likely to be more than 2,500 g.

Fetal kidney and bladder: The fetal kidneys are regularly seen when transverse cross-section of the fetus is done [85]. They appear to be situated on either side of the fetal spinal column (Fig. 19).

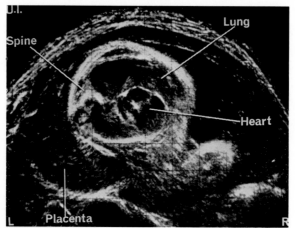

Fig. 18 Fetal heart (Courtesy of Dr. W.J. GARRETT, Mr. G. KOSSOFF and Mr. D.E. ROBINSON, Sydney).

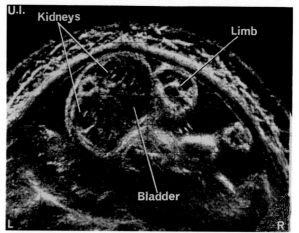

Fig. 19 Fetal kidneys and bladder (Courtesy of Dr. W.J. GARRETT, Mr. G. KOSSOFF and Mr. D.E. ROBINSON, Sydney).

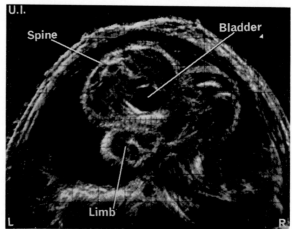

Fig. 20 Fetal urinary bladder (Courtesy of Dr. W.J. GARRETT, Mr. G. KOSSOFF and Mr. D.E. ROBINSON, Sydney).

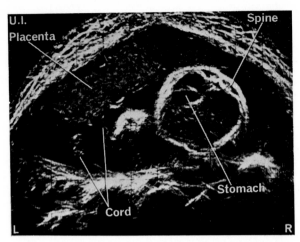

Fig. 21 Fetal stomach (Courtesy of Dr. W.J. GARRETT, Mr. G. KOSSOFF and Mr. D.E. ROBINSON, Sydney).

GARRETT and his colleagues [88] made a prenatal diagnosis of fetal polycystic kidney by demonstrating gross enlargement of the kidney together with fetal ascites, extreme oligohydramnios and cystic spaces in the kidney in the echograms.

The fetal urinary bladder, when full, is seen as a light circle close to the anterior abdominal wall of the fetal lower abdomen [85], as is clearly demonstrated by the grey scale ultrasonography in Fig. 20. It is distinguished from the heart by the absence of pulsation [85].

CAMPBELL and his colleagues [56] developed an ultrasonic method of assessing the hourly fetal urine production rate (HFUPR) and confirmed the relationship (r=0.8955) between HFUPR and the menstrual age of the fetus. There was a gradual rise in the mean HFUPR from 12.2 ml at 32 weeks to 28.2 ml at 40 weeks.

Fetal liver: The fetal liver is difficult to clearly delineate without experience. GARRETT and ROBINSON [85] described two patterns of fetal liver ultrasonogram: (1) characteristic appearance of two short lines in a position corresponding to the gall bladder, and (2) a y-shaped echo running from the region of the porta hepatis to the region of the neck of the gall bladder.

Fetal meningocele: Ultrasonograms of meningocele have been reported [89]. In some cases, meningocele can be diagnozed by the double ring outline produced by the double sac of the meningocele.

Fetal duodenal atresia: HOULTON and colleagues [90] encountered a case of fetal duodenal atresia, and suggested that in the presence of polyhydramnios the ultrasonic appearance of distended abdomen showing a normal fetal soft-tissue outline and an absence of opacified amniotic fluid in the fetal gastrointestinal tract or lungs was strongly suggestive of fetal duodenal atresia.

Fetal stomach: GARRETT, KOSSOFF and ROBINSON of Sydney further explored the fetal anatomy and demonstrated the fetal stomach as shown in Fig. 21.

6. FETAL DEATH

The characteristic features of sonographic finding of fetal death are chiefly limited to the most prominent, clearly defined part of the fetus, namely, the head.

Since the fetal head starts to be seen sometime between the 13th and the 15th week as was previously described, the positive finding of fetal death can be obtained after this period.

Sonographic findings of the head in the presence of fetal death

(1) *Double line of the fetal head contour:* This is the most striking finding that B-scan can pick up in the presence of fetal death. The earliest time that this sign has been detected is 4 days after the fetal death (unpublished data). This sign is seen in larger heads.

(2) *Deformed or collapsed fetal head:* This sign is seen in smaller heads of relatively early stage of pregnancy.

(3) *Cessation of head growth by serial cephalometry:* This may either be an alarming sign of impending fetal death or indicate the fetal death that has just recently taken place.

(4) *Overlapping of the skull bones:* This is not so common.

When scanning for evidence of fetal death, one may detect some noticeable change in the position of the fetal head on the oscilloscope screen at the first and second scans, moments apart (Fig. 22). This is obviously the sign of fetal life and is seen in relatively small or medium-sized heads. Similarly, fetal extremities may be noticed to move.

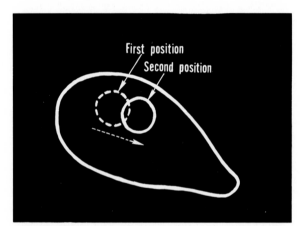

Fig. 22 Identification of fetal movement (From KOBAYASHI, M.: Illustrated Manual of Ultrasonography in Obstetrics and Gynecology. Igaku Shoin, Tokyo, 1974).

Sonographic findings other than the fetal head

The Denver group [91, 92] described the changes in echo pattern within a few hours after fetal death and a coarse brush-stroke appearance of the fetal thoracic outline along with some flattering of the head some twelve hours after death [93].

The Sydney group [85] could not find any specific features associated with fetal death until the occurrence of fetal maceration. With this present, the fetal skull began to collapse, the fetal thorax lost its normal contour and developed the brush-stroke appearance described by the Denver group. In addition, the Sydney group described the displacement of fetal organs with advanced maceration.

CONCLUSION

We are going deeper into the infrafetal structures with sonar technique to understand various aspects of fetal anatomy and physiology. It is hoped that with more refinement and sophistication of the ultrasonic equipment we shall be able to study a great deal more about the fetus and its intrauterine development.

REFERENCES

1. DONALD, I., MacVICAR, J. and BROWN, T.G.: Investigation of abdominal masses by pulsed ultrasound. Lancet 1; 1188, 1958.
2. DONALD, I. and BROWN, T.G.: Localisation using physical devices, radioisotopes and radiographic methods. Brit. J. Radiol. 34; 539, 1961.
3. DONALD, I.: Diagnostic uses of sonar in obstetrics and gynaecology. J. Obstet. Gyneac. Brit. Cwlth. 72; 907, 1965.
4. DONALD, I. and ABDULLA, U.: Further advances in ultrasonic diagnosis. Ultrasonics 5; 8, 1967.
5. DONALD, I. and ABDULLA, U.: Ultrasonics in obstetrics and gynaecology. Brit. J. Radiol. 40; 604, 1967.
6. DONALD, I. and ABDULLA, U.: Placentography by sonar. J. Obstet. Gynaec. Brit. Cwlth. 75; 993, 1968.
7. DONALD, I.: Sonar in obstetrics and gynecology. In: Year Book of Obstetrics and Gynecology 1967–1968. Greenhill, J.P. (ed.) Year Book, Chicago, p. 242.
8. DONALD, I.: Ultrasonics in obstetrics. Brit. Med. Bull. 24; 71, 1968.
9. DONALD, I.: Sonar as a method of studying prenatal development. J. Pediatrics 75; 326, 1969.
10. DONALD, I.: On launching a new diagnostic science. Amer. J. Obstet. Gynec. 103; 609, 1969.
11. DONALD, I.: Sonar—further scope and prospects. Proc. Roy. Soc. Med. 64; 991, 1971.
12. DONALD, I.: Diagnostic sonar in obstetrics and gynecology. In: Obstetrics and Gynecology Annual 1972. Wynn, R.M. (ed.) Appleton-Century-Crofts, New York, 1972, p. 245.
13. DONALD, I., MORLEY, P. and BARNETT, E.: The diagnosis of blighted ovum by sonar. J. Obstet. Gynaec. Brit. Cwlth. 79; 304, 1972.
14. MacVICAR, J. and DONALD, I.: Sonar in the diagnosis of early pregnancy and its complications. J. Obstet. Gynaec. Brit. Cwlth. 70; 387, 1963.
15. HELLMAN, L.M., KOBAYASHI, M., FILLISTI, L. and LAVENHAR, M.: Growth and development of the human fetus prior to the twentieth week of gestation. Amer. J. Obstet. Gynec. 103; 789, 1969.
16. HELLMAN, L.M., KOBAYASHI, M., FILLISTI, L. and LAVENHAR, M.: Sources of error in sonographic fetal mensuration and estimation of growth. Amer. J. Obstet. Gynec. 99; 662, 1967.
17. ROBINSON, H.P.: Sonar in the management of abortion. J. Obstet. Gynaec. Brit. Cwlth. 79; 90, 1972.
18. VARMA, T.R.: The value of ultrasonic B-scanning in diagnosis when bleeding is present in early pregnancy. Amer. J. Obstet. Gynec. 114; 607, 1972.
19. HELLMAN, L.M., KOBAYASHI, M. and CROMB, E.: Ultrasonic diagnosis of embryonic malformations. Amer. J. Obstet. Gynec. 115; 615, 1973.
20. KOHORN, E.I. and KAUFMAN, M.: Sonar in the first trimester of pregnancy. Obstet. Gynec. 44; 473, 1974.
21. ANDERSON, G.V. and NISWONGER, J.W.: Cephalometry by ultrasound. Amer. J. Obstet. Gynec. 91; 563, 1965.
22. CAMPBELL, S.: An improved method of fetal cephalometry by ultrasound. J. Obstet. Gynaec. Brit. Cwlth. 75; 568, 1968.
23. CAMPBELL, S.: The prediction of fetal maturity by ultrasonic measurement of the biparietal diameter. J. Obstet. Gynaec. Brit. Cwlth. 76; 603, 1969.
24. CAMPBELL, S.: Ultrasonic fetal cephalometry during the second trimester of pregnancy. J. Obstet. Gynaec. Brit. Cwlth. 77; 1057, 1970.

25. CAMPBELL, S. and NEWMAN, G.B.: Growth of the fetal biparietal diameter during normal pregnancy. J. Obstet. Gynaec. Brit. Cwlth. **78**; 513, 1971.

26. CAMPBELL, S. and DEWHURST, C.J.: Diagnosis of the small-for-dates fetus by serial ultrasonic cephalometry. Lancet **2**; 1002, 1971.

27. CAMPBELL, S. and KURJAK, A.: Comparison between urinary oestrogen assay and serial ultrasonic cephalometry in assessment of fetal growth retardation. Brit. Med. J. **4**; 336, 1972.

28. CAMPBELL, S.: Ultrasonic cephalometry. Lancet **2**; 1145, 1973.

29. CAMPBELL, S.: Ultrasonic cephalometry. Lancet **1**; 69, 1974.

30. CHRISTIE, A.D.: Fetal cephalometry. Lancet **1**; 177, 1974.

31. DAVISON, J.M., LIND, T., FARR, V. and WHITTINGHAM, T.A.: The limitations of ultrasonic fetal cephalometry. J. Obstet. Gynaec. Brit. Cwlth. **80**; 769, 1973.

32. DAVISON, J.M., LIND, T., FARR, V. and WHITTINGHAM, T.A.: Ultrasonic cephalometry. Lancet **2**; 1329, 1973.

33. DEWHURST, C.J., BEAZLEY, J.M. and CAMPBELL, S.: Assessment of fetal maturity and dysmaturity. Amer. J. Obstet. Gynec. **113**; 141, 1972.

34. DURKAN, J.P. and RUSSO, G.L.: Ultrasonic fetal cephalometry: Accuracy, limitations, and applications. Obstet. Gynec. **27**; 399, 1966.

35. GARRETT, W.J. and ROBINSON, D.E.: Assessment of fetal size and growth rate by ultrasonic echoscopy. Obstet. Gynec. **38**; 525, 1971.

36. GOLDBERG, B.B., ISARD, H.J., GERSHON-COHEN, J. and OSTRUM, B.J.: Ultrasonic fetal cephalometry. Radiology **87**; 328, 1966.

37. IANNIRUBERTO, A. and GIBBONS, J.M.: Predicting fetal weight by ultrasonic B-scan cephalometry. Obstet. Gynec. **37**; 689, 1971.

38. KOHORN, E.I.: An evaluation of ultrasonic cephalometry. Amer. J. Obstet. Gynec. **97**; 553, 1967.

39. LEE, B.O., MAJOR, F.J. and WEINGOLD, A.B.: Ultrasonic determination of fetal maturity at repeat cesarean section. Obstet. Gynec. **38**; 294, 1971.

40. LUNT, R.M. and CHARD, T.: Reproducibility of measurement of fetal biparietal diameter by ultrasonic cephalometry. J. Obstet. Gynaec. Brit. Cwlth. **81**; 682, 1974.

41. MARTIN, C.B., MURATA, Y. and RABIN, L.S.: Diagnostic ultrasound in obstetrics and gynecology. Obstet. Gynec. **41**; 379, 1973.

42. PYSTYNEN, P., YLOSTALO, P. and JARVINEN, P.A.: Foetal cephalometry by ultrasound. Annales Chirurgiae et Gynaecologiae Fenniae **56**; 114, 1967.

43. SABBAGHA, R.E., TURNER, H., ROCKETTE, H., MAZER, J. and ORGILL, J.: Sonar BPD and fetal age. Obstet. Gynec. **43**; 7, 1974.

44. SCHER, E.: Evaluation of cephalometry by ultrasound in breech presentation. Amer. J. Obstet. Gynec. **103**; 1125, 1969.

45. STONE, M.L., WEINGOLD, A.B. and LEE, B.O.: Clinical applications of ultrasound in obstetrics and gynecology. Amer. J. Obstet. Gynec. **113**; 1046, 1972.

46. TAYLOR, E.S., HOLMES, J.H., THOMPSON, H.E. and GOTTESFELD, K.R.: Ultrasound diagnostic techniques in obstetrics and gynecology. Amer. J. Obstet. Gynec. **90**; 655, 1964.

47. THOMPSON, H.E., HOLMES, J.H., GOTTESFELD, K.R. and TAYLOR, E.S.: Fetal development as determined by ultrasonic pulse scho techniques. Amer. J. Obstet. Gynec. **92**; 44, 1965.

48. VARMA, T.R.: Prediction of delivery date by ultrasound cephalometry. J. Obstet. Gynaec. Brit. Cwlth. **80**; 316, 1973.

49. VARMA, T. R.: Fetal growth and placental function in patients with placenta praevia. J. Obstet. Gynaec. Brit. Cwlth. **80**; 311, 1973.

50. WILLOCKS, J.: The use of ultrasonic cephalometry. Proc. Roy. Soc. Med. **55**; 640, 1962.

51. WILLOCKS, J., DONALD, I., DUGGAN, T. C. and DAY, N.: Foetal cephalometry by ultrasound. J. Obstet. Gynaec. Brit. Cwlth. **71**; 11, 1964.

52. WILLOCKS, J., DONALD, I., CAMPBELL, S. and DUNSMORE, I. R.: Intrauterine growth assessed by ultrasonic foetal cephalometry. J. Obstet. Gynaec. Brit. Cwlth. **74**; 639, 1967.

53. DONALD, I.: Diagnostic ultrasonic echo sounding in obstetrics and gynaecology. Transactions of the College of Physicians, Surgeons and Gynaecologists of South Africa. **11**; 61, 1967.

54. CAMPBELL, S. and KOHORN, E. I.: Placental localization by ultrasonic compound scanning. J. Obstet. Gynaec. Brit. Cwlth. **75**; 1007, 1968.

55. CAMPBELL, S. and DEWHURST, C. J.: Quintuplet pregnancy diagnosed and assessed by ultrasonic compound scanning. Lancet **1**; 101, 1970.

56. CAMPBELL, S., WLADIMIROFF, J. W. and DEWHURST, C. J.: The antenatal measurement of fetal urine production. J. Obstet. Gynaec. Brit. Cwlth. **80**; 680, 1973.

57. SCHIFFER, M. A., ERTEL, N. H., HELLMAN, L. M. and KOBAYASHI, M.: Combined method for evaluating fetal well-being by plasma estriol measurements and ultrasonography. Am. J. Obstet. Gynec. **108**; 1277, 1970.

58. HAMILTON, L. A., SZUJEWSKI, P. F. and PATEL, M. K.: Combined sonographic and biochemical estimation of fetal maturity in high-risk pregnancy. Obstet. Gynec. **41**; 837, 1973.

59. GOTTESFELD, K. R., THOMPSON, H. E., HOLMES, J. H. and TAYLOR, E. S.: Ultrasonic placentography—a new method for placental localization. Amer. J. Obstet. Gynec. **96**; 538, 1966.

60. KOBAYASHI, M., HELLMAN, L. M. and FILLISTI, L.: Placental localization by ultrasound. Amer. J. Obstet. Gynec. **106**; 279, 1970.

61. KOBAYASHI, M., HELLMAN, L. M. and CROMB, E.: Atlas of Ultrasonography in Obstetrics and Gynecology. Appleton-Centry-Crofts, New York, 1972.

62. KOBAYASHI, M.: Illustrated Manual of Ultrasonography in Obstetrics and Gynecology. Igaku Shoin, Tokyo, 1974.

63. KOHORN, E. I., SECKER WALKER, R. H., MORRISON, J. and CAMPBELL, S.: Placental localization. Amer. J. Obstet. Gynec. **103**; 868, 1969.

64. MISKIN, M., DORAN, T. A., RUDD, N., GARDNER, H. A., LIEDGREN, S. and BENZIE, R.: Use of ultrasound for placental localizaion in genetic amniocentesis. Obstet. Gynec. **43**; 872, 1974.

65. RAMPONE, J.F., SANDERS, R.C. and NIEBYL, J.R.: Ultrasonic aspiration transducer for management of Rh incompatibility. Obstet. Gynec. **43**; 780, 1974.

66. ROBINSON, D.E., GARRETT, W.J. and KOSSOFF, G.: Ultrasonic echoscopy in clinical obstetrics and gynaecology. C.A.L. report No. 40. Commonwealth Acoustic Laboratories, Sydney, 1967.

67. SCHEER, K.: Ultrasonic diagnosis of placenta previa. Obstet. Gynec. **42**; 707, 1973.

68. TUTERA, G. and NEWMAN, R.L.: Placental localization and diagnosis of antepartal hemorrhage by ultrasonography. Obstet. Gynec. **42**; 684, 1973.

69. ADULLA, U., CAMPBELL, S., DEWHURST, C.M., TAILBERT, D., LUCAS, M. and MULLARKEY, M.: Effect of diagnostic ultrasound on maternal and fetal chromosomes. Lancet **2**; 829, 1971.

70. BOBROW, M., BLACKWELL, N., UNRAU, A.E. and BLEANEY, B.: Absence of any observed effect of ultrasonic irradiation on human chromosomes. J. Obstet. Gynaec. Brit. Cwlth. **78**; 730,1971.

71. BOYD, E., ABDULLA, U., DONALD, I., FLEMING, J.E.E., HALL, A.J. and FERGUSON-SMITH, M.A.: Chromosome breakage and ultrasound. Brit. Med. J. May 29, 501, 1971.

72. COAKLEY, W.T., HUGHES, D.E., SLADE, J.S. and LAURENCE, K.M.: Chromosome aberrations after exposure to ultrasound. Brit. Med. J. January 9, 109, 1971.

73. HELLMAN, L.M., DUFFUS, G.M., DONALD, I. and SUNDEN, B.: Safety of diagnostic ultrasound in obstetrics. Lancet **1**; 1133, 1970.

74. LOCH, E.G., FISCHER, A.B. and KUWERT, E.: Effect of diagnostic and therapeutic intensities of ultrasonics on normal and malignant human cells in vitro. Amer. J. Obstet. Gynec. **110**; 457, 1971.

75. MCCLAIN, R.M., HOAR, R.M. and SALTZMAN, M.B.: Teratologic study of rats exposed to ultrasound. Amer. J. Obstet. Gynec. **114**; 39, 1972.

76. MERMUT, S., KATAYAMA, K.P., CASTILLO, R.D. and JONES, H.W.: The effect of ultrasound in human chromosomes in vitro. Obstet. Gynec. **41**; 4, 1973.

77. ROBINSON, H.P., SHARP, F., DONALD, I., YOUNG, H. and HALL, A.J.: The effect of pulsed and continuous wave ultrasound on the enzyme histochemistry of placental tissue in vitro. J. Obstet. Gynaec. Brit. Cwlth. **79**; 821, 1972.

78. SMYTH, M.G.: Animal toxicity studies with ultrasound at diagnostic power levels. In: Diagnostic Ultrasound. Grossman, C.C., Holmes, J.H., Joyner, C. and Purnell, E.W. (eds.) Plenum Press, New York, 1966. p. 296.

79. SUNDEN, B.: On the diagnostic value of ultrasound in obstetrics and gynaecology. Acta Obstet. Gynec. Scan. **43**; Suppl. 6, 1964.

80. WATTS, P.L. and STEWARDT, C.R.: The effect of fetal heart monitoring by ultrasound on maternal and fetal chromosomes. J. Obstet. Gynaec. Brit. Cwlth. **79**; 715, 1972.

81. BANG, J. and NORTHEVED, A.: A new ultrasonic method for transabdominal amniocentesis. Amer. J. Obstet. Gynec. **114**; 599, 1972.

82. HELLMAN, L.M., KOBAYASHI, M., TOLLES, W.E. and CROMB, E.: Ultrasonic studies on the volumetric growth of the human placenta. Amer. J. Obstet. Gynec. **108**; 740, 1970.

83. MORRISON, J., KOHORN, E.I. and BLACKWELL, R.J.: Ultrasonic scanning in obstetrics. 4. The diagnosis of multiple pregnancy. Aust. N.Z. J. Obstet. Gynaec. **10;** 4, 1970.

84. GARRETT, W.J., KOSSOFF, G. and ROBINSON, D.E.: Ultrasonic echoscopic examination in late pregnancy. Obstet. Gynec. **28;** 164, 1966.

85. GARRETT, W.J. and ROBINSON, D.E.: Ultrasound in Clinical Obstetrics. Charles C Thomas, Springfield, Ill., 1970.

86. GARRETT, W.J. and ROBINSON, D.E.: Fetal heart size measured in vivo by ultrasound. Pediatrics **46;** 25, 1970.

87. SUZUKI, K., MINEI, L.J. and SCHNITZER, L.E.: Ultrasonographic measurement of fetal heart volume for estimation of birthweight. Obstet. Gynec. **43;** 867, 1974.

88. GARRETT, W.J., GRUNWALD, G. and ROBINSON, D.E.: Prenatal diagnosis of fetal polycystic kidney by ultrasound. Aust. N.Z. J. Obstet. Gynaec. **10;** 7, 1970.

89. MICHELL, R.C. and BRADLEY-WATSON, P.J.: The detection of fetal meningocoele by ultrasound B scan. J. Obstet. Gynaec. Brit. Cwlth. **80;** 1100, 1973.

90. HOULTON, M.C.C., SUTTON, M. and AITKEN, J.: Antenatal diagnosis of duodenal atresia. J. Obstet. Gynaec. Brit. Cwlth. **81;** 818, 1974.

91. THOMPSON, H.E.: Clinical use of pulsed echo ultrasound in obstetrics and gynecology. Obstet. Gynec. Survey **23;** 903, 1968.

92. THOMPSON, H.E.: Ultrasonic diagnostic techniques. In: Davies' Gynecology and Obstetrics. III, 26N:1, 1974, Harper and Row, New York.

93. GOTTESFELD, K.R.: The practical application of ultrasound in obstetrics and gynecology. In: Diagnostic Ultrasound. Grossman, C.C., Holmes, J.H., Joyner, C. and Purnell, E.W. (eds.) Plenum Press, New York, 1966, p. 428.

Prenatal diagnosis with amniotic fluid

Taiso TSUCHIMOTO, M.D.* and Erika M. BÜHLER, M.D.

Department of Genetics, Basle University Children's Hospital, Basle

INTRODUCTION

Early studies of amniotic fluid cells were directed mainly at sexing of the fetus, where X-linked disorders were suspected. In the mid-1950's several groups independently reported the accurate prediction of the sex of the fetus by X-chromatin analysis of uncultured amniotic fluid cells [1–5]. It was middle 1960's, however, when needle aspiration of fluid from the amnotic cavity (amniocentesis) first gained widespread acceptance for the management of Rh incompatibility [6, 7]. Maternal and fetal morbidity and mortality were reported to be minimal when this procedure was used after the 28th week of gestation to follow the level of bilirubin-like pigments in the amniotic fluid of erythroblastic fetuses [8, 9].

Within the past several years, advances in cell culture techniques have permitted the growth of amniotic fluid cells [10–12], obtained as early as the 12th week of gestation, in sufficient quantity such that both chromosome studies of the fetus and an increasing number of chemical and enzymatic assays could be done to diagnose antenatally a wide range of genetic diseases [12–18]. Since selective abortion of an affected fetus is now possible in many countries, development of these methods has become a very useful adjunct in genetic counseling.

Prenatal diagnosis using amniotic fluid has been performed in Basle University Children's Hospital since 1971. In this chapter, we will briefly review our experience in this field and discuss usefulness and problems of the procedure in prenatal detection of genetic disorders.

INDICATIONS FOR AMNIOCENTESIS

Amniocentesis for purposes of genetic counseling is recommended to those who are at risk of bearing a child with genetic defects. Indications for the procedure are (Tables 1 and 2):

1) **Chromosomal Disorders**
   a. High Risk Group: One parent is a carrier of a chromosomal translocation (G/G, D/G, or reciprocal); A woman with trisomy 21.

---

* *Present Adress:* Sandoz LTD, Medical and Biological Research Division, 4002 Basle, Switzerland.

Table 1 Indications for prenatal diagnosis.

1. Chromosome disorders:
   Chromosomal translocation carrier
   Maternal trisomy 21
   Previous child with a chromosomal aberration
   Advanced maternal age
2. X-linked disorders:
   Maternal heterozygotes
3. Metabolic disorders:
   Both parents heterozygous for the same autosomal recessive disorders
4. Neural-tube defects:
   Open defects of the neural-tube such as anencephaly and spina bifida

Table 2 Risks of chromosomal disorders.

Indications	Risks (%)
1. Translocation carrier	
D/G (13/21)	
Male	3.7
Female	8.6
G/G	
21/21	100
21/22	5.6
D/D (13–15/13–15)	less than 1
Reciprocal	33
2. Maternal trisomy 21	50
3. Preivous child with Down's syndrome	1.6(?)
4. Advanced maternal age	
35–39	0.2–0.5
40–44	0.5–1.0
45–49	1–2

b. Moderate Risk Group: Women over 40 years of age, where the risk of Down's syndrome alone is 0.5–1 per cent and 1–2 per cent at the ages of 40–44 and 45–49, respectively [18–22]. Women who have previously borne a child with Down's syndrome [19, 23, 24].

c. Low Risk Group: Women over 35 years of age in whom the risk of chromosomal disorder is 0.2–0.5 per cent [18–22].

2) **X-linked Disorders**

Known maternal carriers of X-linked diseases such as hemophilia and Duchenne muscular dystrophy, in which the risk is 25 per cent.

3) **Metabolic Disorders**

Both parents heterozygous for an autosomal recessive disorder which is prenatally detectable. The risk is 25 per cent.

4) **Neural-tube Defects**

Most of our material has been obtained at Basle University Women's Hospital, where transabdominal amniocentesis is generally performed as an outpatient procedure [25], mainly at between 15th and 18th week of gestation. Puncture is made routinely under observation with ultrasound to estimate the size of the uterus, the amount of the amniotic fluid, fetal position and the location of the placenta and the needle. The uterus is palpated bimanually to locate its position, then the lower abdominal wall, anterior to the uterus, is cleansed with an antiseptic solution. Local anesthetic is injected over the site to be punctured. During manual elevation of the uterus from below, a No. 22 stylet needle is introduced into the amniotic cavity and 10–20 ml of yellowish transparent, occasionally somewhat cloudy and/or hemorrhagic, fluid is withdrawn. This fluid is immediately brought to our laboratory, usually within two hours after the puncture. At the time of amniocentesis chromosome preparations using peripheral blood are made from the couple involved and kept.

HANDLING OF THE AMNIOTIC FLUID

The amniotic fluid thus obtained is placed in a siliconized sterile tube and centrifuged at 150 g for 5 minutes. The supernatant is used for *alpha*-fetoprotein assays in every case [25], and may also be used for other examinations [27–31].

AMNIOTIC FLUID CELL CULTURE AND RESULTS

The pellet of cells obtained by centrifuging the amniotic fluid is resuspended in 2 ml of F-10 medium (Difco) supplemented with 20% fetal calf serum and antibiotics, and cultivated by a method modified from CONSCIENCE et al [32]. The suspended cells are layered in one to three Leighton tubes containing a coverglass on the flat surface. This glassware is sterilized before use. The cells are then incubated at 37 °C in 5% CO_2 atmosphere with medium changes generally being required every three or four days, depending on pH of the medium and the rate of cell proliferation. At the time of the first medium change cells obtained from the waste medium are processed for Y-chromatin examinations.

The cultured cells grow in monolayer. Actually, the cultures may consist entirely of fibroblastoid, epithelioid or pleomorphic cells, or may be mixtures of these types. In general, within two to four weeks after initiation of culturing, the cells have grown to confluence up to one-third or one-half of the surface of the coverglass and may be harvested for cytogenetic examinations and/or subcultured. The cells are trypsinized for subculturing and are treated as typical monolayer cultures. The cultured cells are used for chromosome examinations [32], analyses of sex chromations [33], biochemical and enzymatic assays [34–36], histochemical [37], ultrastructural [38] and autoradiographic studies [37].

When the number of mitotic cells increases—most frequently seen 18–24 hours after medium change—the culture may be processed for chromosome preparation following five hours' treatment with Colcemid (Ciba, 1 μg/ml). The coverglass is transferred from the Leighton tube to a Petri dish. 4 ml of 0.17% NaCl solution (37 °C) is added slowly along the side of the dish which is then incubated at 37 °C for 20 minutes. The hypotonic solution is slowly removed and replaced by drop-wise addition of acetic acid/methanol fixative; 1 : 3 v/v. The cells are allowed to stand for one to two hours; the fixative is removed, and the coverglass is dried at room temperature. This preparation is stained with Giemsa and mounted on a slide-glass. The same preparation is destained after karyotypic analyses, then stained with quinacrine dihydrochloride.

A total of 77 amniocenteses were carried out in 67 cases in our study (Table 3): 63 were at risk of chromosomal aberrations. Two were an obligate and another a possible carrier

Table 3   Disorders at risk.

Disorders	No. of Cases
Chromosomal	63
X-linked	3
Metabolic	1
Neural-tube defects	0

of Duchenne muscular dystrophy. The remaining case was at risk of an inborn error of metabolism. Of 63 women carrying fetuses at risk of chromosome disorders, three were translocation carriers; two of these had previously born a child with Down's syndrome or trisomy 13, one of whom was also of advanced maternal age. 32 of the 63 were of advanced maternal age over 35, and one was of advanced age and had a previous child with Down's syndrome; another group of 18 had already had a child with Down's syndrome or another autosomal trisomy. The other 10 cases had questionable indications such as history of repeated spontaneous abortions and a previous child with multiple malformations.

Amniotic fluid cells were successfully cultivated and chromosome diagnoses were made from the initial samples in 54 cases. A repeated tap was made in 6 out of 13 cases in which cell growth was poor; in one case a third tap was necessary. In one instance, the woman was known to be a carrier of X-linked muscular dystrophy. Because the growth of amniotic fluid cell culture was slow in this case, the cells were processed for fetal sex determination using X and Y chromatin staining. The interval between the tap and chromosome diagnosis was 2–3 weeks.

47 women out of 67 studied have terminated the pregnancies. The outcome was: 38 normal full-term births, three premature birth, one still-birth at 24th week of gestation, and one therapeutic and four spontaneous abortions. Two out of the four women who developed spontaneous abortions had a previous history of repeated abortions, while the third woman had a hydatidiform mole. Amniocentesis was performed in the fourth women at 11th week of pregnancy because of advanced age. All of these four abortions occurred 3–6 weeks after the puncture.

CHROMOSOMAL DISORDERS

To date, detection of fetal chromosomal abnormality represents the main application of intrauterine diagnosis, although this pattern is changing in some countries where neural-tube defects have been more frequently screened recently for [39, 40]. Since the first report of STEELE and BREG of successful culturing and karyotypic analysis of amniotic fluid cells [10], cytogenetic studies of cultured amniotic fluid cells have become an established and practical diagnostic method for prenatal sex determination and detection of fetal chromosomal errors [12, 17, 41–53]. So far antenatal detection of various fetal chromosomal conditions have been reported, e.g., balanced and unbalanced translocations [12, 44, 47–49], Down's syndrome [17, 41, 42], other autosomal trisomies [43–45, 50–53], and sex chromosome abnormalities [42, 46, 49, 52].

63 cases in the present series were studied for fetal chromosomal disorders as shown in Table 3. One case was detected to have trisomy 21 *in utero*, which was later confirmed by the examination of the therapeutically aborted fetus. In three cases one parent was a balanced D/D translocation carrier. Chromosome analysis of cultivated amniotic fluid

cells disclosed D/D translocation, presumably balanced, in two of these three cases; the outcome was the delivery of a healthy child with balanced D/D in both cases. In another instance, both parents had relatives with Down's syndrome, and fetal karyotype obtained at the 17th week of gestation revealed 46, XX, +F, −G [54]. Down's syndrome with G/G translocation was first suspected in the fetus, however chromosome banding methods demonstrated one of the F group chromosome to be one of the No. 22 chromosomes with prominent satellites. Maternal lymphocyte metaphases showed a similar chromosome No. 22. As there was no evidence that the fetus was abnormal, the parents elected to continue the pregnancy; the mother was delivered of an apparently healthy girl at full term. In two further cases, fetal karyotypes showed enlarged satellites on one of the D chromosomes; the outcome was deliveries of healthy children. There was one case in which one out of 22 cells analyzed had a ring chromosome, and the woman delivered a healthy full-term child.

X-LINKED DISORDERS

Prenatal sex determination has been accurately made in majority of reported cases by means of karyotypic analyses of cultivated amniotic fluid cells [46, 48]. In our study the predicted sex was correct in all 41 cases in which a child included in the present study has already been born. In one case fetal karyotype showed apparent 46, XY but without intense quinacrine fluorescence in any of five small acrocentric choromosomes. A rare possibility of 46, XO, +G was excluded since the father also lacked intense Q-fluorescence in his Y chromosome (Fig. 1).

It is possible to identify the sex of the fetuses in women heterozygous for X-linked di-

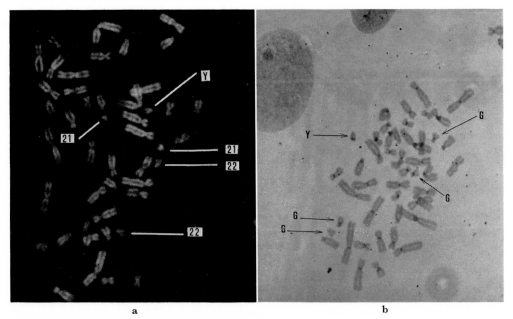

a   b

Fig. 1 Quinacrine staining did not show intense fluorescence of the Y chromosome (a), while C-banding demonstrated the Y (b).

seases. However, only 50 per cent of the male fetuses will be affected by the disease in question, and cytogenetics alone can not be used to distinguish between the affected and non-affected. This renders the decision to abort difficult. As yet hemophilia and Duchenne muscular dystrophy, two of the more common X-linked disorders, have not yet been specifically detected *in utero*. There are, however, less common X-linked metabolic disorders such as Lesch-Nyhan, Fabry's disease and Hunter's syndrome which can now be specifically diagnosed prenatally [37, 55–57].

We observed three cases at risk of X-linked disorders: two with hemophilia A and one with Duchenne muscular dystrophy. Prenatal sexing disclosed one of each sex in the former and a female in the latter. All these pregnancies were continued and the outcome was in agreement with the prediction. The female child whose mother was an obligate heterozygote for Duchenne muscular dystrophy started developing symptoms at the age of two which were indistinguishable from those seen in X-linked Duchenne muscular dystrophy.

METABOLIC DISORDERS

Introduction of biochemical and enzymatic analyses to amniocentesis has greatly extended its value as a method of intrauterine diagnosis; the list of indications has grown rapidly. Not only the X-linked disorders described above, but also many other autosomal recessive disorders can now be diagnosed prenatally by assays of specific enzymes or chemical constituents in the cell-free amniotic fluid [30, 31] and cultured and uncultured amniotic fluid cells [13–17, 31, 58–64]. Studies of absent or diminished enzyme activity or excess storage material have been done extensively on cultivated skin fibroblasts derived from individuals with various inborn errors of metabolism as well as from normal controls [65], upon which biochemical and enzymatic studies in prenatal diagnosis using amniotic fluid cells are mainly based. Differences have been observed between activities of certain enzymes in skin fibroblasts as compared to those in cultivated amniotic fluid cells [66].

Among other biochemical disorders detected prenatally are: Gaucher's disease [62]; Globoid cell leukocystrophy (Krabbe's disease) [64]; GM_1-gangliosidosis, type 1 [63]; GM_2-gangliosidosis, type 1 and 2 (Tay-Sachs disease and Sandhoff's disease, respectively) [31, 61, 67]; Metachromatic leukodystrophy [17]; Niemann-Pick disease [60]; Hurler's syndrome [37, 68]; Sanfilipo syndrome A [69]; Cystinosis [70]; Maple-syrup-urine disease [71]; Methylmalonic aciduria [30, 72]; Galactosemia [13, 73]; Glycogen-storage disease, type II (Pompe's disease) [15, 59]; Lysosomal acid phosphatase deficiency [17]; and Xeroderma pigmentosum [74].

We had a case of obligate heterozygote parents for cystinosis. Cultured amniotic fluid cells were sent to Dr. J. A. SCHNEIDER, University of California. The uptake amount of ^{35}S-cystine by these cells showed that the fetus was either healthy or heterozygous for cystinosis. A female child was born as predicted at full term, and she has so far been healthy.

NEURAL-TUBE DEFECTS

The association between neural-tube defects and high *alpha*-fetoprotein levels in the amniotic fluid has been well established [25, 75]. Since technical problems involved in the assay of this protein and false positives are minimal, neural-tube defects such as anencephaly and spina bifida have become the main indication for prenatal diagnosis in Great Britain [39, 40].

Until the present day we have had neither cases which were specifically indicated for these disorders, nor affected fetuses with neural-tube defects found *in utero*, yet *alpha-fetoprotein* levels in the amniotic fluid have been routinely determined in every case where amniocentesis has been done.

COMMENTS

1) AMNIOCENTESIS

Transabdominal amniocentesis appears to be a reasonably safe procedure after the 20th week of gestation to control Rh incompatibility; maternal and fetal complications reported are very low [8, 9]. Major maternal morbidity includes hemorrhage [76]. Fetal death or abortion has been observed following abruptio placentae, amnionitis and fetal hemorrhage [76, 77], but the risk is less than 1 per cent [8, 9, 76–78]. Puncture of the fetus has occurred in a few cases [9, 79, 80]. The risk of the procedure may also be very low when it is performed in early mid-trimester. GERBIE et al. [81] found no evidence of increased maternal or fetal complications among 408 women in whom the procedure was performed during the second trimester of pregnancy. Studies done by MILUNSKY and ATKINS [82] disclosed similar results. In our series of 67 cases on which 77 amniocenteses were carried out, four spontaneous abortions occurred between 3 and 6 weeks after the puncture. Except for one case we have not been able to demonstrate the direct correlation between the tap and abortions, since two of these abortions occurred in women who had had previous history of repeated abortions and another who had hydatidiform mole.

Amniocentesis may well be safe to both mothers and fetuses, yet, considering fetal and uterine size and the amount of the amniotic fluid present [83, 84], the procedure may still be too hazardous to the fetus before the 13th week of gestation. The number of viable amniotic fluid cells is too small for culturing and subsequent harvesting in time before the 12th week of pregnancy, but increased steadily with advancing pregnancy from the 12–15th week up to the 20th gestational week [85, 86]. In view of these factors, i.e., number of viable cells, time necessary for cell culturing, and optimal timing of possible therapeutic abortions, the most advantageous moment for amniocentesis appears to be between the 15th and 18th week of gestation.

Although immediate risk to both mother and fetus has been claimed very low by a few groups, experience with amniocentesis as a prenatal diagnostic tool is still limited. Long-term follow-up of children who were exposed to this procedure during the fetal life is justified to detect any possible late-effects of the tap. We collect and keep the data concerning personal history of the mother and child involved, physical examination up to several years after birth and results of prenatal evaluation. Until safety of the procedure is proven, amniocentesis should be limited to use in women who have higher risks of bearing a child with a detectable disorder or who have moderate or low risks of chromosomal disorders but strong anxiety of having an affected child.

2) AMNIOTIC FLUID CELLS

The exact origin of the amniotic fluid being yet unknown, amniotic fluid cells are of fetal origin and derived from fetal skin, buccal mucosa, vagina, urinary and respiratory tracts, and amnion [87–92]. When cultivated, the cells transform into fibroblastoid or epithelioid cells, or into more pleomorphic cells [93].

A number of variations of the technique of amniotic fluid cell culturing have appeared in the literatures [10–13, 32, 44, 85, 94–103]. The basic principle, however, is to grow the cells to confluence, or close to it, as rapidly as possible, since induced abortion becomes more complex with advancing pregnancy. The average reported interval between amnio-centesis and chromosome diagnosis is one to two weeks [17, 85, 95, 97, 98, 102, 103]. Culti-vation of amniotic fluid cells which are several days old may be successful [104], thus allowing the shipment of samples to tissue culture laboratories.

3) CHROMOSOME DISORDERS

When the risk of amniocentesis has been confirmed as negligible to both the fetus and mother, amniocentesis could be recommended to all pregnant women over 35 years old, since the risk of Down's syndrome as well as of other chromosomal abnormalities increases with advancing maternal age [20, 105–108]. Such a "screening" may prenatally identify about half of those afflicted with Down's syndrome [23]. Since the opportunity for thera-peutic abortions is available in a number of countries, a sizeable saving of both institutional costs and emotional burden to parents may be achieved. MILUNSKY et al. [105] further suggested that this procedure might, in the future, be offered to all pregnant women, as serious chromosomal disorders occur with a frequency of one in 200 live births [106]. However, such wide-spread routine use of amniocentesis will be dependent on the number of qualified and experienced laboratories available to process the samples, and the number of cases capable of being handled in each laboratory. At present, such a screening ap-proach appears to be far from being practical [107].

Evidence has been presented that women who have born one child with Down's syndrome have a higher risk of this disorder occurring in a later child [19, 23, 24, 109], although the exact figure has not yet been calculated. In the report by LITTLEFIELD et al. [110], three fetuses with trisomy 21 were found among 182 pregnancies (1.6%, compared to 0.11–0.19% in overall live births [23]) in women who had previously had a child with the same disorder. Moreover, such individuals have a strong anxiety whether they might have another similarly affected child. Therefore, previous delivery of a child with Down's syndrome seems justified to be an added indication for amniocentesis.

There are certain pitfalls in prenatal chromosome diagnosis. The possibility of sampling only one amniotic sac in cases of multiple pregnancies may lead to an erroneous interpre-tation of the findings [111, 112]. Ultrasonic scanning or fetal ECG should be routinely used prior to puncture, and, in the event of twins, two taps may be made with the aid of a compound contact scanner with storage oscilloscope or a linear waterbath sector scanner [113].

In utero detection of fetal chromosomal mosaicism has been reported, yet this chromosome condition may provide another problem in prenatal diagnosis [114–117]. In one reported case the first amniotic fluid sample showed 45, XO [114]. The fetus was therapeutically aborted, and a postmortem examination disclosed a phenotypically normal male with normal testicular tissue. The second amniotic fluid specimen obtained at the time of abortion revealed 46,XY. Although they considered that the fetus might have had two cell lines, it was not confirmed. Mosaicism probably occurring *in vitro* has been described for fetuses with normal chromosome complements [116–118], which suggests necessity of a careful interpretation of chromosome examination.

In our laboratory amniotic fluid cells are cultivated on a coverglass until they form several cell colonies on it. The cells are hypotonically treated and fixed *in situ*, and karyotypes are made from as many different cell colonies as possible. This procedure appears to reflect fetal chromosome condition more closely, since each of the colonies often starts from a single cell [116].

Maternal cell overgrowth in amniotic fluid cell cultures has been reported. NADLER and GERBIE [17] suggested that maternal cell contamination must be suspected when rapid cell growth occurred within a few days after initiation of culturing, and that chromosome analyses should be carried out in at least two cultures at different stages of cultivation in order to prevent a misdiagnosis. Others described successful fetal karyotypic analyses using uncultivated amniotic fluid cells [119–121], thus avoiding a possible contamination with maternal cell mitoses. However, the reliability of uncultured cells for karyotypic analyses is still questionable [71, 122].

Occasional appearance of tetraploid cells in amniotic fluid cell cultures [117, 123, 124] may be partly due to an artifact of *in vitro* culture conditions and partly due to the presence of cells which are derived from the amnion, an organ in which tetraploidy is common [125]. Tetraploidy has been noted in abortuses [126, 127], but very few cases have been recorded in the literature as having had tetraploid/diploid or triple mosaicism and multiple malformations [128–130]. The occurrence of polyploidy in cultured amniotic fluid cells has so far been consistent with the birth of a healthy child with a normal karyotype [117, 123, 124], and the appearance of such cells in culture should not be a reason for terminating a pregnancy.

Variant chromosomes may provide another problem [54, 131]. Acrocentric chromosomes with enlarged satellites can be misdiagnosed as D/G or G/G translocations. In such cases chromosome banding methods are of particular value [54, 131].

MACINTYRE [132] reported two patients who had congenital malformations and reciprocal translocations of autosomes. The father and two sibs in the first patient and the mother in the second, all of whom were phenotypically normal, had karyotypes which were morphologically indistinguishable from those of the respective patients. These cases, especially the first, indicate the care which must be taken in interpreting inherited fetal reciprocal translocations.

4) X-LINKED DISORDERS

The reliability of sex prediction by means of sex chromatin examination of uncultured cells is still open to question [71, 131, 133]. Should sex chromatin analyses be used for fetal sexing due to poor cell growth, both X- and Y-chromatin must be examined. However, X-chromatin examination of amniotic fluid cells is often of little practical value because of technical reasons [71, 131]. When Y-chromatin alone is used, the interpretation may be erroneous in cases of abnormal sex chromosome constitutions such as 45,XO and 47,XXY, and delection of Y long arm [134]. In addition, certain autosomes may have brightly fluorescing segments after quinacrine staining [134], which, in interphase nuclei, may be interpreted as Y-chromatin. Thus, karyotypic analyses of cultured amniotic fluid cells are currently considered to be the most convincing way of predicting fetal sex. Great care should be taken in cases of multiple pregnancies and maternal cell overgrowth in culture as previously mentioned.

Hemophilia and Duchenne muscular dystrophy, which are more common X-linked disorders, can not be specifically diagnosed *in utero*. Comparable coagulation factor VIII (AHG)-like activity has been found in cultured skin fibroblasts from both hemophilia and normal individuals [135, 136] and in amniotic fluid cells [110] which was equally active in both normal and hemophiliac cells. Hemophiliac fetuses are unlikely to be distinguishable from the normal using this criterion.

The genetic loci for hemophilia A and glucose-6-phosphate dehydrogenase (G6PD) are known to be closely linked to each other on the X chromosome; and the chance is lower than 4 per cent that a cross-over between these two loci will occur [137]. When a woman is heterozygous for both G6PD A and B, and hemophilia A genes, and when she has already born a hemophiliac son, prenatal detection of a hemizygote and heterozygote of hemophilia A can be made with a high probability by examining G6PD pattern of the affected son and of amniotic fluid cells [138]. A similar approach can be applied to autosomal dominant myotonic dystrophy whose gene locus is closely linked to that for secretor status [139]. The secretor status of a fetus can be determined by examination of the amniotic fluid [140, 141]. Such procedures may become more valuable as more informations concerning more number of gene loci become available.

Muscular dystrophy, presumably autosomal recessive, has been described in the literature [142], the clinical picture of which is similar to Duchenne muscular dystrophy. We had one such case occurring in a female child, and this suggested a need for careful history taking for this X-linked disorder.

5) METABOLIC DISORDERS

Intrauterine diagnosis of metabolic disorders is one of the most promising areas, witthess the growing list of such conditions detectable by amniocentesis. Until now about 60 inherited metabolic disorders are potentially diagnosable *in utero* [131]. To this approach, enzymatic activities or metabolic functions in question must be expressed in the amniotic fluid or in its cultivated or uncultivated cells.

A few cases of adrenocortical hyperplasia have been predicted prenatally by determining the levels of 17-ketosteroids and pregnanetriol in the amniotic fluid at term or of estriol in maternal urine [143–146]. However, these diagnostic methods are presently considered of no value in the prenatal diagnosis of adrenogenital syndrome [71]. Cultivated fibroblasts from patients with cystic fibrosis contained metachromatic granules when stained with toluidine blue O [147], so that detection of this disease *in utero* seemed feasible, although this later turned out to be unreliable [148].

Direct analyses of various enzymes and biochemical constituents of the amniotic fluid and uncultured cells have been done, which will avoid problems of and time necessary for cell culturing and may facilitate a rapid diagnosis [149–151]. However, the value of using the amniotic fluid and uncultivated cells in diagnosing metabolic disorders remains open to question: the number of cells available on each tap may be insufficient for precise assays; or the fluid may be contaminated with maternal blood or enzymes of undetermined origin [151]. Cultivated cells are considered more appropriate toward this end.

There are several limitations and problems in prenatal diagnosis of metabolic disorders by means of cultivated amniotic fluid cells. A few prerequisites must be established before considering the prenatal diagnosis of a metabolic diseases [66].

1)   The enzymatic deficiency or metabolic defects in question must be clearly demonstrable in skin fibroblasts from affected individuals. This prerequisite would eliminate certain disorders in which defects are localized in specific organs such as von Gierke's disease and phenylketonuria.

2)   Heterozygotes must be clearly differentiated from homozygotes.

3)   The enzyme activity or metabolic function in question must be quantitatively assessed in cells grown from normal amniotic fluid samples obtained during early mid-gestation. Certain enzymes may be undetectable or have very low activities in cultured normal amniotic fluid cells, although they are clearly demonstrable in skin fibroblasts [152]. Other enzymes may have activities which vary according

to the phase of gestation [66].

4) Normal range of specific activities of enzymes must be established in normal fetal tissues obtained at 18–24 weeks of gestation. When positive intrauterine diagnoses are established and pregnancies are interrupted, corroboration of amniotic fluid cell fiindings must be made with aborted fetal tissues.

It has been noticed that different types of amniotic fluid cells in culture may have different enzyme activities [153, 154], and detection of certain fetal metabolic disorders requires cultured cell of the appropriate type. Enzyme activity may vary according to the degree of cell confluency [155, 156], length of culture time [156] and the stage of the cell growth cycle in culture [155–160]. Variable concentrations of nutrients in the culture medium may lead to changes in enzyme activities [159]. Mycoplasma contamination, even if not apparent, may alter biochemical functions [161] as well as chromosomal structure of the cells. Enzymatic properties may also be affected by viral transformation of the cells. All of these factors taken together suggest the complexity of interpreting enzyme assay results, and indicate that better understanding of the numerous biochemical and culture conditions is required. Furthermore, the range of normal values for each enzyme and chemical in the cultured amniotic fluid cells obtained at different stages of gestation must be established along with standardization of assay methods and cell culture techniques. It is anticipated that automated analysis system may be introduced in the future to perform multiple simultaneous analyses of enzyme and biochemical costituents and concentrations of many metabolites from a small aliquot of cells.

Heterozygous carriers are usually asymptomatic and are generally indentified only after the delivery of an affected child. However, methods for the detection of heterozygotes of several inborn errors of metabolism have recently been developed using direct measurement of gene products such as enzyme activities in blood cells, skin fibroblasts, serum, urine or other tissue samples as well as amniotic fluid cells [162–164]. When carrier screening of a large scale becomes simple and reliable, intrauterine detection of homozygotes will be feasible, thus offering the possibility of preventing the tragedy of having an affected child.

6) OTHERS

In the cases of neural-tube defects, *alpha*-fetoprotein enters the amniotic fluid probably by leakage of cerebrospinal fluid through the exposed neural tissue. Recently, it was shown that the level of this protein was raised in both the amniotic fluid [25, 75] and maternal serum [165, 166] in cases where the fetus had spina bifida or anencephaly. It will be possible, in the future, to monitor all pregnancies for these types of neural-tube defects by using maternal blood.

It is worth emphasizing that couples at risk who agree to this procedure should be informed well in advance that technical failure may occur in obtaining the fluid or in cell culturing, and that the diagnosis can never assure the birth of a normal child.

Most parents will elect interruption of pregnancies in which the fetus is known to be affected with a serious disorder; however, there is no consensus available in regard to the management of a fetus with 47, XYY for which the pathological significance is yet unknown, or where one of a twin pair found *in utero* is severely affected either chromosomally or metabolically. Some couples might choose to abort less seriously affected fetuses or those with disorders that are amenable to therapy or require extensive treatment. Prenatal diagnosis, in connection with selective abortion, has raised new types of important medical, ethical, moral, religious and legal questions.

CONCLUSION

Prenatal diagnosis based on analyses of the amniotic fluid has provided a powerful and valuable tool for genetic counseling of high risk pregnancies where cytogenetic, X-linked or metabolic disorders, or neural-tube defects are suspected. However, before this procedure can be widely accepted, transabdominal amniocentesis must be definitely shown to be without immediate or long-term risks to the fetus and mother. Clarification of the biochemical conditions of tissue culture should be sought along with standardization and, where possible, automation of the assay methods and culture techniques involved.

REFERENCES

1. SEER, D.M., SACHS, L. and DANON, M.: Diagnosis of sex before birth using cells from the amniotic fluid. Bull. Res. Council Israel 58; 137, 1955.
2. FUCHS, F. and RIIS, P.: Antenatal sex determination. Nature (London) 177; 330, 1956.
3. SHETTLES, L.B.: Nuclear morphology of cells in human amniotic fluid in relation to sex of infant. Amer. J. Obstet. Gynec. 71; 834, 1956.
4. MAKOWSKY, E.L., PREM, K.A. and KAISER, I.H.: Detection of sex of fetuses by the incidence of sex chromatin body in nuclei of cells in amniotic fluid. Science 123; 542, 1956.
5. JAMES, F.: Sexing foetuses by examination of amniotic fluid. Lancet 1; 202, 1956.
6. FREDA, V.J.: The Rh problem in obstetrics and a new concept of its management using amniocentesis and spectrophotometric scanning of amniotic fluid. Amer. J. Obstet. Gynec. 92; 341, 1965.
7. QUEENAN, J.T. and ADAMS, D.W.: Amniocentesis for prenatal diagnosis of erythroblastosis fetalis. Obstet. Gynec. 25; 302, 1965.
8. QUEENAN, J.T.: Amniocentesis and transamniotic fetal transfusion for Rh disease. Clin. Obstet. Gynec. 9; 491, 1966.
9. CREASMAN, W.T., LAWRENCE, R.A. and THIEDE, H.A.: Fetal complication of amniocentesis. J.A.M.A. 204; 949, 1968.
10. STEELE, M.W. and BREG, W.R., Jr.: Chromosome analysis of human amniotic-fluid cells. Lancet 1; 383, 1966.
11. THIEDE, H.A., CREASMAN, W.T. and METCALFE, S.: Antenatal analysis of the human chromosomes. Amer. J. Obstet. Gynec. 94; 589, 1966.
12. JACOBSON, C.B. and BARTER, R.H.: Intrauterine diagnosis and management of genetic defects. Amer. J. Obstet. Gynec. 99; 796, 1967.
13. NADLER, H.L.: Antenatal detection of hereditary disorders. Pediatrics 42; 912, 1968.
14. NADLER, H.L.: Prenatal detection of genetic defects. J. Pediat. 74; 132, 1969.
15. NADLER, H.L. and MESSINA, A.M.: In-utero detection of type II glycogenosis (Pompe's disease). Lancet 2; 1277, 1969.
16. NADLER, H.L. and EGAN, T.J.: Deficiency of lysosomal acid phosphatase. A new familial metabolic disorder. New Eng. J. Med. 282; 302, 1970.
17. NADLER, H.L. and GERBIE, A.B.: Role of amniocentesis in the intrauterine detection of genetic disorders. New Eng. J. Med. 282; 596, 1970.
18. ØSTER, J.: The causes of mongolism. Danish Med. Bull. 3; 158, 1956.
19. CARTER, C.O. and EVANS, K.A.: Risk of parents who have had one child with Down's syndrome (mongolism) having another child similarly affected. Lancet 2; 785, 1961.
20. COLLMANN, R.D. and STOLLER, A.: A survey of mongoloid births in Victoria, Australia, 1942–57. Amer. J. Public Health 52; 813, 1962.
21. STEVENSON, A.C., JOHNSTON, H.A., STEWART, M.I.P. and GOLDING, D.R.: Congenital malformations. A report of a study of series of consecutive birth in 24 centres. WHO, Geneva, 1966.

22. STENE, J.: Statistical inference on segregation ratios for D/G translocations when the families are ascertained in different ways. Ann. Hum. Genet. **34**; 95, 1970.

23. PENROSE, L.S. and SMITH, G.F.: Down's Anomaly. J. & A. Churchill, London, 1966.

24. HAMERTON, J.L., BRIGGS, S.M., GIANNELLI, F. and GARTER, C.O.: Chromosome studies in detection of parents with high risk of second child with Down's syndrome. Lancet **2**; 788, 1961.

25. BROCK, D.J.H. and SUTCLIFFE, R.G.: Alpha-fetoprotein in the antenatal diagnosis of anencephaly and spina bifida. Lancet **2**; 197, 1972.

26. HINSELMANN, M., HINDEMANN, P. and KUBLI, F.: Placental localisation by B-scan ultrasound in transabdominal amniocentesis. Ann. Obstet. Gynec. **92**; 503, 1970.

27. MARKS, J.F., BAUM, J., KAY, J.L., TAYLOR, W. and CURRY, L.: Amniotic fluid concentration of uric acid. Pediatrics **42**; 359, 1968.

28. NELSON, F.M.: Amniotic fluid phopholipid patterns in normal and abnormal pregnancies. Amer. J. Obstet. Gynec. **105**; 1072. 1969.

29. EMERY, A.E.H., BURT, D., NELSON, M.M. and SCRIMGEOUR, J.B.: Antenatal diagnosis and aminoacid composition of amniotic fluid. Lancet **1**; 1307, 1970.

30. MORROW, G., III, SCHWARTZ, R.H. and HALLOCK, J.A.: Prenatal detection of methylmalonic acidemia. J. Pediat. **77**; 120, 1970.

31. SCHNECK, L., FRIEDLAND, J., VALENTI, C., ADACHI, M., AMSTERDAM, D. and VOLK B.W.: Prenatal diagnosis of Tay-Sachs disease. Lancet **1**; 582, 1970.

32. CONSCIENCE, J.-F., SCHMID, W., GYSEL, J., STAMM, H. and SCHREINER, W.: Gewebekultur von Amnionzellen aus Fruchtwasserproben des Fruhen Schwangerschaft. Archiv Genet. **45**; 17, 1972.

33. MUKHERJEE, A.B., BLATTNER, P.Y. and NITOWSKY, H.M.: Sex-chromatin fluorescence in human amniotic-fluid cells. Lancet **2**; 709, 1971.

34. NADLER, H.L.: Patterns of enzyme development utilizing cultivated human fetal cells derived from amniotic fluid. Biochem. Genet. **2**; 119, 1968.

35. SHIH, V.E. and LITTLEFIELD, J.W.: Argininosuccinase activity in amniotic-fluid cells. Lancet **2**; 45, 1970.

36. SHIH, V.E. and SCHULMAN, J.D.: Ornithine-ketoacid transaminase activity in human skin and amniotic fluid cell culture. Clin. Chim. Acta **27**; 73, 1970.

37. FRATANTONI, J.C., NEUFELD, E.F., UHLENDORF, B.W. and JACOBSON, C.B.: Intrauterine diagnosis of the Hurler and Hunter syndromes. New Eng. J. Med. **280**; 686, 1969.

38. HUG, G., SCHUBERT, W.K. and SOUKUP, S.: Prenatal diagnosis of type-II glycogenosis. Lancet **1**; 1002, 1970.

39. LAWRENCE, K.M.: Fetal malformations and abnormalities. Lancet **2**; 939, 1974.

40. BROCK, D.J.H.: Changing pattern of antenatal diagnosis. Lancet **2**; 1077, 1974.

41. VALENTI, C., SCHUTTA, E.J. and KEHATY, T.: Prenatal diagnosis of Down's syndrome. Lancet **2**; 220, 1968.

42. GERTNER, M., HSU, L.Y.F., MARTIN, J. and HIRSCHHORN, K.: The use of amniocentesis for prenatal genetic counselling. Bull. New York Acad. Med. **46**; 916, 1970.

43. KERSEY, J.H., YUNIS, J.J., LEE, J.C. and BENDEL, R.P.: Antenatal detection of partial C (6–12) trisomy. Lancet **1**; 702, 1971.

44. MILUNSKY, A., ATKINS, L. and LITTLEFIELD, J.W.: Amniocentesis for prenatal genetic studies. Obstet. Gynec. **40**; 104, 1972.

45. HSU, L.Y., STRAUSS, L., DUBIN, E. and HIRSCHHORN, K.: Prenatal diagnosis of trisomy 18. Pathologic findings 20-week conceptus. Amer. J. Dis. Child. **125**; 290, 1973.

46. NADLER, H.L.: Indications for amniocentesis in the early prenatal detection of genetic disorders. Birth Defects: Original Article Series **7**; 5, 1971.

47. EBBINS, A.J., WILSON, M.G., TOWNER, J.W. and SLAUGHTER, J.P.: Prenatal diagnosis of an inherited translocation between chromosomes No. 9 and 18. J. Med. Genet. **10**; 65, 1973.

48. WAHLSTRÖM, J., BARTSCH, F.K. and LUNDBERG, J.: Prenatal chromosome determination. A study of 219 cases. Clin. Genet. **6**; 184, 1974.

49. LINDSTEN, J., THERKELSEN, A.J., FRIEDRICH, U., JONASSON, J., STEENSTRUP, O.R. and WIQUIST, N.: Prenatal cytogenetic diagnosis. Int. J. Gynaecol. Obstet. **12**; 101, 1974.

50. BUTLER, L.J., REISS, H.E., FRANCE, N.E. and BRIDDON, S.: Antenatal diagnosis of Patau's syndrome (trisomy 13) including a detailed pathological study of the fetus. J. Med. Genet. **10**; 367, 1973.

51. GORDON, G., SUTHERLAND, G.R., BAULD, R. and BAIN, A.D.: The antenatal diagnosis of trisom3 18. Clin. Genet. **5;** 110, 1974.

52. SCHMID, W., BÜHLER, E., WIECZOREK, V., GEISLER, M., MIKKELSEN, M. and KNÖRR-GÄRTNER, H.: Data from 520 cases of prenatal genetic diagnoses in Germany, Denmark and Switzerland. MRC Prenatal Diagnosis Newsletter **3;** 2, 1974.

53. YUNIS, J.J. and SANCHEZ, O.: A new syndrome resulting from partial trisomy for the distal third of the long arm of chromosome 10. J. Pediat. **84;** 567, 1974.

54. OSZTOVICS, M., BÜHLER, E.M., MÜLLER, H. and STALDER, G.S.: Banding techniques in the evaluation of human chromosomal variants. Humangenetik **18;** 123, 1973.

55. DEMARS, R., SARTO, G., FELIX, J.S. and BENKE, P.: Lesch-Nyhan mutation: prenatal detection with amniotic fluid cells. Science **164;** 1303, 1969.

56. BOYLE, J.A., RAIVIO, K.O., ASTRIN, K.H., SCHULMAN, J.D., GRAF, M.L., SEEGMILLER, J.E. and JACOBSON, C.B.: Lesch-Nyhan syndrome: preventive control by prenatal diagnosis. Science **169;** 688, 1970.

57. BRADY, R.O., UHLENDORF, B.W. and JACOBSON, C.B.: Fabry's disease: antenatal detection. Science **172;** 174, 1971.

58. ANGELINI, C., ENGEL, A.G. and TITUS, J.L.: Adult acid maltase deficiency: abnormalities in fibroblasts cultured from patients. New Eng. J. Med. **287;** 948, 1972.

59. COX, R.P., DOUGLAS, G., HUTZLER, J., LYNFIELD, J. and DANCIS, J.: In-utero detection of Pompe's disease. Lancet **1;** 893, 1970.

60. EPSTEIN, C.J., BRADY, R.O., SCHNEIDER, E.L., BRADLEY, R.M. and SHAPIRO, D.: In utero diagnosis of Niemann-Pick disease. Amer. J. Hum. Genet. **23;** 533, 1971.

61. O'BRIEN, J.S., OKADA, S., FILLERUP, D.L., VEATH, M.L., ADORNATO, B., BRENNER, P.H. and LEROY, J.G.: Tay-Sachs disease: prenatal diagnosis. Science **172;** 61, 1971.

62. SCHNEIDER, E.L., ELLIS, W.G., BRADY, R.O., McCULLOCH, J.R. and EPSTEIN, C.J.: Infantile (type II) Gaucher's disease: in utero diagnosis and fetal pathology. J. Pediat. **81;** 1134, 1972.

63. LOWDEN, J.A., CUTZ, E., CONEN, P.E., RUDD, N. and DORAN, T.A.: Prenatal diagnosis of GM₁-gangliosidosis. New Eng. J. Med. **288;** 225, 1973.

64. SUZUKI, K., SCHNEIDER, E.L. and EPSTEIN, C.J.: *In utero* diagnosis of globoid cell leukodystrophy. Biochem. Biophys. Res. Commun. **45;** 1363, 1971.

65. KROOTH, R.S.: Genetics of cultured somatic cells. Med. Clin. N. Amer. **53;** 795, 1969.

66. KABACK, M.M., LEONARD, C.O. and PARMLEY, T.H.: Intrauterine diagnosis: comparative enzymology of cells cultivated from maternal skin, fetal skin, and amniotic fluid cells. Pediat. Res. **5;** 366, 1971.

67. DESNICK, R.J., KRIVIT, W. and SHARP, H.L.: *In utero* diagnosis of Sandhoff's disease. Biochem. Biophys. Res. Commun. **51;** 20, 1973.

68. CRAWFURD, M. D'A., DEAN, M.F., HUNT, D.M., JOHNSON, D.R., MacDONALD, R.R., MUIR, H., PAYLING WRIGHT, E.A. and PAYLING WRIGHT, C.R.: Early prenatal diagnosis of Hurler's syndrome with termination of pregnancy and confirmatory findings on the fetus. J. Med. Genet. **10;** 144, 1973.

69. HARPER, P.S., LAURENCE, K.M., PARKES, A., WUSTEMAN, F.S., KRESSE, H., FIGURA, K. VON, FERGUSON-SMITH, M.A., DUNCAN, D.M., LOGAN, R.W., HALL, F. and WHITEMAN, P.: Sanfilippo A disease in the fetus. J. Med. Genet. **11;** 123, 1974.

70. SCHNEIDER, J.A., VERROUST, F.M., KROLL, W.A., GARVIN, A.J., HORGER, E.O., III, WONG, V.G., SPEAR, G.S., JACOBSON, C., PELLETT, O.L. and BECKER, F.L.A.: Prenatal diagnosis of cystinosis. New Eng. J. Med. **290;** 878, 1974.

71. MILUNSKY, A.: The Prenatal Diagnosis of Hereditary Disorders. Charles C Thomas, Illinois, 1973.

72. GOMPERTZ, D., GOODEY, P.A., SAUDUBRAY, J.M., CHARPENTIER, C. and CHIGNOLLE, A.: Prenatal diagnosis of methymalonic aciduria. Pediatrics **54;** 511, 1974.

73. FENSOM, A.H., BENSON, P.F. and BLUNT, S.: Prenatal diagnosis of galactosaemia. Brit. Med. J. **4;** 386, 1974.

74. RAMSAY, C.A., COLTART, T.M., BLUNT, S., PAWSEY, S. and GIANNELLI, F.: Prenatal dsagnosis of xeroderma pigmentosum. Report of the first successful case. Lancet **2;** 1109, 1974.

75. ALLAN, L.D., FERGUSON-SMITH, M.A., DONALD, I., SWEET, E.M. and GIBSON, A.A.M.: Amniotic fluid alpha-fetoprotein in the antenatal diagnosis of spina bifida. Lancet **2;** 522, 1973.

76. BURNETT, R.G. and ANDERSON, W.R.: The hazards of amniocentesis. J. Iowa Med. Soc. **58;** 130, 1968.

77. LILEY, A.W.: The technique and complications of amniocentesis. New Zeal. Med. J. **59**; 581, 1960.

78. FREDA, V.J.: Recent obstetrical advances in the Rh problem: antepartum management, amniocentesis, and experience with hysterotomy and surgery in utero. Bull. New York Acad. Med. **42**; 474, 1966.

79. WILTCHIK, S.G., SCHWARZ, R.H. and EMICH, J.P., Jr.: Amniography for placental localization. Obstet. Gynec. **28**; 641, 1966.

80. BERNER, H.W., Jr.: Aminography, an accurate way to localize the placenta: a comparison with soft-tissue placentography. Obstet Gynec. **29**; 200, 1967.

81. GERBIE, A.B., NADLER, H.L. and GERBIE, M.V.: Amniocentesis in genetic counselling. Amer. J. Obstet. Gynec. **109**; 765, 1971.

82. MILUNSKY, A. and ATKINS, L.: Prenatal diagnosis of genetic disorders. An analysis of experience with 600 cases. J.A.M.A. **230**; 232, 1974.

83. ABRAMOVICH, D.R.: The volume of amniotic fluid in early pregnancy. J. Obstet. Gynaec. Brit. Cwlth. **75**; 728, 1968.

84. FUCHS, F.: Volume of amniotic fluid at various stages of pregnancy. Clin. Obstet. Gynec. **9**; 449, 1966.

85. HAHNEMANN, N.: Possibility of culturing foetal cells at early stages of pregnancy. Clin. Genet. **3**; 286, 1972.

86. WAHLSTRÖM, J.: The quality of viable cells at various stages of gestation. Humangenetik **22**; 335, 1974.

87. AUSTIN, C.R.: Sex chromatin in embryonic and fetal tissue. Acta Cytol. **6**; 61, 1962.

88. VAN LEEUWEN, L., JACOBY, H. and CHARLES, D.: Exfoliative cytology of amniotic fluid. Acta Cytol. **9**; 442, 1965.

89. VOTTA, R.A., DE GAGNETEN, C.B., PARADA, O. and GIULIETTI, M.: Cytologic study of amniotic fluid in pregnancy. Amer. J. Obstet. Gynec. **102**; 571, 1968.

90. HUISJES, H.J.: Origin of the cells in the liquor amnii. Amer. J. Obstet. Gynec. **106**; 1222, 1970.

91. WACHTEL, E., GORDON, H. and OLSEN, E.: Cytology of amniotic fluid. J. Obstet. Gynaec. Brit. Cwlth. **76**; 596, 1969.

92. HUSAIN, O.A. and SINCLAIR, L.: Estimation of maturity in the foetus and newborn. Studies on the cytology of amniotic fluid and of the newborn infant's skin in relation to maturity of the infant. Proc. Roy. Soc. Med. **64**; 1213, 1971.

93. HOEHN, H., BRYANT, E.M., KARP, L.E. and MARTIN, G.M.: Cultivated cells from diagnostic amniocentesis in second trimester pregnancies. I. Clonal morphology and growth potential. Pediat. Res. **8**; 746, 1974.

94. VALENTI, C. and KEHATY, T.: Culture of cells obtained by amniocentesis. J. Lab. Clin. Med. **73**; 355, 1969.

95. SANTESSON, B., ÅKESSON, H.-O., BÖÖK, J.A. and BROSSET, A.: Karyotyping human amniotic-fluid cells. Lancet **2**; 1067, 1969.

96. ABBO, G. and ZELLWEGER, H.: Prenatal determination of fetal sex and chromosomal complement. Lancet **1**; 216, 1970.

97. GREGSON, N.M.: A technique for culturing cells from amniotic fluid. Lancet **1**; 84, 1970.

98. LISGAR, F., GERTNER, M., CHERRY, S., HSU, L.Y. and HIRSCHHORN, K.: Prenatal chromosome analysis. Nature (London) **225**; 280, 1970.

99. LEE, C.L.Y., GREGSON, N.M. and WALKER, S.: Eliminating red blood cells from amniotic fluid samples. Lancet **2**; 316, 1970.

100. BUTLER, L.J. and REISS, H.E.: Antenatal detection of chromosome abnormalities. J. Obstet. Gynaec. Brit. Cwlth. **77**; 902, 1970.

101. KNÖRR-GÄRTNER, H. and HÄRLE, I.: A modified method of culturing human amniotic fluid cells for prenatal detection of genetic disorders. Humangenetik **14**; 333, 1972.

102. THERKELSEN, A.J., PETERSEN, G.B., STEENSTRUP, O.R., JONASSON, J., LINDSTEN, J. and ZECH, L.: Prenatal diagnosis of chromosome abnormalities. Acta Paediat. Scand. **61**; 397, 1972.

103. NAKAGOME, Y., IINUMA, K. and MATSUNAGA, E.: Polyploidy in cultured amniotic-fluid cells. Lancet **2**; 387, 1972.

104. WAHLSTRÖM, J., BROSSET, A. and BARTSCH, F.: Viability of amniotic cells at different stages of gestation. Lancet **2**; 1037, 1970.

105. CARTER, C.O. and MACCARTHY, D.: Incidence of mongolism and its diagnosis in the newborn. Brit. J. Soc. Med. **5**; 83, 1951.

106. TAYLOR, A.I.: Autosomal trisomy syndromes: a detailed study of 27 cases of Edwards' syndrome and 27 cases of Patau's syndrome. J. Med. Genet. **5**; 227, 1968.

107. COURT BROWN, W.M., LAW, P. and SMITH, P.G.: Sex chromosome aneuploidy and parental age. Ann. Hum. Genet. **33**; 1, 1969.

108. TURPIN, R. and LEJEUNE, J.: Human Afflictions and Chromosomal Aberrations. Pergamon Press, London, 1969.

109. STENE, J.: Detection of higher recurrence risk for age-dependent chromosome abnormalities with an application to trisomy G_1 (Down's syndrome). Hum. Hered. **20**; 112, 1970.

110. LITTLEFIELD, J.W., MILUNSKY, A. and JACOBY, L.B.: Prenatal genetic diagnosis: present and future development. In: Human Genetics. DE GROUCHY, J., EBLING, F.J.G. and HENDERSON, I.W. (eds.) Excerpta Medica, Amsterdam, 1972.

111. NADLER, H.L. and GERBIE, A.: Present status of amniocentesis in intrauterine diagnosis of genetic defects. Obstet Gynec. **38**; 789, 1971.

112. LÁSZLO, J., GAÁL, M. and BÖSZE, P.: Source of error in prenatal sex determination. Lancet **2**; 1367, 1972.

113. PERRY, T.B. and PATRICK, J.E.: Error in prenatal sex determination. Lancet **1**; 371, 1973.

114. KARDON, N.B., CHERNAY, P.R., HSU, L.Y.F., MARTIN, J.L. and HIRSCHHORN, K.: Problems in prenatal diagnosis resulting from chromosomal mosaicism. Clin. Genet. **3**; 83, 1972.

115. BLOOM, A.D., SCHMICKEL, R., BARR, M. and BURDI, A.R.: Prenatal detection of autosomal mosaicism. J. Pediat. **84**; 732, 1974.

116. COX, D.M., NIEWCZAS-LATE, V., RIFFELL, M.I. and HAMERTON, J.L.: Chromosomal mosaicism in diagnostic amniotic fluid cell cultures. Pediat. Res. **8**; 679, 1974.

117. ATKINS, L., MILUNSKY, A. and SHAHOOD, J.M.: Prenatal diagnosis: detailed chromosomal analysis in 500 cases. Clin. Genet. **6**; 317, 1974.

118. KAJII, T.: Pseudomosaicism in cultured amniotic-fluid cells. Lancet **2**; 1037, 1971.

119. HUGHES, D.T., RINK, E., GRIFFITHS, S. and PAINTIN, D.B.: Fetal karyotype from amniotic cells without culturing. Lancet **2**; 1319, 1971.

120. HUGHES, D.T. and RINK, E.: Prenatal diagnosis from uncultured amniotic-fluid cells. Lancet **1**; 270, 1972.

121. QUAYLE, S., CHITHAM, R.G. and CRAFT, I.: Prenatal diagnosis from uncultured amniotic-fluid cells. Lancet **1**; 269, 1972.

122. HAMERTON, J.L.: Fetal karyotype of amniotic cells without culturing. Lancet **1**; 203, 1972.

123. KOHN, G. and ROBINSON, A.: Tetraploidy in cells cultured from amniotic fluid. Lancet **2**; 778, 1970.

124. WALKER, S., LEE, C.L.Y. and GREGSON, N.M.: Polyploidy in cells cultured from amniotic fluid. Lancet **2**; 1137, 1970.

125. SCHLEGEL, R.J., NEU, R.L., CARNEIRO LEAO, J., FARIAS, E., ASPILLAGA, M.J. and GARDNER, L.I.: Observations on the chromosomal, cytological and anatomical characteristics of 75 human conceptuses. Cytogenetics **5**; 430, 1966.

126. CAR, D.H.: Chromosome studies in abortuses and stillborn infants. Lancet **2**; 603, 1963.

127. WAXMAN, S.H., ARAKAKI, D.T. and SMITH, J.B.: Cytogenetics of fetal abortions. Pediatrics **39**; 425, 1967.

128. KOHN, G., MAYALL, B.H. and MILLER, M.E.: Tetraploi-diploid mosaicism in a surviving infant. Pediat. Res. **1**; 461, 1967.

129. ATNIP, R.L. and SUMMITT, R.L.: Tetraploidy and 18-trisomy in a six-year-old triple mosaic boy. Cytogenetics **10**; 305, 1971.

130. KELLY, T.E. and RARY, J.M.: Mosaic tetraploidy in a two-year-old female. Clin. Genet. **6**; 221, 1974.

131. HSU, L.Y.F. and HIRSCHHORN, K.: Prenatal diagnosis of genetic disease. Life Sci. **14**; 2311, 1974.

132. MACINTYRE, M.N.: Chromosome problems of intrauterine diagnosis. Birth Defects: Original Article Series **7**; 10, 1971.

133. OLSON, C., PRESCOTT, G.H., PERNOLL, M.L. and HECHT, F.: Danger in nuclear-sexing the fetus. Lancet **2**; 226, 1974.

134. MACINTYRE, M.N., RUSTAD, R.C. and TURK, K.B.: Prenatal evaluation in a case of familial Y chromosome long arm deletion (Yq-). J. Med. Genet. **11**; 367, 1974.

135. ZACHARSKI, L.R., BOWIE, E.J.W. and TITUS, J.L.: Cell-culture synthesis of a factor VIII-like activity. Mayo Clin. Proc. **44**; 784, 1968.

136. GREEN, D., RYAN, C., MALANDRUCCOLO, N. and NADLER, H.L.: Characterization of the coagu-
      lant activity of cultured human fibroblasts. Blood **37**; 47, 1971.
137. BOYER, S.H. and GRAHAM, J.B.: Linkage between the X chromosome loci for glucose-6-
      phosphate dehydrogenase electrophoretic variation and hemophilia A. Amer. J. Hum. Genet.
      17; 320, 1965.
138. McCURDY, P.: Use of genetic linkage for the detection of female carriers of hemophilia. New
      Eng. J. Med. **285**; 218, 1971.
139. RENWICK, J.H., BUNDEY, S.E., FERGUSON-SMITH, M.A. and IZATT, M.M.: Confirmation of
      linkage of the loci for myotonic dystrophy and ABH secretion. J. Med. Genet. **8**; 407, 1971.
140. HARPER, P., BIAS, W.B., HUTCHINSON, J.R. and McKUSICK, V.A.: ABH secretor status of the
      fetus: a genetic marker identifiable by amniocentesis. J. Med. Genet. **8**; 438, 1971.
141. SCHROTT, H.G., KARP, L. and OMENN, G.S.: Prenatal prediction in myotonic dystrophy:
      guidelines for genetic counseling. Clin. Genet. **4**; 38, 1973.
142. IONASESCU, V. and ZELLWEGER, H.: Duchenne muscular dystrophy in young girls? Acta Neu-
      rol. Scandinav. **50**; 619, 1974.
143. JEFFCOATE, T.N.A., FLIEGNER, J.R.H., RUSSEL, S.H., DAVIS, J.C. and WADE, A.P.: Diagnosis
      of adrenogenital syndrome before birth. Lancet **2**; 553, 1965.
144. NICHOLS, J.: Antenatal diagnosis of adrenocortical hyperplasia. Lancet **1**; 1151, 1969.
145. NICHOLS, J. and GIBSON, G.G.: Antenatal diagnosis of the adrenogenital syndrome. Lancet
      2; 1068, 1969.
146. NICHOLS, J.: Antenatal diagnosis and treatment of the adrenogenital syndrome. Lancet **1**;
      83, 1970.
147. DANES, B.S. and BEARN, A.G.: A genetic cell marker in cystic fibrosis of the pancreas. Lancet
      1; 1061, 1968.
148. NADLER, H.L., SWAE, M.A., WODNICKI, J.M. and O'FLYNN, M.E.: Cultivated amniotic-
      fluid cells and fibroblasts derived from families with cystic fibrosis. Lancet **2**; 84, 1969.
149. MATALON, R., DORFMAN, A., NADLER, H.L. and JACOBSON, C.B.: A chemical method for the
      antenatal diagnosis of mucopolysaccharidoses. Lancet **1**; 83, 1970.
150. NADLER, H.L. and GERBIE, A.B.: Enzymes in noncultured amniotic fluid cells. Amer. J.
      Obstet. Gynec. **103**; 710, 1969.
151. SUTCLIFFE, R.G. and BROCK, D.J.H.: Enzymes in uncultured amniotic fluid cells. Clin. Chim.
      Acta **31**; 363, 1971.
152. KABACK, M.M. and HOWELL, R.R.: Infantile metachromatic leukodystrophy: heterozygote
      detection in skin fibroblasts and possible applications to intrauterine diagnosis. New Eng. J.
      Med. **282**; 1336, 1970.
153. MELANCON, S.G., LEE, S.Y. and NADLER, H.L.: Histidase activity in cultivated human amnio-
      tic fluid cells. Science **173**; 627, 1971.
154. GERBIE, A.B., MELANCON, S.B., RYAN, C. and NADLER, H.L.: Cultivated epithelial-like cells
      and fibroblasts from amniotic fluid: their relationship to enzymatic and cytologic analysis.
      Amer. J. Obstet. Gynec. **114**; 314, 1972.
155. DeMARS, R.: Some studies of enzymes in cultivated human cells. US Nat. Cancer Inst.
      Monogr. **13**; 181, 1964.
156. De LUCA, C. and NITOWSKY, H.M.: Variations in enzyme activities during the growth of
      mammalian cells *in vitro*: lactate and glucose-6-phosphate dehydrogenases. Biochim. Biophys.
      Acta **89**; 208, 1964.
157. PAN, Y. and KROOTH, R.S.: The influence of progressive growth on the specific catalase
      activity of human diploid cell strains. J. Cell Physiol. **71**; 151, 1969.
158. BUTTERWORTH, J., SUTHERLAND, G.R., BROADHEAD, D.M. and BAIN, A.D.: Lysosomal enzyme
      levels in human amniotic fluid cells in tissue culture. I. *alpha*-glucosidase and *beta*-glucosidase.
      Life Sci. **13**; 713, 1973.
159. SUTHERLAND, G.R., BUTTERWORTH, J., BROADHEAD, D.M. and BAIN, A.D.: Lysosomal enzyme
      levels in human amniotic fluid cells in tissue culture. II. *alpha*-galactosidase, *beta*-galactosidase
      and *alpha*-arabinosidase. Clin. Genet. **5**; 351, 1974.
160. BUTTERWORTH, J., SUTHERLAND, G.R., BROADHEAD, D.M. and BAIN, A.D.: Lysosomal enzyme
      levels in human amniotic fluid cells in tissue culture. III. *beta*-glucuronidase, N-acetyl-*beta*-D-
      glucosaminidase, *alpha*-mannosidase and acid phosphatase. Clin. Genet. **5**; 356, 1974.
161. HAYFLICK, L.: The mycoplasmatales and the L-Phase of Bacteria. Appleton-Century-Croft,
      New York, 1969.

162. BEUTLER, E., KUHL, W., TRINIDAD, T., TEPLITZ, R. and NADLER, H.: *Beta*-glucosidase activity in fibroblasts from homozygotes and heterozygotes for Gaucher's disease. Amer. J. Hum. Genet. **23**; 62, 1971.

163. HSIA, D.Y.Y.: The detection of heterozygous carriers. Med. Clin. N. Amer. **53**; 857, 1969.

164. FUJIMOTO, W.Y., SEEGMILLER, J.E., UHLENDORF, B.W. and JACOBSON, C.B.: Biochemical diagnosis of an X-linked disease in utero. Lancet **2**; 511, 1968.

165. BROCK, D.J.H., BOLTON, A.E. and SCRIMGEOUR, J.B.: Prenatal diagnosis of spina bifida and anencephaly through maternal plasma-alpha-fetoprotein measurement. Lancet **1**; 767, 1974.

166. WALD, N.J., BROCK, D.J.H. and BONNAR, J.: Prenatal diagnosis of spina bifida and anencephaly by maternal serum-alpha-fetoprotein measurement. A controlled study. Lancet **1**; 765, 1974.

Normal and abnormal human development in the early prenatal stage

Takashi TANIMURA, M.D.

Department of Anatomy, Faculty of Medicine, Kyoto University, Kyoto

HUMAN EMBRYONIC AND FETAL SPECIMENS FOR STUDIES OF NORMAL AND ABNORMAL DEVELOPMENT

Human conceptuses (embryos, fetuses and their fetal membranes) are very precious and valuable materials not only for embryology but also for teratology, and collection of excellent human embryonic and fetal specimens and their detailed description is the first essential step for the studies of human congenital anomalies.

Tremendous effort has been directed to this problem since the end of the last Century. His [1], Keibel [2] and Mall [3] are just a few of the early contributors worthy of special mention. Keibel's Normentafeln described the detailed series of early human development based on the individual cases. Later, Dr. George L. Streeter, late director of the Carnegie Institute of Washington, Baltimore, U.S.A., and his associates established the staging system at embryonic age. The proposed criteria for staging conceptuses by mostly remarkable differentiation of external and internal features furnished us the method of a more accurate description of human embryos as compared to previously used criteria for staging such as crown-rump length and clinically determined age using menstrual record, and thus facilitated the comparison of isolated case reports by different investigators. Moreover, they showed estimated ovulation age of the embryos at each stage by comparison with the monkey specimens at the similar developmental stage. The term "horizon" was adopted to emphasize the importance of thinking of the embryo as a living organism which in its time assumes many guises, always progressing from the smaller and simpler to the larger and more complex [4]. Twenty-three horizons were assigned for fertilized ova and embryos up to 30 mm crown-rump length. Characteristic features of embryos at each horizon from X to XXIII have been presented [4–8]. The unique study of Hertig et al. [9] fairly disclosed the most early phase of human development up to 17 days of conceptional age. Very recently, O'Rahilly [10] first systematically described a detailed account of human embryonic development in the first three weeks which was based primarily on the materials housed in Carnegie Collection, the world most famous collection of human embryonic specimens. It is announced that a revision of later stages (3 to 8 postovulatory weeks) is to be followed by the same author. Accordingly, the new term to describe the developmental stages of human embryos revised by O'Rahilly is to be called Carnegie stage instead of the formerly used Streeter's horizon. However, most of the materials ever reported including those in the Carnegie Collection were usually derived from abnormal course of pregnancy such as spontaneous abortions or ectopic pregnancies and, therefore, can not be regarded as the representative of the true intrauterine population.

As for the abnormal development in the early human prenatal stage, the work by HERTIG et al. [9] should be again emphasized. They found about 40 per cent of those conceptuses in the first 17 days of fertilization were abnormal, and estimated that it would have been impossible for them to survive or to be born alive. However, no systematic epidemiological studies on the embryos at three to eight weeks of age have been done, although there were reported a considerable number of cases of malformed embryos at this stage which were found incidentally (Examples of such cases reported before 1966 were summarized in our previous paper, NISHIMURA et al. [11]). Caution should be paied for those early case reports, because such specimens were obtained mainly form abnormal pregnancy such as spontaneous abortion and ectopy, and it was very difficult clearly to distinguish developmental anomalies existing in utero from post-mortem changes and artificial damages during and after the operation and fixation. As a matter of fact, some earlier authors presented a very doubtful case allegedly as a true malformation.

It should be added here that spontaneous abortion occurs more frequently in cases with anomalies than in normal cases from the established fact that aborted conceptuses show very high frequency of structural anomalies (reviewed by STRATFORD [12]). Therefore, the malformations detected in the perinatal stage are only a residual part of the whole range of maldevelopments. The real prevalence of malformation may be found only by studying specimens in the overall early intrauterine population.

Since 1961, Dr. HIDEO NISHIMURA, Professor of Anatomy, Faculty of Medicine, Kyoto University and his group have been engaged in collecting human embryos and early fetuses for studies of normal and abnormal development. This program was realized by a special circumstance of Japan after the Second World War. Under the revision of the Japanese Eugenic Protection Law in 1952, a large number of induced abortions have been performed mainly for socioeconomic indication by the discretion of qualified obstetricians in response only to the request of both husband and wife concerned. No permission from the public authorities was to be requested. This revision has resulted in more than a million of induced abortions and, accordingly, a sharp decrease in birth rate. The number of reported induced abortions had been about an equal number of births, although in recent years they are reported to be sharply declining in number partly due to the developments of various contraceptive measures.

In more than 90 per cent of cases of induced abortions, the interruption of pregnancies has been conducted in the period from the second to the fourth month of pregnancy by means of dilatation and curettage whereas a small number of induced abortions have been done in the later stages by means of induced premature labor, usually by the insertion of instruments into the uterine cavity such as bougie and metreurynter. The time when the majority of induced abortion is performed corresponds incidentally to the period of major organogenesis, the most important stage for embryology and teratology. Moreover, the induced abortions are generally performed at small private clinics rather than large public hospitals. Therefore, it was presumed that unselected cases could be obtained if we could get the cooperation of a large number of those obstetricians at private clinics. There is, however, one technical difficulty that in more than 95 per cent of cases the embryonic specimens are crushed after dilatation and curettage, and unfortunately unsuitable for morphological study, and acquisition of undamaged embryos usually depends on a chance. However, with the collaboration of more than 1,000 obstetricians, we have been able to collect a large number of normal and abnormal embryonic and fetal specimens which could be regarded as approximately a non-selected sample of the total early human prenatal population. Our laboratory engaged in the human embryo study is called the Human Embryo Center, and it is now to be claimed that this holds one of the largest collection of human embryonic and early fetal specimens in the world. The outline of the conceptuses collected and histological specimens prepared in our laboratory is as follows:

a. Specimens obtained in the Human Embryo Center
Embryos (crown-rump length approximately less than 30 mm): ca. 35,000 (About one fourth are undamaged and about 500 malformed cases have been detected.); Fetuses: 4,000

b. Histological embryonic and fetal specimens stored in the Human Embryo Center
Normal embryos (serial): 686 cases; Abnormal embryos (serial): 351 cases; Non-serial section of normal and abnormal embryos and fetuses: ca. 1,000 cases.

The studies to be described in the following are a summary of the collaborative works by Dr. NISHIMURA and his associates including the author himself during these 15 years. The author has served the collection and studies of those embryos since the beginning of the project as he had a career of obstetrician and has been a key staff in Dr. NISHIMURA's team. As described above, in order to get a sufficient number of undamaged embryonic specimens for the studies of abnormal development, it is necessary to get in touch with a very large number of cooperative obstetricians. In fact, such obstetricians are widely distributed mostly in large cities throughout the central areas of Japan. This situation inevitably leads to the fact that majority of the embryonic specimens should be fixed and stored for some period of time by obstetricians concerned. Accordingly, most of the embryonic specimens are first fixed in Bouin's fluid, transferred on the next day into 10% formalin and then stored, while majority of the fetal specimens are simultaneously fixed and stored in 10% formalin. Bouin's fluid was selected because the embryos can keep in it some hardness suitable for the examination under stereomicroscope and excellent state of histological specimens is maintained. However, for special occasions and purposes fresh embryos and fetuses have been obtained through the obstetricians in Kyoto City area, and also same frozen specimens have been furnished by several obstetricians. They are used in most cases in non-epidemiological studies shown in Fig. 1.

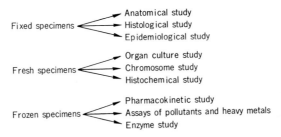

Fixed specimens ← Anatomical study / Histological study / Epidemiological study

Fresh specimens ← Organ culture study / Chromosome study / Histochemical study

Frozen specimens ← Pharmacokinetic study / Assays of pollutants and heavy metals / Enzyme study

Fig. 1 Study areas using human embryonic specimens in Kyoto University.

A record form with respect to 1) menstruation and coital date if known; 2) parental age; 3) parental consanguinity; 4) obstetric history such as parity, frequency of the past spontaneous or induced abortion, and period after previous delivery; 5) contraceptive measures, 6) complications during the present pregnancy (acute infections, chronic diseases, genital bleeding, no matter either due to threatened abortion or any others, etc.); 7) medical treatments (operations, radiations, drug exposures, vaccinations, etc.); and 8) other items such as parental occupation, maternal smoking and drinking was filled in for each case by the cooperating obstetricians. In the cases at and above the fourth month of pregnancy, the permission of parents for dissection and preservation of the fetal materials was obtained through the obstetricians. We have asked the collaborative obstetricians to preserve the fetal specimens up to the 20th week of gestation, because the fetuses in the later stage are too large to be fixed and stored as a whole and they tend to be more biased materials selected by the obstetricians themselves.

At our laboratory, careful examination was made under the stereomicroscope to determine the developmental stage. In embryos the criteria developed in our laboratory [13] primarily based on the STREETER's horizon system [4–8] and the revised Carnegie stage system [10] were used for determining the developmental stage only by the external examination. Then, examination for malformations or indication of intrauterine death was carefully made. And finally, the measurement of crown-rump length and other necessary items is performed. The major findings were described in the punch card. For further studies, histological examination, microdissection or macrodissection was performed for detection of any internal anomalies, and in some cases the specimens were cleared and stained for observation of skeletal development.

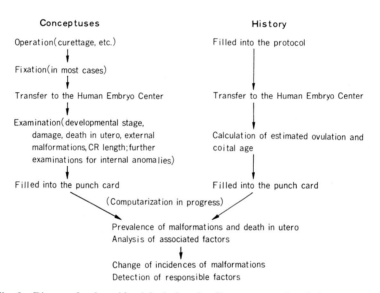

Fig. 2   Diagram for the epidemiological study of human normal and abnormal development using fixed embryos in Kyoto University. (From TANIMURA, T.: The use of induced abortuses for monitoring. In: Shepard, T.H. et al. (eds.) Methods for Detection of Environmental Agents that Produce Congenital Defects. pp. 197–201, North-Holland, Amsterdam, 1975)

Since we have concentrated our efforts to the systematic studies of the human embryonic specimens (up to 30 mm crown-rump length) for various reasons mentioned above, the summary of the studies mainly on embryos such as 1) establishment of normal standards in development; 2) prevalence of abnormal development and associated factors, monitoring for detection of teratogens; 3) pathogenesis of malformations will be described in the following chapters. Flow of examination of conceptuses and analysis of their history is schematically given in Fig. 2.

NORMAL DEVELOPMENT

Every student or scientist who reads the textbooks of embryology may be embarrassed more or less with the confusion of the criteria in development. Crown-rump length is the simplest and fairly accurate item for comparison throughout the prenatal period. Menstrual age or estimated ovulation age calculated from the menstrual age is the only item accessible clinically. Staging of the embryonic specimens by various developmental features is the best accurate way for description and the horizon system proposed by STREETER has greatly contributed to the understanding of each specimen. However, the reliable relationship between these three criteria has not been systematically reported and thus aroused much confusion in reading the literature.

NISHIMURA et al. [14] reported the results of observation of 675 specimens singled out using the following criteria: mothers with menstrual cycles of 27–32 days within a range of 2 days, no history of genital bleeding during the terminated pregnancy, and the specimens showing no signs of death *in utero* or external malformations. The relations between various variables such as ovulation age, developmental stage, crown-rump length and body weight were examined. The ovulation age was estimated by substracting the period (menstrual cycle — 14 days) from the menstrual age in days. Recently, several precious cases of early embryonic specimens at the neural groove and early somite period (stage 7 to 12) were added to our standard [15]. One of the earliest specimens at stage 6 is illustrated in Fig. 3. A series of photographs showing the external forms of normal embryos at some selected stages is given in Fig. 4. An example of histology in the embryo at stage 16 is shown in Fig. 5.

Fig. 6 shows the relationship between the developmental stage and the ovulation age. A fairly wide range in developmental stage was noted for any ovulation age. For instance, embryos at about 6 weeks of age showed stages ranging from 14 to 22. This fact gives the very important lesson when one considers clinically the critical period (or sensitive stage) for malformations. The real sensitive stage for production of a specific type of anomalies

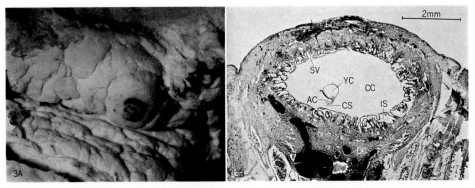

Fig. 3   A conceptus at stage 6 obtained by hysterectomy at the 30th day after the last menstrual period.
  A.   Surface view of the implantation site.
  B.   Histology.
     AC, Amniotic cavity; CC, Chorionic cavity; CS, Connecting stalk; DC, decidua; FC,
     Fibrin coagulum; IS, Intervillous space; SV, Secondary stem villus; TS, Trophoblastic
     shell; YC, Yolk sac cavity.

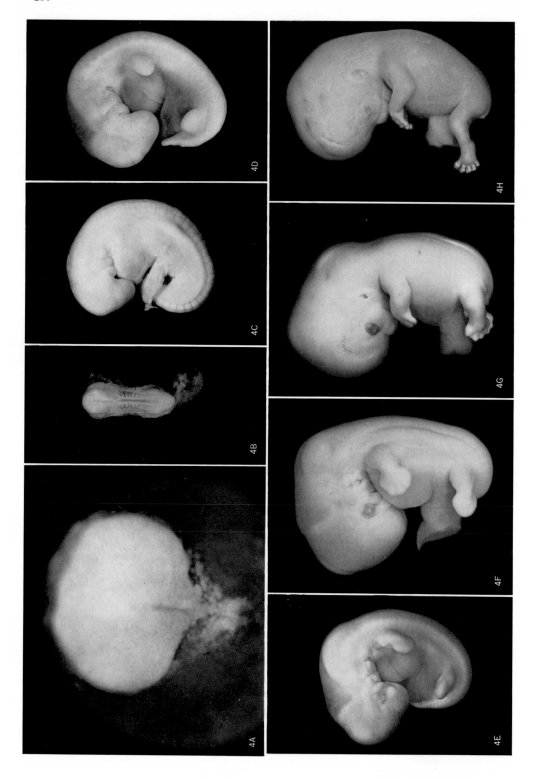

Fig. 4 External form of normal embryos at stages 7 to 23. (A and B, dorsal view; C through H, lateral view)

A. Stage 7 (average length at this stage, ca. 0.4 mm; average age, ca. 16 days). Developmental characteristics at this stage: neural plate, primitive groove, allantois, notochordal process (neural groove, notochordal and neurenteric canal at stage 8). (From NISHIMURA, H. et al.: Teratology **10**; 1, 1974)

B. Stage 10 (ca. 2–3.5 mm, ca. 22 days). Developmental characteristics at this stage: 4–12 somites (somites first appear at stage 9), neural folds begin to fuse, otic placode, optic sulcus, anterior hypophysis, two branchial arches, heart tube fuses and beat begins (possibly at stage 9), formation of fore-, mid- and hind gut, nephrogenic cord (mesonephric duct at stage 11), primordium germ cells in yolk sac. (From NISHIMURA, H. et al.: Teratology **10**; 1, 1974)

C. Stage 12 (ca. 4 mm, ca. 28 days). Developmental characteristics at this stage: 21–29 somites, closure of anterior neuropore (posterior neuropore closes at stage 13), deep otic pit (pit appears at stage 11 and closes at stage 13), oropharyngeal membrane ruptures, three branchial arches, thyroid diverticulum, upper limb buds just appearing, septum primum, liver cord, gallbladder and dorsal pancreas, mesonephric duct reaches cloaca.

D. Stage 14 (ca. 6 mm, ca. 34 days). Developmental characteristics at this stage: about 38 somites, cerebral vesicle, cerebellar plate, optic cup, invagination of optic lens (closes at stage 15), olfactory placode, cervical sinus deepens, thymus, parathyroid, ultimobranchial body, septum secundum, sixth aortic arches develop, primary bronchi (lung bud appears at stage 13), ventral pancreas, gonadal ridge, ureteric bud, primordium germ cells to genital ridge, lower limb buds fin-like.

E. Stage 16 (ca. 10 mm, ca. 38 days). Developmental characteristics at this stage: first cortical region in hippocampi and fiber tracts in the hypothalamus, retinal pigment, semicircular canals, auricular hillocks, nasal pit faces ventral, hand plate (appearing at stage 15) divided into carpus and digital plate, ostium primum obliterated, atrioventricular cushions fuse, secondary bronchial diverticula, stomach completes rotation, spleen, three centers of proliferation in leg bud, genital tubercle.

F. Stage 18 (ca. 14 mm, ca. 42 days). Developmental characteristics at this stage: eyelids beginning, nasal tip, sex differentiation in gonad, chondrification, interdigital notches in hand, partitioning of heart and truncus arteriosus completed, nipples, paramesonephric duct develops (it appears at stage 17), cloacal membrane ruptures (or at stage 19).

G. Stage 20 (ca. 19 mm, ca. 46 days). Developmental characteristics at this stage: superficial vascular plexus halfway between eye-ear level and vertex, upper limbs bent at elbows, hands are curved over heart and reach edge of nose, ossification beginning, metanephros shifted to abdominal cavity, interdigital notches in foot.

H. Stage 23 (ca. 28 mm, ca. 52 days). Embryonic period ends when bone marrow formation begins in humerus. Major organogenesis is completed but palate is not closed. Developmental characteristic at this stage: superficial vascular plexus near vertex, eyelids encroach on eyeballs, full cochlea coiling, hair primordia in eyebrow, complete separation of Rathke's porch, primordia of all salivary glands, renal tubules of fourth or fifth orders, paramesonephric duct fuses, anal membrane ruptures.

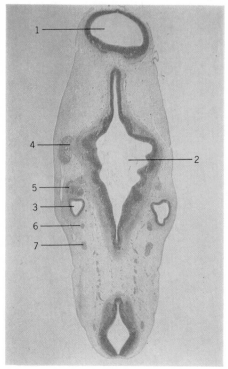

A

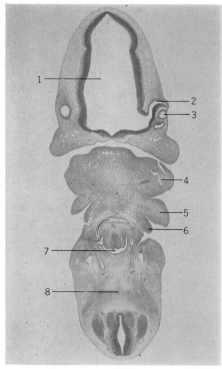

B

Fig. 5 Histology of the human embryo at stage 16 (10 mm, 38 days).
(A through E, transverse section; F, sagittal section)

A. Section through otocyst
    1. mesencephalon; 2. myelencephalon; 3. otic vesicle; 4. ganglion n. V; 5. ganglion n. VII and n. VIII; 6. ganglion n. IX; 7. ganglion n. X.

B. Section through eye
    1. diencephalon; 2. optic cup; 3. lens; 4. branchial arch I; 5. branchial arch II; 6. branchial arch III; 7. pharynx; 8. notochord.

C. Section through heart
    1. telencephalon; 2. olfactory pit; 3. ventricle; 4. endocardial cushion; 5. atrium, 6. spetum primum; 7. trachea; 8. esophagus.

D. Section through liver
    1. tail; 2. A. umbilicalis, 3. liver; 4. ductus venosus; 5. bronchus; 6. posterior cardinal vein; 7. dorsal aorta; 8. upper limb bud.

E. Section through metanephros
    1. dorsal aorta; 2. coelom; 3. mesonephros; 4. mesonephric duct; 5. A. umbilicalis; 6. metanephros; 7. lower limb bud.

F. Paramedian section
    1. myelencephalon; 2. Rathke's pouch; 3. tongue; 4. telencephalon; 5. spinal ganglion; 6. truncus arteriosus; 7. atrium; 8. ventricle; 9. lung; 10. mesonephros; 11. stomach; 12. pancreas; 13. liver; 14. V. umbilicalis; 15. A. umbilicalis; 16. metanephros; 17. spinal cord.

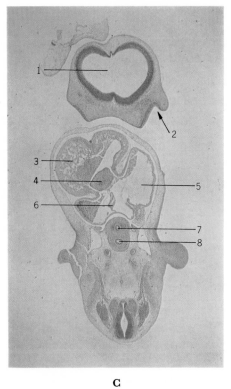

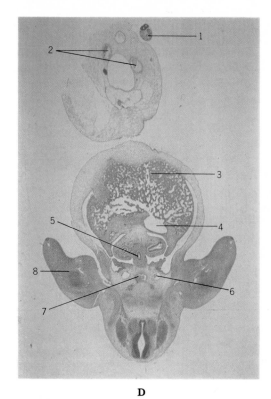

C

D

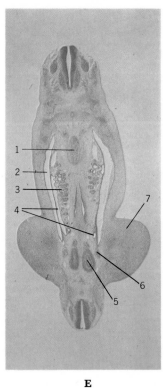

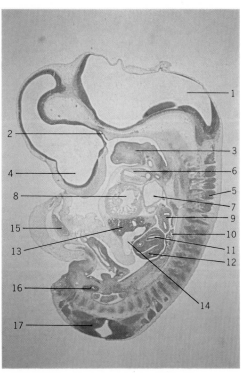

E

F

such as polydactyly by teratogens may be short for each embryo but collectively it has a long range. Therefore, it is virtually impossible clinically to predict the definite critical period in an individual case. Such a remarkable individual variability was also noted by KOBYLETZKI and GELLEN [16] in their series of embryos from induced abortion. Sources for these large variations are difficult to determine, but may partly be due to the inaccuracy of memory of the last menstrual period by patients, uncorrect history taking by doctors, irregularity of ovulation time in respect to the terminated pregnancy, aging of the gamete before ovulation, individual difference in time of fertilization and implantation, and in the rate of early development after implantation.

It should be noted that the lines for mean age relative to the developmental stage presented by STREETER and his associates [4–8] and ours are almost parallel but our line represents about 5 day older age than STREETER's for any given stages after 12. This indicates that the mean ovulation age for each stage of our embryos was 5 days more than STREETER's. Several investigators also reported a similar finding that the STREETER's standards of age for each stage in the middle and late embryonic period may be slightly too young (Table 1). This might be partly due to the facts that STREETER's human

Table 1 Estimated ovulation age in human embryos.

Carnegie stage	STREETER and associates (1942, 1945, 1948, 1951) [4–8]	Kyoto University* (1964, 1974) [14, 15]	OLIVER and PINEAU (1961) [17]	IFFY et al. (1961) [18]	JIRÁSEK (1971) [19]
11	24	27	24	—	23–26
12	26	30	26	—	26–30
13	28	32	28	28	28–32
14	29	34–35	32	32	31–35
15	31.5	36	33	34.5	35–38
16	33	38	37	37	37–42
17	35	40	41	40	42–44
18	37	42	44	43	44–48
19	39	44	47.5	45	48–51
20	41	46	50.5	47	51–53
21	43	48	52	48.5	53–54
22	45	50	54	50	54–56
23	47	52	56.5	52	56–60

* The curve for the actual mean at each stage is smoothened and the number is rounded by the author.

series included pathological specimens obtained from spontaneous abortion or ectopy and that they were supplemented with data obtained from rhesus monkeys.

Another interesting finding in Fig. 6 is that a remarkable variation and fairly older age (more than 20 days of conceptional age in most cases) of embryos are at the earliest stage (7 to 10). It may presumably be due to the clinical limitation that the pregnant women visited obstetricians seeking for induced abortion at least one week after the missed period suspecting being pregnant. Therefore, the real standard curve should be lower because our materials do not include many cases of postconceptional age less than 20 days. Indeed, an embryo at stage 6 incidentally obtained by hysterectomy was only 14 days old from the menstrual record (Fig. 3).

Fig. 7 shows the crown-rump length in relation to age. The most striking is the fact that large length variations existed for any given age. The reason is the same as described in the stage-age relationship, that is the difficulties of clinical estimation of ovulation age and the presence of some factors after ovulation. Moreover, deformities at the fixation intensify

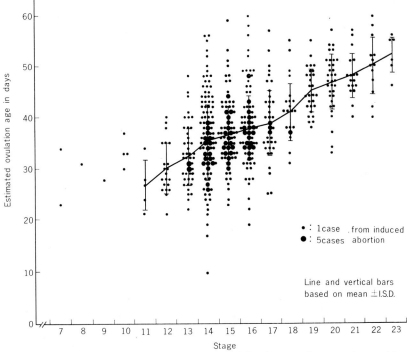

Fig. 6   Relation between estimated gestation age and developmental stages of normal human embryos. (Modified from NISHIMURA, H. et al.: Teratolcgy **10**; 1, 1974)

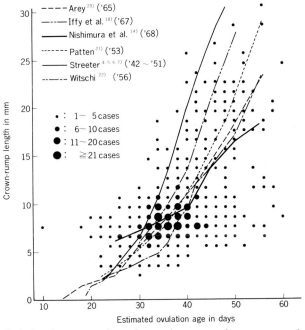

Fig. 7   Relation between estimated gestation age and crown-rump length of normal human embryos. (From NISHIMURA, H. et al.: Teratology **1**; 281, 1968)

the variations. Compared with reports by other investigators our mean line is inclined more horizontally. This indicates that mean length increases more gradually with age in our series.

STREETER's staging system based on the developmental features of various organ system is a quite useful and convenient method for description of embryos. We adopted his criteria on external features only [13]. This modified method enables us to determine the stage of embryos without resorting to internal microdissection or histology and specimens thus diagnosed can be followed immediately by the subsequent necessary studies other than histology.

Following STREETER's criteria, however, we have often encountered the dissociation of stages among some regions and even between the side. Among the regions, the limb is one of the quite variably developed organs. Therefore, we scored the points in each of the regions and the stage in which the majority of regions correspond is assigned for the specific embryo [13]. Cases which needed to be determined by "decision by the majority" were found most frequently in embryos at stages 14 and 15. Some asymmetric progress of the embryonic development was occasionally noted in the following features: appearance of vascular plexus of the head; closure of the invaginated lens placode; appearance of the retinal pigment; fusion of the eyelids; number of the pharyngeal arches; formation of the definite external ear; formation of the limb buds or digital rays. As for the internal development, there were observed quite a great variations among organs. It was already pointed out by STREETER [7] that the determination of stage in late embryos (stages 19–23) should be based on the scores of the representing histological features of some selected organs. In our study [23], such variations in the development of internal organs in an individual embryo as well as among different embryos are also remarkably noted in younger specimens below stage 18. However, it was also noted that the developmental state of various organ primordia is in general most closely correlated with the developmental stage based on our modified Carnegie staging system, the summarized evaluation of the external development.

Unfortunately, a useful criterion by developmental features in early and late fetuses has not been developed. This is largely due to the fact that only a few remarkable changes in the external and internal features occur at fetal stage. Some of the developmental changes on the surface of early fetal period to be used practically and their relationship with crown-rump length are being examined in our group (YAMANAKA et al., unpublished). The items currently evaluated for external developmental features in the early fetal stage are: superficial vascular plexus, vortex of scalp hairs, eyebrow, philtrum, tuberculum labii superior, hair in the trunk, palmar flexure lines, finger print in thumb and the first toe and gluteal cleft. However, at present, the simple and useful criteria for development are still crown-rump length and body weight. Caution should be paid on the effects of fixation. Using our materials, the relationship between crown-rump length and menstrual age is shown in Fig. 8. Range of standard deviation is fairly constant through the fetal period, indicating larger variations in the smaller specimens. Standards of organ weights for the fetuses of the whites and negroes below 500 grams were designated by the author [24], with some references on Japanese fetuses. A fairly large number of references on late fetuses especially after 28 weeks of pregnancy (from LMP) have been recently offered as the increased interests on perinatalogy, but this is out of the author's present scope.

Another practical method to evaluate the fetal development without destroying the specimens is examination of the skeletal development by means of X-ray. There have been published some references on this topic (HILL [25]; FLECKER [26]; NOVACK [27]; NOVACK and ROBERTSON [28]; O'RAHILLY and MEYER [29]; in Japanese fetuses, NOZAKI [30]; SHIMIZU [31]). However, the uniform comparison of many fetal specimens with one or two

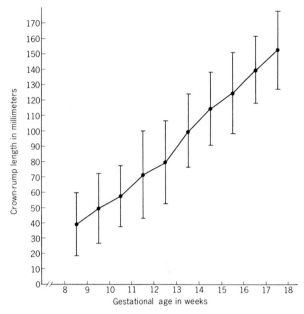

Fig. 8 Relation between estimated gestation age and crown-rump length of normal human fetuses up to the 18th week. (From Tanimura, T. and Tanioka, Y.: Comparison of embryonic and foetal development in man and rhesus monkey. In: Perkins, E.T. and O'Donoghue, P. N. (eds.) Breeding Simians for Developmental Biology. pp. 205–233, Laboratory Animals Ltd., London, 1975)

photographs is difficult because of many factors involved such as fixatives and torsion of the fixed specimens. In our laboratory, Tanaka and Nishimura [32] established the relationship of ossification centers in fetuses and crown-rump length by examining the alizarin red S stained cleared specimens. This method allows the quite complete examination of the fetal skeleton, but the specimens are not suitable for other studies. The comparative study of both methods is in progress in our laboratory for the purpose of finding an easy and reliable criterion of ossification by X-ray photograph.

Finally, it is of course important to study the normal histogenesis in the fetuses in order to understand the abnormal development in the fetal period. Histological differentiation of various organs of human fetuses from the 9th week of gestation to term was compared with that of the rheses macaques from days 50 to 100 [33]. Some other pertinent references on histogenesis in Japanese fetuses were also included. Some organs show the quite similar pattern of differentiation between the two species, while others such as adrenals and testis demonstrate remarkable differences on histological development.

ABNORMAL DEVELOPMENT

By abnormal development it implies the developmental processes which deviate outside the normal range of variations. Abnormal development originating in the prenatal stage is called congenital anomalies or birth defects. Death *in utero*, gross structural anomalies (malformations), growth retardation, and other microscopic, biochemical or functional abnormalities should be included even at the human embryonic stage just as used in the later stage or in the experimental embryology. For the epidemiological study using the fixed embryonic specimens, however, death *in utero* and malformations are the essential and most important items to be examined. These two are occasionally called developmental or pregnancy wastage. Sometimes growth retardation is also referred to.

Establishment of the criteria for death *in utero* and malformations is the first step in the embryo study. The structural abnormalities detected in the embryos may be classified into the following three categories. 1. The established malformations similar to those seen in newborns (eg. polydactyly). 2. Minor anomalies or variations as frequently seen also in newborns (eg. accessory nipples). 3. Transitionary anomalies particularly seen in the specific stage of embryos, the final destiny of which is not always certain because no corresponding type of malformation has been confirmed in newborns or the affected region itself is usually regenerated in the later course of development (eg. tubercle in the branchial region). Since the embryos are on the way to rapid differentiation and growth, that is in the period of organogenesis, diagnosis of malformations should always be made by taking into consideration the developmental stage of the specimen and the completed definite form found in fetuses or newborns. One should be cautions in determining an anomalous state as belonging to definite malformation. It may just merely represent a localized growth retardation since many of the malformations are regarded to originate in developmental arrest or unusual delay of the development. Typical examples are unfused nasal processes (cleft lip) and non-fusion of interventricular septum (ventricular septal defect).

Among 6,936 undamaged embryos or embryonic sacs, 1,103 (15.9%) are diagnosed to be dead *in utero*. Some details on morphology are given in the section A.

Among 5,833 undamaged embryos at stage 7 to 23 (alive *in utero*), 113 (1.93%) are found to have external malformations. As the appearance of malformations depends on the stage of embryos, we arbitrarily classified these stages into the three subgroups (Table 2). The prevalence in the earlier phase (stages 7–15) is distinctly low as compared with the other two advanced stages. This is self-evident because some malformations such as hand and foot anomalies are not to be detected in the earlier stages.

The more important is the comparison of the rate of a certain specific type of malformations between the embryos and the newborns. The embryonic specimens only at and over the stage when the definite form in the region concerned is established, are to be checked and compared. Since embryos slightly damaged but intact in the questioned region may be added, the increased number of specimens definitely improve the efficiency for the analysis. Prevalences of some representative types of malformations in the embryos in comparison with the data in newborns are listed in Table 3. It is clear from this comparison that the prevalence of most types of common malformations at the embryonic stage is fairly higher (often ten times or more) than that found in newborns. A common-sensed explanation for this finding is that many of such malformed embryos are lost in spontaneous abortions during the later course of pregnancy. It is supported also by many reports that anomalies are more often found in the spontaneously aborted specimens. Another explanation is that some of the malformations at the embryonic stage only indicate a sign of intrauterine growth retardation and may be repaired later, or slight deviations in the embryonic stage may not progress so that such alternations are hidden by the rapidly growing surrounding tissues and lost in the later course of the development.

Yearly change of the prevalence of malformed embryos in the present study is shown in Table 4. The prevalence at each year has been fairly constant between 1965 and 1970 except in 1968 when the prevalence was significantly higher as compared with the mean between 1965 and 1967. This was found to be due to a slight increase of total limb defects at this period as described later more in details. Another significant and striking finding in

Table 2   Prevalence of externally malformed embryos by developmental stage and corresponding figures in newborns.

Embryos			Newborns
Carnegie stage	Total no.	Prevalence of malformed (%)	Prevalence of malformed (%)
7–15	1,778	1.29	0.66 (MORIYAMA, 1964) [34] 0.78 (TSUKAMOTO, 1956) [35]
16–18	2,334	2.27	0.83 (MITANI and KITAMURA, 1968) [36] 0.91 (BABA et al., 1967) [37]
19–23	1,679	2.20	1.02 (NEEL, 1958) [38] 1.11 (MORIYAMA and MINAGAWA, 1974) [39]

Table 3   Prevalence of certain malformations in embryos compared with that in newborns.

Type	Prevalence (%)		
	Embryos (Stage*)	Newborns	P. Embryos/P. Newborns
Holoprosencephaly	0.73 (14–23)	0.01	73
Exencephaly or anencephaly	0.27 (11–23)	0.06	ca. 5
Myeloschisis or spina bifida	0.34 (12–23)	0.02	17
Cleft lip	0.43 (18–23)	0.17	ca. 3
Polydactyly hand	1.41 (17–23)	0.093	ca. 15
foot	0.37 (18–23)	0.043	ca. 9
Cardiac malformations	3.49 (21–23)	0.8	ca. 4

* By Carnegie stage.

Table 4   Yearly change of prevalence of malformed embryos.**

Year	No. of undamaged embryos	No. of malformed	%
1965	720	13	1.81
1966	952	15	1.58
1967	862	13	1.51
1968	871	23	2.64*
1969	790	9	1.14
1970	557	11	1.97
1971	418	16	3.83*
1972	490	15	3.06*
1973	242	9	3.72*
Total	5,902	124	2.10

 * $p < 0.05$ as compared to the mean 1965–1967 and 1969–1970.
** From TANIMURA, T.: The use of induced abortuses for monitoring. In: Shepard, T. H. et al. (eds.) Methods for Detection of Environmental Agents that Produce Congenital Defects. pp. 197–201, North-Holland, Amsterdam, 1975.

Table 4 is the higher prevalence of total malformations in the recent 3 years (1971–1973). It was noted that the prevalences of neural tube defects (exencephaly and myeloschisis) and holoprosencephaly are fairly constant during these 9 years, while the prevalence of limb defects in 1971 and 1972 is higher than that in the previous years (Table 5). The prevalence of the preaxial polydactyly in hand is especially high in 1971. However, no specific environmental agents have been identified as factors associated with these high prevalences due to a smallness of the sample size.

Analysis of the factors associated with the occurrence of the congenital malformations is one of the final goals in this epidemiological study. It is very important as the findings are expected to contribute directly to the prevention of malformations. Since the number of the specific type of malformation is not yet sufficient, only general survey for the correlation of the maternal factors with total malformation or death *in utero* will be described in the following. It should be emphasized here that the methods and findings are still preliminary, and it is hoped that when a sufficient number of the malformed or *in utero* dead specimens are obtained, the data will be put into the computor and more refined methods as multivariate analysis will be applied.

1) GENITAL BLEEDING DURING PREGNANCY

Table 6 shows that malformation or death *in utero* occurs more frequently in women with a history of genital bleeding during early pregnancy than in those without, and particularly so in cases of the patients who were performed curettage due to threatened abortion. The higher prevalence in death *in utero* is quite concordant with the data shown in the older fetuses or newborns. Controversial results have been yielded whether bleeding in early pregnancy is associated with malformations in infants. KNÖRR [40], SAKAKURA [41], JUNG [42], KRAUS and SABBAGH [43], WALLNER et al. [44], RUMEAN-ROUQUETTE et al. [45], and WALLNER et al. [46] reported the positive association while some others (eg. MAU and NETTER [47]) did not find such association. One fact should be noted from this table that almost half of the cases terminated for threatened abortions resulted in externally normal live embryos. It is quite interesting to investigate whether these externally normal embryos are perfectly normal also in internal structures and from the cytogenetic point of view. This would give some suggestions to the way to treat patients under threatened abortion so as to relieve some innocent embryos.

2) PARAMETERS DIRECTLY RELATED TO REPRODUCTION

a. Maternal age

The prevalences of death *in utero* and malformation at the embryonic stage were compared between median aged cases (20–35) classified into the three subgroups (Table 7). In case of malformation, a possible tendency, although not significant, that increased age may be associated with higher prevalence of malformations, while for embryos dead *in utero* no such relation was seen. In order to examine the effects of extreme maternal ages on early conceptuses, the prevalences of malformed embryos and those dead *in utero* among the youngest (less than 20) and the oldest (over 41) were compared with the above mentioned median aged group. There is no significant difference in prevalence of malformed embryos or embryos dead *in utero* between the youngest and the median aged group. This may be partly due to the fact that very young mothers of less than 17 years old were not included in the present study. As for the old aged group, a significant increase of the death *in utero* was shown as compared to the median aged group, but age effects on prevalence of malformations were not recognized. This is in contrast to the results of several observation in newborns. The main reason for such discordance may be due to the facts that firstly there is a difference between the observed types of anomalies in the present study and those in others, and secondly, the cases of the aged group in the present study consisted of multigravidas with good reproductive capability and did not include any of primigravid cases.

b. Parity

Parity in this analysis refers to frequency of previous pregnancies (prior to the terminated one) which were maintained for 28 weeks of the menstrual age or more regardless of the live birth or stillbirth. Comparison of average parity among the normal live, malformed live and dead *in utero* groups demonstrated that mothers with the embryos dead *in utero* show parity lower than those of the normal group. Parity of the mother with malformed

Table 5   Yearly change of prevalences of some representative types of malformations in embryos.**

Year	Limb defect (stage 17 and over)			Exencephaly and myeloschisis (stage 12 and over)		Holoprosencephaly (stage 13 and over)	
	No. of specimens examined	Total limb malformations Prevalence(%)	Preaxial poly- dactyly(hand) Prevalence(%)	No. of specimens examined	Prevalence (%)	No. of specimens examined	Prevalence (%)
1965	244	0.82	0.41	715	0.98	700	0.71
1966	304	0.99	0.33	945	0.63	933	0.43
1967	381	1.31	1.05	858	0.35	852	0.70
1968	474	2.11	0.84	861	0.70	853	0.82
1969	432	0.69	0.23	787	0.13	779	0.39
1970	311	0.96	0.32	555	0.18	553	0.72
1971	229	5.68*	3.06*	413	0.73	413	0.48
1972	280	3.21*	1.07	487	0.62	486	0.82
1973	144	2.78	1.39	240	0.42	235	1.28
Total	2,799	1.86	0.82	5,861	0.53	5,804	0.65

 * p<0.05 as compared to the mean 1966–1970.
** From Tanimura, T.: The use of induced abortuses for monitoring. In: Shepard, T. H. et al. (eds.) Methods for Detection of Environmental Agents that Produce Congenital Defects. pp. 197–201, North-Holland, Amsterdam, 1975.

Table 6   Maternal genital bleeding and pathological embryos.

Genital bleeding	Total no.	No. of malformed (%)[+]	No. of dead *in utero* (%)[++]
−	2,771	44 (1.6)	76 (2.7)
+	395	13 (3.6)**	38 (9.6)**
++*	390	24 (9.8)**	145 (37.2)**

 * With symptoms of threatened abortion at the time of operation.
** p<0.05.
 [+] Per cent of live embryos,   [++] Per cent of total embryos.

Table 7   Maternal age and pathological embryos.

Maternal age	Total no.	No. of malformed (%)[+]	No. of dead *in utero* (%)[++]
17–19	153	1 (0.8)	27 (17.7)
20–24	1,271	14 (1.3)	215 (16.9)
25–29	1,874	30 (2.0)	339 (18.1)
30–34	1,789	42 (2.8)	276 (15.4)
41–	405	5 (1.6)	84 (20.7)*

 * p<0.05 as compared with the age group 20–34.
 [+] Per cent of live embryos;   [++] Per cent of total embryos.

Table 8   Pathological embryos and previous induced abortion.

Maternal age	Normal live			Malformed live			Dead *in utero*		
	20–24	25–29	30–34	20–24	25–29	30–34	20–24	25–29	30–34
Parity	0.35	1.35	1.97	0.36	0.93 ↓ *	1.95	0.25 ↓	0.93 ↓	1.51 ↓
Spontaneous abortion	0.07	0.21	0.27	0.14	0.23	0.36	0.21 ↑ **	0.43 ↑	0.51 ↑
Induced abortion	0.70	1.00	1.42	0.93	0.63 ↓	1.07	0.48 ↓	0.69 ↓	1.06 ↓
Gravidity	1.12	2.56	3.66	1.43	1.79 ↓	3.38	0.94 ↓	2.05 ↓	3.07 ↓

 * Arrow (↓) indicates the value is significantly lower as compared with the corresponding one.
** Arrow (↑) indicates the value is significantly higher as compared with the corresponding one.

embryos was lower only in the age group 25–29 than that of the normal group (Table 8). It is also disclosed that nulliparous women have higher frequency of having embryos dead *in utero* than the parous (eg. 2.69% vs 1.56% in the 20–24 aged group), and that the probability of having embryos dead *in utero* increases as the age advances in the nulliparous patients.

c. Spontaneous abortion

Overall prevalence of the externally malformed embryos among the mothers who experienced spontaneous abortion is 2.83% and slightly higher, though not significantly different, than those (1.94%) without history of the previous spontaneous abortion. Prevalence of death *in utero* (12.4%) is naturally higher among the women with history of spontaneous abortion than those (7.4%) without such history.

d. Induced abortion

Late sequalae of induced abortion, especially possible effects on subsequent fertility and pregnancy outcome have been issues of complicated discussion. Increased risk of spontaneous abortion especially after the operation on the primigravida and subsequent ectopic pregnancy has been seriously debated. In Japan, Nakajima et al. [48] raised the question and many discussions followed without consensus. WHO Experts Committee [49] did not disclose any conclusion on the possible harmful effects on the subsequent pregnancy.

Analysis of the specimens and their records in our collection revealed that risk of having malformed embryos is not related to the number of the previous induced abortions. Prevalence of dead embryos *in utero* is significantly reduced as the number of the previous abortions increases. This negative correlation was remarkable among the cases in which mothers were operated for the presence of threatened abortion, but it was not observed in cases with no maternal genital bleeding (Table 9). A case-controlled study between the

Table 9 Frequency of previous induced abortion and dead embryos as classified by the presence of genital bleeding.

Genital bleeding	Induced abortion	Maternal age		
		20–24	25–29	30–34
Threatened abortion	0	70.5%* ⎫	73.6% ⎫	64.8% ⎫
	1–2	56.5% ⎬ $\chi^2=4.7$	48.5% ⎬ $\chi^2=41.9$	60.4% ⎬ $\chi^2=13.0$
	≥ 3	44.4% ⎭	17.2% ⎭	29.0% ⎭
No genital bleeding	0	8.3% ⎫	6.7% ⎫	8.3% ⎫
	1–2	6.7% ⎬ $\chi^2=1.5$	6.3% ⎬ $\chi^2=0.4$	5.1% ⎬ $\chi^2=3.8$
	≥ 3	4.2% ⎭	7.9% ⎭	6.5% ⎭

* Dead cases % of the total induced cases.

group of embryos dead *in utero* and the normal live embryos matched for maternal age and gravidity also showed the negative association. Such an effect might be partly due to higher fertility of mothers who had more frequent induced abortions. Conclusively, so far, induced abortion did not show clear-cut adverse effects on embryonic development of the subsequent pregnancy.

e. Use of some contraceptive measures around the establishment of the present pregnancy

The control was matched for maternal age, gravidity and season of conception. Our materials included very few cases with the history of use of IUD, pill and jelly possibly because of their efficacy and their limited use by Japanese women. Therefore, the data are not sufficient to be analyzed for possible adverse effects in early conceptuses obtained as unsuccessful outcome. Seventy two cases in which pregnancy was established despite the use of rhythm method (Ogino method) were compared with 233 cases without the experience of rhythm method around the conception. No significant difference was obtained between the two groups as for malformations and death *in utero*.

f.   Coital date

We have obtained 83 cases of the embryonic specimens in which a fruitful coital date is definitely known. It was shown that pregnancy can be established at any phase of menstrual cycle as far as the coital date is concerned: 23 cases at precycle, 46 cases at midcycle and 14 cases at postcycle. Among these 14 cases in which the pregnancy was established by the coitus at postcycle, conceptuses of 5 cases (35.8%) were found dead *in utero* and one of the dead embryo showed exencephaly. Further large scaled studies are needed to confirm if the pregnancies arising from the possible aged ovum by the coitus at postcycle may result in higher rate of pregnancy wastage, because it will give an important information on the potential adverse effects on the progeny by the failure of contraception with rhythm method.

g.   Season at conception

No evidence was shown of association between season of conception and the malformation or death *in utero*.

3)   GENETIC FACTORS

Our protocols include very few items on genetic items, because asking questions on heredity by obstetricians in private clinics is difficult and seems not uniform among doctors. Frequency of stated consanguinity is (2.3%) is somewhat lower than the reported general incidence in Japan. The association of parental consanguinity with the prevalence of embryos dead *in utero* was examined and the preliminary analysis showed that in the group of threatened abortion, the consanguineous group showed a significantly higher prevalence of death *in utero* compared with the non-consanguineous group.

4)   SOME OTHER ENVIRONMENTAL FACTORS

Preliminary analysis was done with respect to the following 28 items described in the protocol (Maternal smoking, alcohol drinking, common cold, diabetes, hyperthyroidism, tuberculosis, syphilis, anemia, hypertension, cardiac diseases, hepatic diseases, renal diseases, lumbago, radiation, vaccination, and intake of the following drugs: adrenocorticoids, drugs for cold, vitamins, drugs for gastrointestinal organs, analgesia, antibiotics, tranquilizers, hypnotics, antihistamins, antituberculous drugs, emmenagogues, antiemetica, and drug for anemia). A significant positive association was shown between the malformations and hyperthyroidism, and between death *in utero* and each of maternal irradiation, intake of drugs for anemia, antibiotics and vitamins. Of course, further collection of materials is needed and analysis such as separation of association with disease from drug intake should be prudently done.

Finally the possible relationship between the ovulation age and developmental stage of the malformed embryos was examined. A preliminary analysis showed that the majority of malformed embryos had a greater ovulation age than normal embryos. This may account for the theory that embryonic wastage is often associated with aging of ovum. Another possibility is that marked retardation of general development occurs in malformed embryos. The study further examined major four types of malformations. Ovulation age of embryos with holoprosencephaly, exencephaly and myeloschisis, preaxial polydactyly of the hand and cleft lip was compared with the standard [14] for normal Japanese embryos. It was demonstrated that the development of a large proportion of the cases with severe malformations such as holoprosencephaly, and exencephaly and myeloschisis was significantly below the standard, whereas this tendency was not significant among other mild malformations [50].

In the following some noteworthy findings obtained in our laboratory are described separately in accordance with embryonic death *in utero* or types of anomalies.

1) EMBRYONIC DEATH IN UTERO

External signs of resorption or maceration of the embryos may serve as an indication of intrauterine death. Even after fixation, brownish color of skin, soft unelastic property of body, and indistinctness and disorganization of the peripheral parts such as limbs and chin indicate the death *in utero*. In order to confirm whether some dead cases had been over-looked by this macroscopic method, we examined histologically 382 specimens which were considered alive *in utero* under the stereomicroscope. Only one of the cases, obtained from a mother with threatened abortion, showed a slight degenerative change indicating possible embryonic death. Thus, it is concluded that our determination of death by external observation is quite reliable.

Anatomically, most of the cases with embryonic death *in utero* is without embryonic remnant, so-called empty sac (Table 10), followed by severely resorbed or deformed embryos as PATTEN [21] describes cylindrical.

Table 10   Anatomical classification of embryos dead *in utero*.*

Embryo completely resorbed (empty sac)	Embryo being resorbed or macerated		
	Embryonic mass with indistinct external features	Developmental stage determined	
		Roughly	Distinctly
164 (64.0%)	32 (12.7%)	46 (18.2%)	13 (5.1%)

* From NISHIMURA, H.: An analysis of ten thousand induced abortion. Proceedings of the Sixth World Congress on Fertility and Sterility, Tel Aviv 1968. The Israel Academy of Sciences and Humanities, Jerusalem, 1970.

Histologically, such regions as central nervous system and epithelia in the digestive system are most severely affected. Epidermis may be the last tissue which preserves the apparent cell and tissue structure. In embryos dead *in utero,* abnormal proliferations or fold formation of the disintegrated central nervous system is often predominant, although it is not clear that this phenomenon may show the cause of death.

In a small and severely resorbed dead embryonic mass, it is very difficult to differentiate even histologically postmortem changes from changes which took place during the dyeing process in a specific part of the embryo or gross structural defect which already existed while alive *in utero*. Even in the more advanced stage, it is often difficult to distinguish specific type of malformation from postmortem changes or artificial damages at the time of operation. Therefore, we believe that those specimens should be classified collectively into dead *in utero* group, although some others (eg. POLAND [51]) tried to differentiate complete disorganization.

It is an established fact that cytogenetic anomalies are frequently found in the living parts of conceptuses in the spontaneous abortion. Earlier reports did not describe the states of embryos. However, recently, efforts have been initiated to link the morphology of embryos dead *in utero* to cytogenetic findings [52–56]. Although most of our materials are fixed and unfortunately unsuitable for cytogenetic analysis, it is hoped that more efforts will be exerted to clarify the relationship between the embryonic death or developmental defects and cytogenetic anomalies.

Many factors are considered responsible for or associated with embryonic death. One of the fundamental associations is of course is maternal genital bleeding as already described. It should be noted that in about a half of the cases with threatened abortion and about one-third of the cases which terminated in spontaneous abortions, the embryo was considered alive *in utero*. This may give some reasons that the patients with threatened abortion should be treated accordingly, if they wish to have babies.

2) ANENCEPHALY AND SPINA BIFIDA

Anencephaly and spina bifida are two of the most eminent and easily recognizable malformations in the central nervous system. Although the clinical significance of both malformations is very much different, the conditions have been customarily discussed together because of the similar pathogenesis involved.

Anencephaly has especially attracted the attention of teratologists not only for many problems on pathogenesis, etiology, and epidemiology but also from the viewpoint of experimental teratology. Exencephaly, the supposedly equivalent precursor of human anencephaly, is one of the most easily induced malformations in experimental animals. The characteristic form of anencephaly in humans at birth is not to be seen in the human embryos, since the condition observed at term is the result of the secondary degenerative modification in the late intrauterine life. On the contrary, the main type of gross anomalies found in the human embryonic stage is "exencephaly" showing the characteristics of

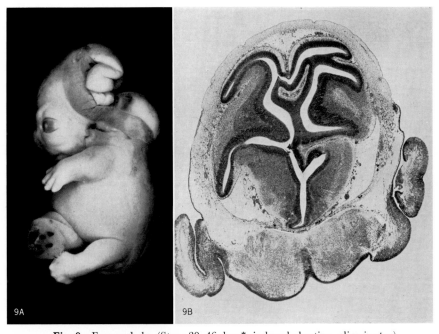

Fig. 9   Exencephaly. (Stage 20, 46 days*, induced abortion, alive *in utero*)
A.   Lateral view. Calvarium is absent in the occipital region and the exposed brain shows overgrowth.
B.   Histology (transverse section). Note the everted overgrown rhombencephalon and complicated foldings in the telencephalon.
*   Average age for normal embryos at the corresponding stage is given.

protruded open neural tube without the covering of the future skull and scalp tissues, just
as seen in the exencephalic rodent fetuses either experimentally induced or spontaneously
observed (Fig. 9 A).

Among 5,835 undamaged embryos exencephaly was in 16 cases (0.27%). This figure is
far higher than the reported figures 0.06 per cent among 144,670 newborns [36].

Histological examination of these exencephalic embryos reveals that these malformed
embryos have in most cases non-closed neural tubes. Some embryos show sign of overgrowth
although it is not a universal feature (Fig. 9 B). HAMERSMA [57] reviewed 41 cases of
human embryos with exencephaly as well as 24 embryos with myeloschisis, and concluded
that anomalies occur if the neural tube does not close. Despite the prevailing cases in favor
of the view that most of human exencephalies are derived from the primary non-closure of
the neural tube, the less popular but attractive theory of secondary reopening of the once
closed neural tube is interesting [58, 59]. Some embryos with nuchal blebs show the rupture
of the central nervous system (see section 9), and it should be prudently discussed whether
these embryos may develop to anencephaly *in utero*. Degenerative hemangiomatous tissue
is a characteristic form of human anencephaly at term and a theory that human anencephaly is a result of vascular malformation should be evaluated by the further studies on development of brain arteries of the human exencephalic and normal embryos.

Spina bifida presents a variety of discussion on the treatment and a more important
clinical entity than anencephaly. The primary phenomenon of human spina bifida is
ascribed to myeloschisis, or the separation of the spinal canal. Non-closure of the posterior
neuropore might be a common feature, because the most frequently affected site in the
embryos is the lumbosacral region, the posterior neuropore. It shows sometimes mound-
like elevation with clear slit for the central canal (Fig. 10). Occasionally the proliferation is
not so manifest and bank-like structures with neural groove something like a gorge between
them are noted. Histologically the neural tissues of these regions are pronounced and

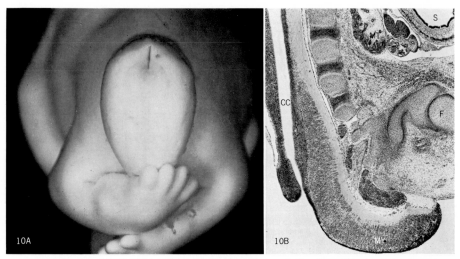

Fig. 10 Myeloschisis. (Stage 22, 50 days, induced abortion, alive *in utero*)
A. Caudal view. (From SWINYARD, C. A. et al.: Pediatric Annals **2**; 26, 1973)
B. Histology (sagittal section). A disc-like elevation showing the overgrowth of the myeloschitic
tissues at the lumbosacral region is observed. Note an open central canal at the cranial end
of the myeloschisis.
CC, central canal; F, femur; MT, metanephros; MY, myeloschitic region; S, stomach.
This case is combined with left cleft lip.

concordant with the overgrowth described by PATTEN [60]. LEMIRE et al. [61] reported a case of caudal myeloschisis in a 5 mm embryo and described a defective external limiting membrane of the neural tube in addition to the overgrowth. Whether this overgrowth is a primary cause of myeloschisis or a secondary phenomenon of the open remained neural tube is difficult to determine. Examination of the large number of the embryos with myeloschisis gives us an impression that the overgrowth may be a result. However, we found a case of the localized overgrowth of the lumbar region of the neural tissues at stage 11, when the neural tube remains open in normal cases (Fig. 11). It should be emphasized that these regions usually do not show degenerative signs such as necrosis and have normally developed neural-crest cells.

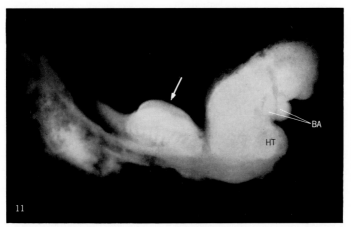

Fig. 11 Myeloschisis. (Stage 11, 24 days, induced abortion, alive *in utero*) Lateral view. The neural tube in the caudal regions remains broadly open as indicated by arrow. Localized overgrowth of the nervous tissues is remarkable.
BA, branchial arches; HT, heart.

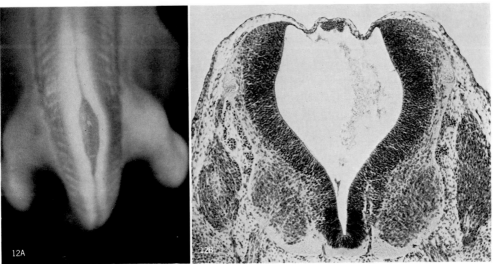

Fig. 12 Hydromyelia. (Stage 17, 40 days, spontaneous abortion, alive *in utero*)
A. Dorsal view.
B. Histology (horizontal section). The central canal is dilated and appears cystic at the lumbar region. No rupture of the skin or meninges is noted. Brain and the ventricles are normal.

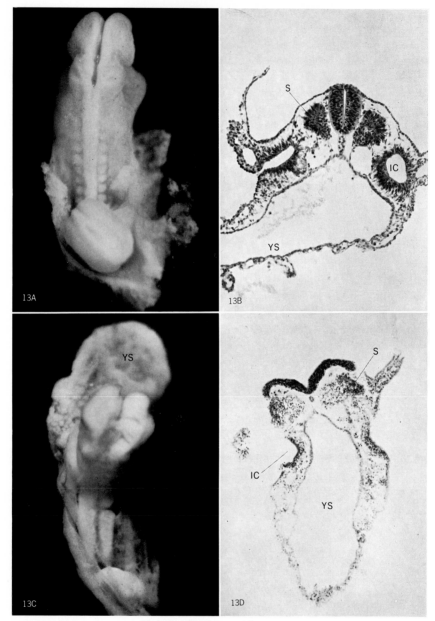

Fig. 13 Total dysraphism.

A. Dorsal view of the normal embryo. (Stage 11, 24 days, induced abortion, alive *in utero*)
   Anterior and posterior neuropores are visible. The neural tube is widely closed.

B. Histology of the normal embryo A. (transverse section)
   The neural tube is closed and the somite (S) and the intraembryonic coelom (IC) is well
   developed.
   YS, yolk sac.

C. Dorsal view of the dysraphic embryo. (Stage 11, 24 days, spontaneous abortion, alive *in utero*)
   The closure of the neural folds is totally absent.
   YS, yolk sac.

D. Histology of the dysraphic embryo. (transverse section)
   Note the open neural fold without overgrowth, the poorly developed somite (S) and the intra-
   embryonic coelom (IC).
   YS, yolk sac.

It might be added that a transparent slit-like area is sometimes seen in the lumbar region, and histologically it is confirmed that this may be an early stage of embryonic hydromyelia, with the thin wall of roof plate and wide space in the central canal but without any rupture (Fig. 12).

Five cases of complete dysraphism (total non-closure of the neural folds) were found among our collection (Fig. 13). DEKABAN and BARTELMEZ [62] reported a case of complete dysraphism in a 14 somite embryo. Three cases of the present cases were 1.5–2.4 mm in length and had 14 to 16 somites corresponding to stage 11 [63]. All five embryos show a few mitotic figures with severe necrosis. Considering the history that the maternal genital bleeding was recorded in four out of the five cases, those embryos are judged to die *in utero* sooner or later. These findings support the view that non-closure of the neural folds has the important role in pathogenesis of certain types of central nervous system malformations in man.

3) HOLOPROSENCEPHALY

Holoprosencephaly, malformations of forebrain associated with related eye and face anomalies, is one of the most common malformations found in embryos and various grades of abnormalities in brain and the related region are observed. Therefore, it is considered to be an adequate material for the study of pathogenesis in the central nervous system malformation. DeMyer et al. [64] classified holoprosencephaly into the five types according to the severity of facial defects (I. cyclopia, II. ethmocephaly, III. cebocephaly, IV. with median cleft lip, V. with median philtrum-premaxilla anlage). The most severe type of holoprosencephaly is cyclopia, the grotesque feature of which attracted the attention of people in the old days and was already cited in the Greek mythology. The unique features are univentricular prosencephalon, defect of olfactory bulbs, and various grades of median facial defects—hypotelorism and fused eyes, nose defect (sometimes proboscis), cleft lip, etc. The anomaly is to be primarily caused by defect of the prechordal mesoderm which results in the deficient separation and morphogenesis of the prosencephalon leading to form single ventricle, absence of corpus callosum, incomplete pituitary, lack of olfactory lobes, etc. Characteristic facial features might be caused by the missing or incomplete midfacial development, especially in the median nasal process. Only about 10 cases of the human embryonic holoprosencephaly have been reported so far, but most of them were dead *in utero* and no detailed histology was presented (LESER [65]; 2 cases by MALL [66]; POLITZER [67]; MITANI and HASHIZUME [68]; LLORCA RODRIGO [69]; 2 cases by ORTS LLORCA [70]; SUZUMURA et al. [71]; ASAMI [72]; ROUX [52]).

Eighty-one cases of holoprosencephaly were found among 11,068 embryos (stages 14–23, 6 to 28 mm crown-rump length and 34 to 52 days of gestation according to our standard (NISHIMURA et al. [14]), in our collection [73]. The prevalence is 0.73 per cent and about 75

Table 11   Prevalence (%) of holoprosencephaly in embryos (stages 14–23).

Maternal history	Total no.	Embryos		
		live *in utero*	dead *in utero*	total
Induced abortion				
Without genital bleeding	8,967	0.25	4.80	0.32
With genital bleeding (not due to threatened abortion)	1,159	0.28	7.29	0.86
Theatened abortion	788	1.53	7.96	3.68
Spontaneous abortion	154	7.90	8.62	8.44
Total	11,068	0.35	7.24	0.73

times higher than that (0.01% by MITANI and KITAMURA [36]) reported in newborns (Table 11). The prevalence is especially high in the group of spontaneous abortion (8.4%) and in that of threatened abortion (3.7%). Forty-five cases (56%) showed signs of intrauterine death. It might be added that diagnosis of holoprosencephaly in embryos dead *in utero* is relatively easy, especially due to hypotelorism determined by long persisted pigments of eyes even in severely resorbed embryos.

By the external examination, they were classified as follows: cyclopia with single lens, 9 cases; cyclopia with double lenses, 32 cases; ethmocephaly, 7; cebocephaly, 22; hypoplasia of nasal process with slight hypotelorism, 11 (Figs. 14 and 15). Some embryos in the last category show median cleft lip. Twenty-nine cases (36%) had combined external malformations outside the face such as polydactyly (17 cases), myeloschisis (7 cases) and hypoplasia of the upper limb (3 cases). Most of polydactylies observed were of preaxial type in hand, although it is stated that holoprosencephaly in newborns due to D trisomy is sometimes combined with postaxial polydactyly. By histological examination of 12 cases of well preserved holoprosencephalic embryos alive *in utero*, only two cases were found to have combined internal anomalies; one is hypoplasia of adrenal cortex and the other focal vesicle in forebrain. Histological examination of holoprosencephalic embryos revealed univentricular hypoplastic telencephalon in all cases, frequently hypoplastic hypophysis primordium, occasional fusion of the oculomotor nerves of both sides, dilatation of the fourth ventricle, and almost normal existence of the V, VII & VIII, IX and X ganglia. Even in an externally perfect cyclopia, the lens showed some incomplete division.

Positive associations with genital bleeding during pregnancy, low parity (1.26 vs 1.71 in the control), and higher menstrual age by 2.5 days compared to the standard age of normal embryos at the same developmental stage were observed. Parental age, consanguinity, maternal diseases and drug uptake were not found significantly associated.

Recently we observed a case of holoprosencephaly at stage 13 when lens vesicle is not formed. It is hoped that some abnormal development of the precordal mesoderm and prosencephalon is detected by histological examination of younger embryos at and before stage 12. Holoprosencephaly is relatively easily produced in lower animals and in mammals by various methods including administration of chemicals (reviewed by ROGERS [74]). Therefore, comparative examination of holoprosencephalic embryos at the various developmental stages is expected to elucidate the mechanism of formation of this interesting midfacial-brain anomaly in man.

4)   CLEFT LIP AND PALATE

Cleft lip and palate is one of the most commonly found anomalies in Japanese. It is generally agreed that the prevalence is higher than that observed in Caucasian or Negro population (reviewed by WARKANY [75]). It is also clinically important to know the etiology and pathogenesis of these anomalies in order to contribute to the prevention and treatment of this face anomaly.

An interesting investigation on the cleft lip and palate in the spontaneously aborted human embryos and fetuses at the age of 6 to 19 weeks by KRAUS et al. [76] showed that 60 specimens with cleft lip and/or palate among 3,216 cases (1.88%). However, the true prevalence in the early human prenatal population has never been investigated, although several incidentally observed cases with cleft and/or palate at the initiating stage have been reported [77–84].

The embryos at stages 18 to 23 (14 to 28 mm, 42 to 52 days), which arose from the pregnancies terminated for socioeconomical indications, were carefully examined under the stereomicroscope. The embryos with cleft lip were decapitated and most of them were

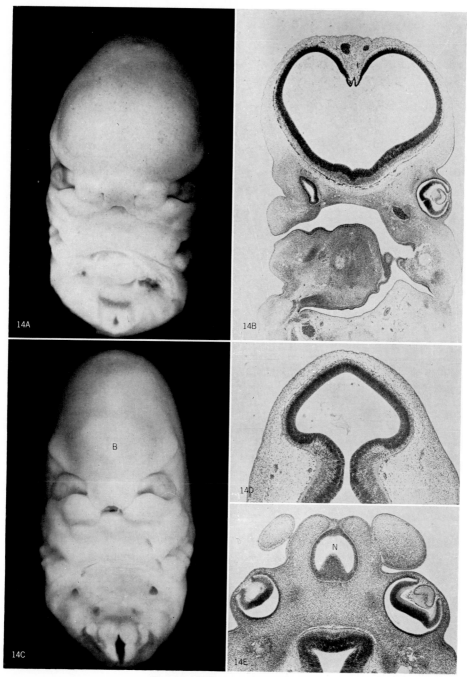

Fig. 14   Holoprosencephaly (I).

A.   Face of the normal embryo. (Stage 18, 42 days, induced abortion, alive *in utero*) Frontal view.
B.   Histology of A. (transverse section) Note the well formed bilateral cerebral vesicles. It happen-
      ed to be obliquely sectioned, the right eye and the left nasal cavity is observed in this section.
C.   Holoprosencephaly (cebocephalic type). (Stage 18, 42 days, induced abortion, alive *in utero*)
      Note the hypotelorism and the hypoplasia of the forebrain (B) and the median nasal region.
D.   Histology of C. (transverse section through telencephalon)
      Note the hypoplastic undivided telencephalon.
E.   Histology of C. (transverse section through eyes)
      Note the incomplete single nasal cavity (N) located in the median.

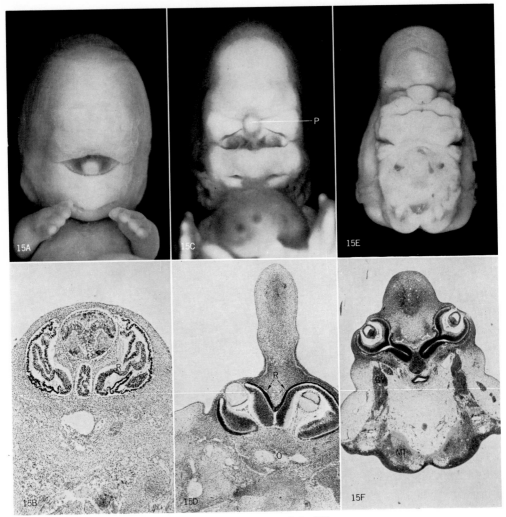

Fig. 15 Holoprosencephaly (II).

A. Cyclopia. (Stage 18, 42 days, spontaneous abortion, dead *in utero*)
     Frontal view.

B. Histology of A. (transverse section)
     Although it is macroscopically the complete cyclopia, a single lens (L) shows the slight indica-
     tion of the division by histology.
     R, retina.

C. Cyclopia with proboscis. (Stage 18, 42 days, induced abortion, alive *in utero*)
     Frontal view.
     Prominent proboscis (P) is visible above the single orbit.

D. Histology of C. (transverse section)
     It has a single nasal cavity and the pigment layer of the retina (R) is common to both eyes. The
     oculomotoric nerve (O) is fused.

E. Ethmocephaly. (Stage 17, 40 days, induced abortion, alive *in utero*)
     Note the microcephaly with a single ventricle of the forebrain and the large proboscis. This
     case is combined with exencephaly.

F. Histology of E. (transverse section)
     Note the hypotelorism. Basis of the metencephalon (MT) is broadly exposed.
     GV, ganglion n. V.

histologically studied. Preliminary results were reported by MATSUDA et al. [85] followed by the detailed report [86]. In addition, the fetuses of crown-rump length ranging from 46 to 160 mm were also examined for facial defects.

Among 5,117 embryos, 22 specimens with cleft lip were found (0.43%) comprising 8 bilateral, 13 unilateral and one median type [86] (Fig. 16). This prevalence is about two

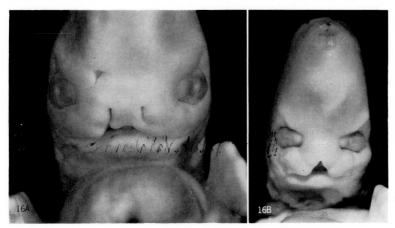

Fig. 16   Cleft lip.
A.   Lateral cleft lip. (Stage 18, 42 days, abortion, alive *in utero*)
     Incomplete fusion between the right maxillary swelling and the medial nasal swelling.
B.   Median cleft lip associated with holoprosencephaly. (Stage 18, 42 days, induced abortion,
     alive *in utero*)
     Note the hypotelorism. No nasal pit is visible. This case is combined with bilateral preaxial polydactyly of the foot.

times or more higher than the figures in newborns (0.17%, KOBAYASHI [87]; 0.21%, NEEL [38]; 0.17%, MITANI and KITAMURA [36]; 0.14%, TANAKA [88]). Moreover, it was demonstrated that 5 specimens (0.81%) exhibited cleft lip with or without palate among 616 early fetuses (46 to 160 mm crown-rump length). This is in good accord with the observations by KRAUS et al. [76] that the spontaneously aborted embryos and fetuses showed far higher prevalence (1.88%) than newborns in live births. A tendency that unilateral cleft is more frequent than bilateral type coincides with the finding in Japanese infants [87, 89]. It has been noted that unilateral cleft lip is more commonly found on the left among infants of both Japanese [87, 89] and Caucasians [90, 91] but the present results do not decidedly reveal this left-side preponderance (10 on the left and 9 on the right). IIZUKA [92] observed some side difference in the early development of the upper lip in 113 embryos at stages 16 to 23, but there was found no consistency. Therefore, it failed to explain the left-side preponderance of the unilateral cleft lip from his embryological study.

IIZUKA [93] studied the human palatal closure and found it begins at 28 mm and is completed at 46 mm in crown-rump length. Earlier works on the time of palate closure also showed side range of individual variations [94–99]. BURDI and SILVEY [100] reported that female embryos delayed in palatal closure as compared with males. This problem is expected to be reconfirmed by our materials.

Among 616 early fetuses (46 to 160 mm in crown-rump length), two cases of cleft lip and palate and two with isolated cleft palate were observed [86]. The prevalence (0.32%) of the isolated cleft palate is also several times higher than that in infants (0.02%, MITANI and KITAMURA [36]; 0.06%, NEEL [38]).

Out of 29 cleft embryos and fetuses, 7 specimens (24.1%) had other external malformations and the defects in the extremities occurred relatively frequently. Although the frequency of associated anomalies is lower than that reported by KRAUS et al. [76] in spontaneously aborted specimens (61.6%), it seems higher than that observed in Japanese newborns (12.0%, HIKITA [101]; 14.9%, KOBAYASHI [87]; 12.9%, NEEL [38]; 17.1%, SANUI [102]; 6.2%, AKASAKA [89]; 16.4%, TANAKA [88]). It should be noted that many statistics in newborns include some of the internal malformations and that umbilical and inguinal hernias undetectable in embryos are fairly commonly associated in newborns. The relationship between sex and the clefts has been long disputed. The sex in the embryos with cleft lip was determined only in 7 cases by histology of gonad and 5 males and 2 females were recoreded by the present author. In addition, 3 males and 2 females among 5 fetuses with cleft lip were ascertained. Although the examined cases are very limited, there is a tendency of the male preponderance in cleft lip in embryos and early fetuses. This also coincides with the reports that cleft lip with or without palate is found more frequently in males in Japanese newborns [87, 88, 101]. Some parental factors such as age were analysed but no particular factors possibly related to the occurrence of cleft lip and/or palate has been identified probably due to the small number of malformed cases.

Pathogenesis of human facial clefts is still under discussion although many studies in experimental animals are available (reviewed by WARKANY [75]). Recently, FREDERIKS [103] called the attention to the role of vascular patterns in the palate region, and suggested hematogenic agents or a general deficiency in oxygen supply may indeed have a chance to play a harmful part in the development of the primary and secondary palate in human embryos. It is expected that the precious materials in our collection will furnish some clues how facial defects are formed.

5) LIMB DEFECTS

Limb defects are one of the most easily recognizable external malformations during the human embryonic period. The arm bud appears at stage 12 (4 mm, 28 days) and the digital rays are observed at stage 17 (12 mm, 40 days). The leg bud appears at stage 13 (5 mm, 32 days), a little later than the arm bud, and the toe rays are detected at stage 18 (14 mm, 42 days). This means that most of the malformations seen at birth can be observed in the embryonic stage and moreover the initiating pathogenesis is fully to be examined. Therefore, monitoring of the malformation in the embryonic stage may present the meaningful data in respect to limbs, except anomalies of joints.

Limb malformations in human embryos at stages 17 to 23 undamaged and alive *in utero* were examined. The materials were classified by the last menstrual period of the mother. The prevalence of limb deformity in the embryonic stage is about five times higher than that observed in newborns (Table 5). Considering the fact that majority of the joint anomalies which are comparatively frequently observed in newborns are not manifested in the embryos, representative types of individual malformation should be compared. Reduction deformities (Fig. 17) were found only in 8 cases during the total period, but 4 cases were detected in 1968. This seems very interesting but further analysis of mother's history including drug intake during pregnancy did not disclose any particular association.

Polydactyly is one of the most common malformations both in the embryos and newborns (Fig. 18). As seen in Table 3, the prevalence of polydactyly is 10 times higher than that in newborns. It is, therefore, presumed that most of the embryos with polydactyly may be aborted during the later stage, or the anomaly be cured or at least not so progressed as recongnizable in the newborns. Although embryos with polydactyly occasionally share severe other internal malformations imcompatible for the later development, this may only

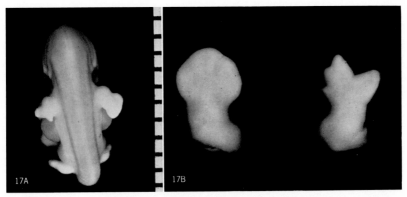

Fig. 17 Reduction deformities of the limbs.
A. Hypoplasia of the upper limb. (Stage 16, 38 days, induced abortion, alive *in utero*)
    Note the hypoplastic left upper limb and the misshaped right hand plate.
B. Split hand. (Stage 18, 42 days, induced abortion, alive *in utero*)
    Note the splitting between the third and the fourth finger of the right hand. The left hand
    is normal.

partially explain why the prevalence of polydactyly is so high in the embryos.

Preaxial (radial side) polydactyly of the hand is the most frequently observed polydacty-lous malformations both in embryos and in newborns. It is quite interesting that they can be recognized even at stage 16 (10 mm, 38 days) when hand plate is well formed but no digital rays are observed. That may mean the preaxial part becomes mature earlier than the postaxial. Hand plates of undamaged embryos at stages 16 to 23 were examined stereomicroscopically in 2,212 cases, and 15 cases with preaxial polydactyly and 2 cases with postaxial polydactyly were observed [104]. These abnormal hands were serially sectioned parallel to volar surface and the initial stage of morphogenesis of polydactyly were examined [105]. Comparison with normal hand plates in the corresponding stage discloses the following findings: (1) Hypertrophy and a delayed involution of the apical ectodermal ridge at the tip of the duplicated thumbs in stages 17 and 18. The apical ecto-dermal ridge is known to appear in stage 12 and disappear in stage 17 [106, 107]. (2) A precocious development of an interdigital notch between the duplicated thumbs in stages 17 and 18. (3) Bifurcation of the distal part of the first digital ray in stage 19. These findings are also reported in case of the polydactyly in animals either experimentally in-duced or genetically determined, and confirm the assumption that the common pathogene-sis exists in humans and animals. A disorder of the interaction between limb ectoderm and mesoderm is considered the pathogenetic event. As *in vitro* culture of the limb buds is relatively easy in terms of the materials and method, it is tempting to recommend that comparative study of pathogenesis in polydactyly or other digital anomalies in man and animals is to be tested. Some promising preliminary results have been shown in our labora-tory [108]. It might be added here that abnormal persistence of the apical ectodermal ridge and precocious formation of the interdigital notches, the characteristic features of preaxial polydactyly, were also seen in the cleft hand of an embryo at stage 18 [109].

Postaxial (ulnar or fibular side) polydactyly is observed in both hands and foot. Among about 5,000 human embryos at stages ranging from stage 17 (12 mm, 40 days) to 23 (28 mm, 52 days), 20 cases of postaxial polydactyly were found [110]. They were classified into the following three types: the complete one with a distinct extra digit, the incomplete one with a small tubercle on the lateral border of the proximal portion of the fifth finger, and the intermediate one. Histological examinations revealed a distinct mesenchymal condensation

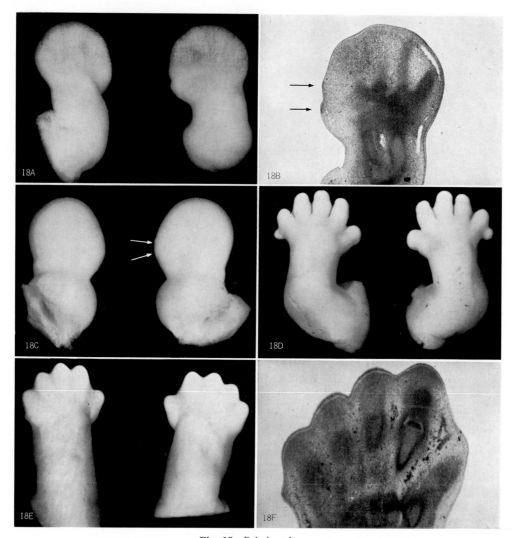

Fig. 18 Polydactyly.

A. Preaxial polydactyly of the right hand. (Stage 17, 40 days, induced abortion, alive *in utero*)
    Note the precocious notch in the duplicated first finger. (From Yasuda, M.: J. Embryol. exp.
    Morph. **33**; 745, 1975)

B. Histology of A. (Parallel to the plane of the hand plate)
    Note the abnormally thick apical ectodermal ridge at the polydactylous site indicated by arrows.

C. Preaxial tubercle of both hands. (Stage 16, 38 days, induced abortion, alive *in utero*)
    Note the tiny tubercles indicated by arrows. Some of the tubercles may be a precursor of the
    preaxial polydactyly.

D. Postaxial polydactyly of both hands. (Stage 20, 46 days, abortion, alive *in utero*)
    This case is combined with holoprosencephaly and postaxial polydactyly of the both feet.

E. Postaxial polydactyly of the left foot. (Stage 20, 46 days, induced abortion, alive *in utero*)
    Note the small extradigit on the fibular side.

F. Histology of E. (Parallel to the plane of the foot plate) No thickening of the apical ectodermal
    ridge is observed.

in the complete extra digits, while mesenchymal cells in those small tubercles were packed less densely. The cytoplasm of ectodermal cells covering the extra digit was rather light, and abnormal persistence of the apical ectodermal ridge, which characterizes the early morphogenesis of preaxial polydactyly, was not observed. These findings suggest that genetically different pre- and postaxial polydactylies are also different in their pathogenesis.

At the stages of digital ray formation, small tubercles at the preaxial or postaxial border of the hand or foot plate are occasionally observed. Sometimes it is very difficult to differentiate them from the established polydactyly. The preaxial tubercles are found only in hand with relatively constant prevalence from stages 16 to 18, where the postaxial tubercles are observed both in hand and in foot but limited only at one or two specific stages (17 in hand and 17 and 18 in foot). Moreover, the preaxial tubercles in hands are observed more often in the right side. The results indicate a strong possibility of the preaxial tubercle to develop into polydactyly, while the postaxial one as a temporary existence of normal regressive phenomenon of the postaxial border [111].

6) CARDIAC ANOMALIES

Development of the circulatory or cardiovascular system is a very complicating process originating intraembryonically and extraembryonically. The heart, especially, begins to form very early at the presomite stage (stage 9, 20 days). This is the first recognizable organ primordium except the central nervous system. The human heart is supposed to be contractile at the 4-somite stage (stage 10, 22 days). Moreover, the heart development is so quick that before the end of the embryonic stage, the major morphogenesis is completed. Therefore, it is agreed that the heart is one of the best organs to be examined for gross malformations at the embryonic stage. However, the classic way of histologically examining the serial section of the heart with complicated chambers or studying with the time consuming reconstruction wax models is not suitable for screening of abnormal specimens. Microdissection, on the other hand, can detect the gross anomalies in a relatively short time, though the great skilfulness is required, and the method has been adopted by Asami [112].

The heart, together with the pulmonary trunk, ductus atriosus and aortic arch, was examined under the stereomicroscope in 1,259 externally normal embryos at stages 18 to 23 (14 mm to 28 mm, 42 days to 52 days) alive *in utero*, and obtained by induced abortion (Semba and others of our group, unpublished). Ventricular septal defect was identified on specimens at and over stage 21 (21 mm, 48 days) (see below). The prevalence of malformed hearts was 8 (1.16%) in 687 embryos at stages 18 to 20 (14 to 19 mm, 42 to 46 days) and 21 (3.5%) in 602 cases at stages 21 to 23 (21 to 28 mm, 48 to 52 days), whereas the corresponding prevalence in live Japanese infants was reported to be 0.14 per cent by Neel [38]. It is to be considered that such types as patent foramen ovale and patent ductus arteriosus which appear in the perinatal stage could not be included in our series. The type of defects and their frequency in our series are as follows: persistent ostium primum: 2, persistent A-V canal: 5, tricuspid valve defect: 1, tricuspid stenosis+pulmonary stenosis+ventricular septum defect: 1, mitral valve defect: 1, ventricular septal defect :10, tetralogy of Fallot: 1 (Fig. 19A), transposition of great vessels+ventricular septal defect: 2, overriding aorta: 2, pulmonary stenosis: 1, aortic valve defect: 2, aortic valve defect+pulmonary valve defect: 1, coarctation of aorta: 1 (Fig. 19B). This result shows that the ventricular septal defect is most common, the fact of which is in accord with the reported findings among the perinatal and clinical cases. The persistent atrioventricular canal is also common on our specimens, while this anomaly has been relatively rare in infants.

The time of closure of the intraventricular foramen has been disputed by several investigators. Kramer [113] and Vernall [114] stated that the foramen is still open at stage 18,

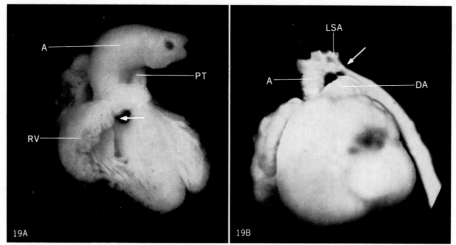

Fig. 19 Cardiac malformations.

A. Tetralogy of Fallot. (Stage 22, 50 days, induced abortion, alive *in utero*)
    Anterior view of the heart after the atria and the right ventricular wall are removed. The arrow
    shows the large ventricular septal defect. The pulmonary trunk (PT) is remarkably smaller
    than the aorta (A). The aorta (A) is straddled above the ventricular septum defect. The right
    ventricular wall (RV) is not hypertrophic at this stage.
B. Coarctation of the aorta. (Stage 23, 52 days, ectopic pregnancy, alive *in utero*)
    Arrow shows portion of the coarctation of the aorta (A) at preductal portion distal to the left
    subclavian artery (LSA).
    DA, ductus arteriosus.

STREETER [6] described it as closed in the older member of stage 18. O'RAHILLY [115] reported that the foramen was found open at stage 18, either open or closed at stage 19, and closed at stage 20. MALL [116] noted it as closed at stage 19. The preliminary report in our group indicates the foramen was not closed in about 30 per cent of the cases at stage 19 and in about 10 per cent at stage 20 [117]. Therefore, at present, we diagnose ventricular septum defect on the cases at and over stage 20 (21 mm, 48 days). It is generally observed that the ventricular septum defects can be closed even in the postnatal life. Whether a slight delay of closure of the interventricular foramen observed in the late embryonic stage is associated with the occurrence of cardiac and other malformations remains to be elucidated.

Among 40 externally normal embryos alive *in utero* at stages 18 to 23 obtained from ectopic pregnancy (mostly tubal), 7 cases (17.5%) with cardiovascular malformations were found [118]. Compared with the corresponding prevalence of 2.3 per cent in the externally normal embryos from intrauterine pregnancy as mentioned above, the occurrence of cardiac malformations in ectopic embryos was obviously higher. This means that the emvironment related to a site of implantation can be a causative factor in cardiovascular development.

Morphogenesis of the heart has been extensively studied by various investigators and was summarized by O'RAHILLY [115] with special reference to the developmental stage. The time and sequence of the critical events in cardiogenesis was presented in tabular form, and the period of determination for the different malformations was analysed [119]. It is hoped that detailed studies of our specimens with malformed heart will verify the stated pathogenesis based on the normal histological differentiation.

7) UROGENITAL ANOMALIES

The urogenital system shows a remarkable growth and differentiation in the embryonic stage and seems a suitable object for the study of the developmental process. Especially, the sexual differentiation with its disorder is a complicated phenomenon and the clue may be obtained through the careful studies on human embryos in the early prenatal stage. JIRÁSEK [19] summarized the normal and abnormal development of the genital system based on his embryological works and clinical observations.

The abdomens of about 2,000 human embryos at stages 18 to 23 (14 mm to 28 mm, 42 to 52 days) were dissected under the stereomicroscope and the development of the urogenital system, especially mesonephros, metanephros, ureter and gonad was minutely examined [120]. Length and width of metanephros were measured under the stereomicroscope. Abnormal organs were then histologically studied.

No gross malformations such as aplasia were detected in mesonephros, although its size was quite variable. As for the metanephros (kidney in future), 11 abnormal cases (0.45%) were found in 2,472 embryos. Of 282 undamaged externally normal embryos, two cases of fused kidney (horseshoe kidney) were found. Of 2,179 partially damaged but externally normal embryos, one case of fused kidney, four cases of hypoplasia and four cases of malposition were detected. It is quite interesting that the prevalence of kidney anomalies is not higher than that reported in the perinatal autopsy population. It may be partly because that the metanephros develops comparatively slower than other internal organs and the establishment of the abnormal development is relatively late. Moreover, neither hydronephrosis nor cystic kidney has been detected in the embryonic stage. However, it is also to be noted that abnormalities in the urinary system are frequently observed in externally malformed embryos.

Fused kidneys are most remarkable anomalies found in the urinary system of embryos. Four cases of the embryonic fused kidney in embryos of 10 to 35 mm crown-rump length were reviewed by ZONDEK [121]. The prevalence is almost similar to that reported in autopsy materials (1: 750, JOLY [122]; 1: 425, CAMPBELL [123]). All the embryonic fused kidneys showed fusion at the lower pole with the ureters located on the anterior surface of the kidney. This is also the commonest type observed postnatally. In addition, a

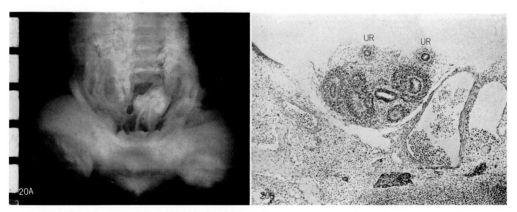

Fig. 20   Crossed ectopic kidney with fusion. (Stage 19, 44 days, induced abortion, alive *in utero*)
  A.   Showing the fused kidney after microdissection. Note the position of the kidneys is lower than normal. Ureters run anterior to the kidneys.
  B.   Histology. Development of the metanephric blastema and collecting tubules are normal.
        A, aorta; UR, ureter.
        This case is combined with cleft lip of both sides and oligodactyly of both hands.

case of crossed ectopic kidney with fusion was found in the embryos at stage 19 (16 mm, 44 days). Cleft lip of both sides and oligodactyly of the both hands were combined [124] (Fig. 20). No gross malformation of the ureter and the urinary bladder has been detected.

The gonads of 1,525 embryos at stages 18 to 23 (14 to 28 mm, 42 to 52 days) were examined under the stereomicroscope [125]. No case of gross malformation in gonad was found. Usually, sex determination was possible by observation under stereomicroscope in cases of the stage at and over 20 (19 mm, 46 days): a testis is of an ellipsoid shape and is smooth on the surface, while an ovary has a cylinder-like shape and is coorse on the surface. The gonads were histologically examined and definite sex determination was made using the following criteria [126, 127].

Male : (1) The existence of short and straight testicular tubules sorrounded by mesenchymal sheath and the rete testis, both of which are darkly stained. (2) The appearance of tunica albuginea which is continuous with coelomic epithelium.

Female : (1) The absence of any cord-like structure in the cortex. (2) The existence of numerous large primitive sex cells intermingled with spindle-shaped mesenchymal cells and intermediate pregranulosa cells. (3) No sign of development of the surface epithelia to tunica albuginea. Sex could not be definitely determined in some of the embryos at stages 18 to 20 due to undifferentiated features.

Of 1,475 cases in which sex was determined, 16 true hermaphrodites (1.05%) were found [125] (Fig. 21). This figure is far higher than the frequency 0.2 to 0.3 per cent in the total postnatal population estimated by OVERZIER [128]. Therefore, it is presumed that most of these embryos will be lost later during intrauterine life, although there is no direct evidence that hermaphrodites are frequently observed in abortuses. No combined malformation in the other parts of body was found in these hermaphrodite specimens. Another possible explanation is that some cases of testis might be unusually retarded in differentiation

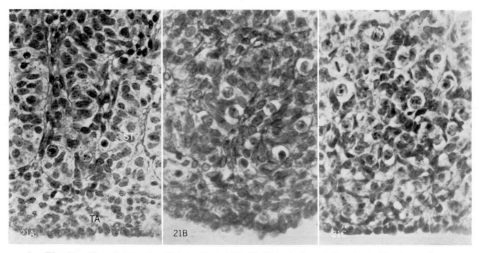

Fig. 21 True hermaphroditism. (Stage 22, 50 days, induced abortion, alive *in utero*).
A. Normal testis at the same developmental stage.
B. Gonad of the true hermaphroditism.
C. Normal ovary at the same developmental stage.
    In the normal testis (A), tunica albuginea (TA) and seminiferous tubules (ST) are clearly observed. On the other hand, in the normal ovary (C), neither tunica albuginea nor cord-formation is visible but the large primordial cells are sporadically recognized. Gonads of both sides in case (B) possess the characteristics of testis and ovary simultaneously and are called ovotestis. Both seminiferous tubules and large primordial cells are present.

and misdiagnosed as female. Types of hermaphrodites are as follows: 9 lateral (one gonad is ovary and the other testis); 4 unilateral (one is ovotestis and the other testis or ovary) and 3 bilateral (both are ovotestes). According to the reports on postnatal population, MERRILL and RAMSEY [129] stated unilateral true hermaphrodites are most common. This may indicate that some of the gonads in lateral hermaphrodites may develop into both ovarian and testicular characteristics. In addition, there was observed a side preposition that the ovarian tissue was more commonly found on the left. This is in accord with the observations on the postnatal hermaphrodites reviewed by OVERZIER [128] and JONES and SCOTT [130]. Some parental factors such as age did not show any association with the occurrence of this anomaly. Unfortunately, Bouin-fixed materials are not suitable for sex chromatin studies. Cytogenetic examination could not be made either. Therefore, it is hoped that further efforts should be made using unfixed specimens to elucidate the detailed pathogenesis in abnormal sex differentiation.

The study of sex determination by gonadal histology naturally leads to the problem on sex ratio in the early intrauterine population. LEE and TAKANO [131] reported that sex ratio (number of males $\times$ 100 divided by number of females) is 153 in the 1,452 embryos at stages 18 to 23 (14 to 28 mm, 42 to 52 days). No definite agreement of sex ratio in embryonic stage has been given by the method of histology of gonad, sex chromosome or sex chromatin; high male preponderance by some (ex. 60, SASAKI et al. [132]) and female predominance by others (ex. 232, SCHULTZE [133]). The number of examined cases in each investigator is relatively small and large scaled investigation on unselected intrauterine population is awaited.

8)   COMBINED INTERNAL ANOMALIES

Recently, the syndromes or multiple defects are of great clinical significance not only from the therapeutical but also from the etiological standpoint. Successive chains of tetratogenesis is expected to be elucidated by analysing the embryological processes of embryos with combined or multiple defects in our collection.

Of 170 cases of externally malformed embryos alive *in utero*, 22 (25.3%) possessed other types of external malformations. It is to be noted that holoprosencephalic embryos alive *in utero* were associated with other external malformations mailny of the central nervous system and of the limbs (51.0%, 25 out of 49 cases).

Twenty-three undamaged externally malformed embryos of stages 14 to 23 (7 to 28 mm, 34 to 52 days), alive *in utero* obtained by curettage or hysterectomy and fixed in Bouin's fluid, and 23 externally normal embryos of the matched stage were used for the study. Histological specimens were examined for the combined internal anomalies. In some cases, reconstruction wax-models were carefully studied [134]. Nine cases (39%) of the externally malformed embryos showed one or more internal anomalies, while no internal malformation was found in the 23 matched externally normal embryos. Organs affected were digestive system (4 cases), urogenital system (3), heart (2), endocrine organs (2), skeletal system (1) and central nervous system (1). No definite association of external malformation with internal anomalies has been identified due to a small number of examined cases. However, it is to be noted that all three embryos with only limb defects disclosed severe malformations in the digestive system (Fig. 22), while holoprosencephaly was less frequently associated with internal anomalies. In addition to these definite malformations, 4 cases of the externally malformed cases and 3 cases of the externally normal cases showed blood stasis in various internal organs such as mesonephros and liver. This may indicate threatened death *in utero* or during operation. Such a high rate of internal anomalies combined with external malformations in the embryonic stage may explain the fact that prevalence of

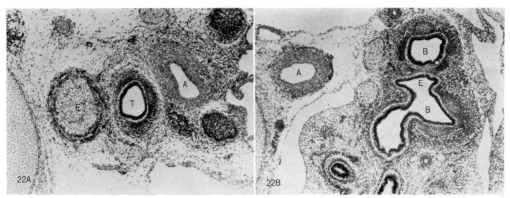

Fig. 22 Esophageal atresia with tracheoesophageal fistula. (Stage 21, 48 days, alive *in utero*)
A. Region of esophageal atresia (transverse section)
B. Region of the initiating caudal esophagus. (ca. 0.9 mm caudal to the section A, just below the bifurcation of the trachea)
A, aorta; B, bronchus; E, esophagus; T, trachea.
This case is combined with oligodactyly of hand and ventricular septum defect.

most types of external malformations in embryos is higher than that in newborns and these malformed embryos are lost during the late course of pregnancy due to severe functional disturbance of malformed internal organs.

9) NUCHAL BLEB

Nuchal bleb, external vesicular projection in the region of the cervical flexure was occasionally found in human embryos at 7 weeks of age, exclusively (as high as about 50%) at stage 21 (21 mm, 48 days) (Fig. 23). Its degree varies from slight diffuse swellings to severe hanging protrusions.

These projections are classified histologically into the following five types [135]: (1) Simple subcutaneous blebs. Central nervous system is intact. (2) Submeningeal blebs. Meningocele is observed. (3) Subcutaneous blebs associated with defects of the skull and the primitive meninx. (4) Subcutaneous blebs with perforation of the roof of the rhombencephalon but without skull defects. The meninx is kept normal. (5) Subcutaneous blebs with brain defects and additional skull defects. No definite correlation has been obtained between the degree of macroscopic projections and histological type of anomalies. Although our histological examination is not extensive, cases with the type (3) are found fairly frequently (about 35%). Moreover, examination of maternal history of these embryos reveals no specific factors associated with the occurrence of the blebs.

TÖNDURY et al. [136] described 12 human embryos of 23–36 mm crown-rump length, characterized by the appearance of external vesicular projections in the region of the cervical and parietal bends. They classified those embryos into three categories (our type 1 to 3). Furthermore, they regarded these blebs as early stages of a pseudencephalus. Among unfixed embryos, preserved with saline for a short time at obstetrician's clinics, we have sometimes observed such an abnormal state. Therefore, the fixation is not an essential factor responsible for the bleb. Judging from the high prevalence of these anomalies among embryos at the specific developmental stage, the nuchal region seems to be transitionally a *locus minoris resistentiae* to be damaged as the cervical flexure gradually extends around this stage. Probably, most of them might have been caused during the course of operation due to mechanical pressure or anoxia or in some cases outside the uterus even in

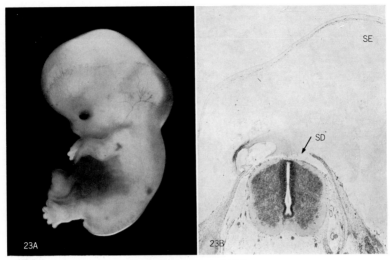

Fig. 23 Nuchal bleb.
A. Nuchal bleb in the fresh (unfixed) state. (Stage 21, 48 days, ectopy, alive *in utero*)
Note the transparent swelling in the nuchal region.
B. Subcutaneous bleb associated with defects of the skull and the primitive meninx. (Nuchal
bleb, Type 3).
Note connection of the submeningeal space with the cervical bleb.
SD, skull defect; SE, subcutaneous edema.

the so-called physiological saline. However, similar changes may exist *in utero* induced by
subtle alternation of uterine environments. Anomalies such as edema may be repaired, but
some of these with affected meninx and/or brain may die during the later course of the
intrauterine development or develop into meningocele or anencephaly. Such anomalies
are interesting in connection with Status Bonnevie-Ullrich [137]. Singh and Carr [138]
described a case of cystic hygroma in the nuchal region with fluid sac in a spontaneously
aborted fetus with XO karyotype (159 menstrual dyas). Therefore, cytogenetic study of
fresh embryos with this abnormality are needed.

Furthermore, it might be added that we observe similar protrusions in frontal and
parietal regions at the late embryonic and early fetal period, although less frequently as
compared with nuchal blebs.

In addition, we have observed crater-like damage formation at the parietal region fairly
frequently in the embryos of stages 18 to 20, (14 to 19 mm, 42 to 46 days). Histological
examination clearly demonstrates the injury of scalp and midbrain associated with bleeding. We believe most of them are artifacts due to the damage at operation and the fixation
procedure although Patten [21] reported a similar embryo as a type of developing ence-
phalocele. Kitasato [139] observed the exposure of diencephalon and mesencephalon in a
12 mm embryo by putting it into Bouin's fixative after 2 mm puncture in parietal region.
However, it can be said the parietal region of human embryos at those stages is another
locus minoris resistentiae as in case of nuchal blebs in the later stage and, in some occasions,
a subtle insult may result in a serious damage of the central nervous system *in utero*.

10) BRANCHIAL ARCH ANOMALIES

Examination of the branchial (pharyngeal) arches on specimens at stages 13 to 16 (5 to
10 mm, 32 to 38 days), before the appearance of recognizable ear auricle and closure of
the cervical sinus, revealed 22 cases with abnormal branchial arch or cleft consisted of 14

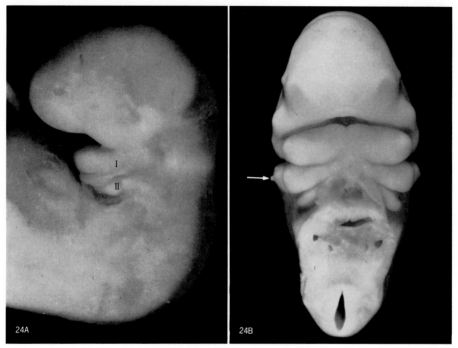

Fig. 24   Pharyngeal arch anomalies.

A.   Hypoplasia of the second pharyngeal arch. (Stage 14, 34 days, induced abortion, alive *in utero*)
     The left first pharyngeal arch (I) is hyperplastic and splitted, and the second arch (II) is hypoplastic. This case is combined with the hypoplasia of the right second arch and of both upper limb buds. (From NISHIMURA, H.: Prenatal versus postnatal malformations based on the Japanese experience on induced abortions in the human being. In: Blandau, R. J. (ed.) Aging Gametes. pp. 349–368, S. Karger, Basel, 1975)

B.   Tubercle in the second pharyngeal arch. (Stage 14, 34 days, abortion, alive *in utero*)
     Note the small tubercle indicated by arrow.

cases with hole like cleft I or II (sometimes histologically perforated), 5 cases with hypoplastic arch I, II (Fig. 24 A) or III and 2 cases with retarded regression of arch III. Twelve cases with those anomalous embryos were accompanied with some of other external malformations. Such anomalies of the early phase of the branchial organs have never been reported, and it is difficult to estimate their definite future development, although some of hypoplastic arch I may be considered a precursor of micrognathia or ear auricle anomalies. In addition, tubercle formations are found on the basal part of the hyoid arch in the embryos at stages 14 to 16 (6 to 10 mm, 34 to 38 days) with the frequency of 14.2 per cent (54 cases in 329) (Fig. 24 B). The future development is not certain but some may remain as auricular appendage seen in postnatal population as often as 1.5 per cent [75]. Some of them are presumably concordant with the description of strong cell proliferation of epidermis in the branchial region by STEINER [140]. At present, no associated factors with these anomalies in our series have been identified. However, since well-known human teratogens, thalidomide and aminopterin, were reported to cause external ear anomalies such as anotia, microtia, low set ear, etc. (in case of thalidomide, KNAPP et al. [141]; KIDA and LENZ [142]; in case of aminopterin, WARKANY et al. [143]; EMERSON [144]; MILUNSKY et al. [145]), detailed systematic survey of branchial arch anomalies may be worthy for detection of another human teratogen in future.

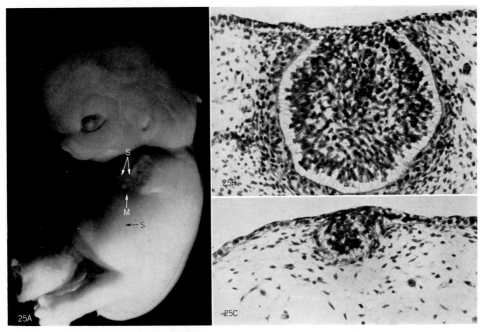

Fig. 25 Supernumerary nipples. (Stage 21, 48 days, induced abortion, alive *in utero*)

A. Showing the primordium of the main gland (M) and several smaller supernumerary nipples (S) around it. Note also an accessory one beneath the main. The left upper limb is resected.

B. Section showing the epithelial primordium of the gland proper.

C. Section showing the smaller similar primordium of the accessory gland.

11) SUPERNUMERARY NIPPLES

Supernumerary nipples (polythelia) or breasts (polymastia) are fairly frequently observed variations. Their phylogenetic significance was once unfruitfully discussed. It is now accepted that supernumerary nipples are mostly found distributed along the so-called embryonic mammary ridge or milk line, and failure of the suppression on the potential breastforming tissue in parts of the line other than the main gland may give rise to multiple formation of the nipples or breasts.

Thickening of the epidermis from the root of the upper limb bud downwards to that of the lower limb bud is observed microscopically in embryos at stage 14 (7 mm, 34 days). At stage 16 (10 mm, 38 days) this thickening is elevated and can be observed under stereomicroscope and at stage 17 (12 mm, 40 days), the ridge is quickly disappearing and leaves a conical elevation with caudal tail at site of the future main mammary gland. At stage 18 (14 mm, 42 days) the main gland is obviously established with deep indentation of epidermis rather than the swelling on the surface. The mammary ridge is completely lost even histologically. However, by examination of late embryos under stereomicroscope, one can usually observe the small circular spots in the lateral thoracic and abdominal wall, particularly around the main gland. Tanimura [146] histologically examined 28 externally normal embryos at stages 18 to 23 (14 to 28 mm, 42 to 52 days), and found such spots to be called supernumerary nipples as they consist of the circumscribed epidermal thickening, miniatures of the main mammary gland primordia (Fig. 25). The supernumerary nipples were found only in one case of 6 examined specimens at stage 18 (14 mm, 42 days), but the prevalence was increased as the embryonic stages advanced (Table 12). No significant side preponderance was found. Moreover, they were fairly widely distributed at the axillar

Table 12 Average number per side of supernumerary nipples of human embryos examined histologically.

Stage	No. of embryos examined	Position related to the main gland		
		Above	Same	Below
18	6	0.2	0.0	0.0
19	4	0.8	0.0	0.8
20	5	1.4	0.3	0.6
21	4	3.8	1.8	2.0
22	5	4.3	1.1	3.0
23	4	5.8	1.4	4.0

region, where even three nipples were identified at the same level, but considerably limited on the mammary ridge in the abdominal region. The study clearly shows that existence of supernumerary nipples is a normal transitionary event of development in the embryonic and early fetal stage. The prevalence of supernumerary nipples in Japanese is not exactly known because of the difference of the diagnostic criteria. Probably it is 2 to 7 per cent in adults [147–150]. The prevalence is generally regarded to be higher in pregnant women because the supernumerary breasts may also function and be easily recognized (15 to 13%, HIRAZAWA [148]; SAKAMOTO [151]; ARAUMI et al. [152]). MORI [153] reported that the prevalence is very high (74% in boys, 79% in girls) at 6 years of age and gradually decreases as the age advances (36% in boys and 41% in girls at 12 years). These surveys may indicate that some of the embryonic supernumerary nipples survive latently and become manifest according to hormonal and other physiological states.

Embryonic supernumerary nipples were described in the last century by SCHMIDT [154, 155]. He found them in all of the embryos and fetuses he examined (28 to 65 mm). He described it as normal hyperthelia of human embryos. His findings were confirmed by another SCHMIDT [156], BERK [157] and LUSTIG [158]. Their descriptions together with the author's findings may indicate that embryonal supernumerary nipples can originate outside the definite mammary ridge. Epidermis in the thoracic and abdominal region may undergo hyperplasia and be transformed into the mammary gland primordia. Most of them will of course be degenerated but some may not be completely regressed.

In addition, it may be worthy to note that localized irregular proliferations of epidermal cells like cumulonimbus are frequently seen in the inguinal region of embryos at later stage (stages 21 to 23). This is considered similar to the findings described by STEINER [140]. The exact nature and significance of this phenomenon remains unknown.

12) SINGLE UMBILICAL ARTERY

Single umbilical artery is one of the anatomical variants but reported to be frequently associated with major malformation, especially of the urogenital system. Anatomists had already shown interests in this anomaly combined with severe malformations such as sympodia in the last and early this century [159]. Since BENIRSCHKE and BROWN [160] pointed out that it could be an external sign suggestive of hidden internal congenital malformations, this anomaly has been considered clinically of significance. Later, it was demonstrated that in babies thalidomide is sometimes associated with single umbilical artery while in malformed monkey fetuses induced by thalidomide sometimes shows this anomaly [161].

The pathogenesis of this anomaly, however, is still unexplained. The genesis of single umbilical artery has been attributed to either primary aplasia [162] or secondary atrophy [163] of one of the umbilical arteries. Recently, MONIE [164] proposed the third possibility

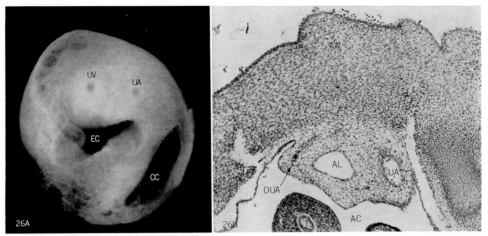

Fig. 26   Single umbilical artery. (Stage 20, 46 days, spontaneous abortion, alive *in utero*)
A.   Transverse section of the umbilical cord near the embryonic end.
B.   Histology of the embryo. (transverse section)
     Note the obliterated rudimentary left umbilical artery in the histological specimen. This case
     is combined with holoprosencephaly and fused kidney.
     AC, abdominal cavity; AL, allantois; AW, abdominal wall; CC, cystic cavity; EC, extraem-
     bryonic coelom; I, intestine; OUA, obliterated umbilical artery; UA, umbilical artery; UV,
     umbilical vein.

that it may also arise from the persistence of the transitionary single artery in the body
stalk with subsequent atrophy of one intra-abdominal umbilical artery as normally occurs
in the rat.

One thousand, five hundred forty-four cords (embryonic end) of human embryos (stages
14 to 23, 6 to 28 mm, 34 to 52 days) were examined under stereomicroscope. Suspected
cases were histologically confirmed [165, 166] (Fig. 26). The frequency of single umbilical
artery was: 1 in 1,471 externally normal embryos alive *in utero*, 1 in 30 externally normal
embryos dead *in utero*, 2 in 31 externally malformed live embryos (both had also internal
anomalies), and 1 in 12 malformed dead embryos. Thus, frequency of cases with single
umbilical artery was higher in the externally malformed embryos than that in the externally normal. Considering the ratio of cases with externally malformed to that of normal
embryos in our collection, the estimated prevalence of single umbilical artery in the early
prenatal population is considered to be 0.1 per cent and probably lower than that reported in Japanese newborns (0.8%, SOMA et al. [167]; 0.2%, NISHIMURA et al. [168]; 0.23%,
KIMURA [169]). Histological examination showed very atrophic artery in most of single
umbilical artery cases of our series. Moreover, in several other cases diagnosed as macroscopically normal, the caliber of one artery was fairly smaller than the other. On the basis of
these findings, it is more likely that single umbilical artery is formed by secondary atrophy
of one of the umbilical arteries during embryonic and even fetal stage. However, the third
explanation raised by MONIE [164] is not to be evaluated by our investigation, because in
our materials it is not always possible to examine the umbilical artery throughout the
whole course of the umbilical cord.

13)   REGRESSION OF THE TAIL

Legends on a tailed race and sporadic case reports on persistence of the tail in the postnatal period have attracted the attention of scientists. On the other hand, embryologists once
had shown interests in the growth and regression of the tail and the most caudal portion of

the neural tube looking for the explanation of pathogenesis in spina bifida. Modern embryologists, however, pay little attention to the destiny of the tail region in human embryos.

Tails of the Japanese embryos in our collection show the full development in size at
stage 17 (12 mm, 40 days). It is in accord with the description by WILLIS [170] that the
human tail reaches its greatest development during the sixth week when the embryo is about
12 mm long. At stages 18 and 19 the tail show remarkable regression. However, the regression after stage 20 (19 mm, 46 days) is relatively slow and quite variable. TANIMURA and
UWABE [171] examined histologically 28 externally normal embryos at stages 20 to 23 (19
to 28 mm, 46 to 52 days) selected at random without prior macroscopic examination of the
tail region. The results were shown in Table 13. Twenty-one (75%) out of 28 specimens
had a small tubercle in the tail region and all but one contained nervous tissues therein.
Usually, the caudal end of the neural tube is associated with the small tubercle, but
occasionally the tip is divided into two parts, one entering the caudal tubercle and the other
approaching towards the vertebral primordium. In 6 cases of these 20 specimens which
possessed tubercle with the neural tissue, the tissue was protruded through the broken
epidermis and exposed on the surface of the body (Fig. 27). This is thought to be a divided
tubercle observed macroscopically. Another case showed an exposed neural tissue without
tubercle. KUNITOMO [172] stated that in 25 and 27 mm embryos the tail is reduced to a
small papilla, called caudal tubercle or tail bud, which contains the caudal end of the
spinal cord and midsacral artery and vein. This is situated dorsal to the coccygeal tubercle,
which possesses vertebral portion. He also described that the tail usually disappears entirely
when the embryos reaches 30 to 35 mm, but the time of disappearance is quite variable.
The youngest embryo without tail was 24 mm in length, but the present author found no
caudal tubercle in some embryos at stage 20 (19 mm, 46 days). Myelocele type structure
at the very end of the tail region is not cited in current textbooks on embryology, but IKEDA
[173] described that the caudal end of the neural tube was expanded in embryos at 25 mm
in length and extruded on the surface with rupture of the epidermis when the embryo
reached about at 30 mm. He designated it as secondary posterior neuropore. POLITZER
[174] observed a similar formation in the embryos of the 8th and 9th weeks. Such a structure
was reported in chicks [175] but not in tailed mammals. Such exposure of the nervous
tissue may be explained that the regression of the nervous tissue in the caudal end is slower
than that of epidermis and vertebral primordium in the tail region, and the spinal cord
persists longer, becomes curved to be finally exposed breaking the covering epidermis.
Most of the secondary neuropore may be closed and recovered by the skin, but its possible
role on causation of the spina bifida is not known at present. A remnant of the caudal portion of the nueral tube, however, can persist beneath the skin of the post-anal pit over the
end of coccyx, as first shown by TOURNEUX and HERMANN [176].

It might be added here that development of the caudal neural tube at stages 14 to 21 is
quite variable, forming canalization, duplication (LEMIRE, [177]; reported earlier by
KUNITOMO [172], STREETER [178], KERNOHAN [179], NAKAGAWA [180]). Such situations
were also frequently observed in our specimens.

14) EMBRYOS FROM ECTOPIC PREGNANCIES

Although our primary aim is not to collect embryonic specimens from ectopic pregnancies, materials furnished by the collaborative obstetricians give the unique opportunity to
compare the embryonic development of the intrauterine pregnancy with that of the extra-
uterine.

Comparison of the prevalence between these two groups clearly shows that a very high
risk of pathological embryos in the conceptuses of the ectopic pregnancy as expected

Table 13 Variation of the caudal end of spinal cord in human embryos (histological examinations).

Carnegie stage	A	B	C	D	E	F	Total
20	2	0	2	4	2	0	10
21	1	0	1	2	1	2	7
22	1	1	0	3	2	0	7
23	1	0	1	1	1	0	4
Total	5(18%)	1(4%)	4(14%)	10(36%)	6(21%)	2(7%)	28(100%)

Table 14 Ectopic pregnancies and pathological embryos.

Pregnancy	Embryos			
	Total	Live normal	Live malformed (%)[+]	Dead (%)[++]
Intrauterine	6,172	5,110	80 (1.5)	982 (19.2)
Ectopic	123	88	5 (5.4)*	30 (24.4)*

* $p < 0.05$
[+] Per cent of live embryos;   [++] Per cent of total embryos.

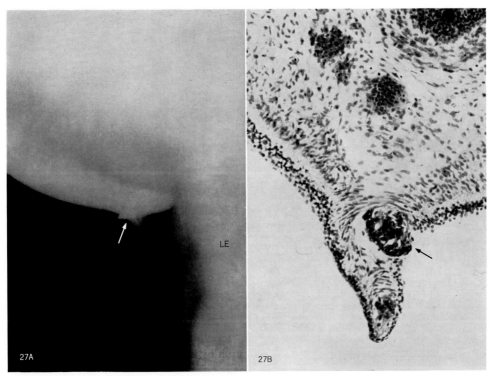

Fig. 27 Bifurcated tip of the tail under regression. (Stage 21, 48 days, induced abortion, alive *in utero*)
A. Lateral view. Arrow indicates the divided tips of the tail portion.
    LE, lower extremity.
B. Histology. Arrow indicates the nervous tissues are protruded through the broken epidermis. Note also the nervous tissues in the tail remnant.

(Table 14). Furthermore, it is to be added that by microdissection of the hearts from the external normal embryos from ectopic pregnancies higher prevalence (17.5%) of cardiac malformation was found as compared to that obtained from intrauterine pregnancy (2.3%, SEMBA et al. [118]). Estimation of ovulation age of the embryos calculated from the menstrual record was compared between the intrauterine and extrauterine pregnancies. Of 103 cases of externally normal live embryos from ectopic pregnancies, 34 showed smaller ovulation age (advanced development) as compared with our standard in the intrauterine pregnancy [14], 37 had similar age to the standard and 32 had greater age (retarded development). Therefore, the surviving embryos can develop as good as in the uterine cavity at least before the rupture of the tuba, although the possible effects from delayed implantation and poor environments in the oviduct should be considered.

As stated earlier, the possible association of the previous induced abortion with occurrence of ectopy in the subsequent pregnancy has been much debated not only in Japan but other countries such as Czechoslovakia and Greece where induced aobrtions by curettage are popular. Ectopic cases are compared with the live normal embryo group in the intrauterine pregnancy matched for maternal age, parity and spontaneous abortion. A significantly lower frequency of the previous induced abortion was noted in the ectopic group. This finding was not observed if compared with the control group matched for maternal age and gravidity. Therefore, at present, it seems unlikely that previous induced abortion plays a great role on the establishment of the ectopic pregnancy.

VARIOUS PROBLEMS OF HUMAN EMBRYO STUDIES IN THE PRESENT AND THE FUTURE

The characteristics of our systematic survey of early conceptuses may be summarized as follows:

1. Majority of the specimens are of three to eight weeks of fertilization, and are called embryos (1 to 30 mm). These weeks correspond to the period of major organogenesis and at the same time the critical period of teratogenesis. In Japan the patient who wishes an interruption of pregnancy may have the operation at the same day of her first visit to the qualified obstetrician. This is a main reason why we can get earlier specimens, while in other countries such as Scandinavia, where the excellent fetal studies have been done, the induced abortions are generally performed a little later than here in Japan.

2. The materials can be regarded as a representative of overall intrauterine population as they are derived mostly from the healthy course of pregnancy. The obstetricians provide the specimens not examining the state of conceptuses as embryos are too small and fragile for them to check before fixation. Therefore, it is expected that unselected and unbiased materials are offered to us.

3. Filing of the maternal history is done just after the operation. Although the survey is a type of retrospective studies, it is expected that memory of mothers in terms of the events during pregnancy, especially during the critical period for teratogenesis, is fresh and precise as compared with the questions usually done at the perinatal period. In addition, as the obstetrician or the patient does not usually know the state of conceptuses, the questions and answers may not be distorted by the existence of anomalies in specimens.

Data presented here is believed to have added a useful knowledge of normal standards on human embryonic and early fetal development. It is expected to continue to supply the newer data to correct or supplement the description of modern textbooks of embryology. Despite a fairly large number of malformed embryos collected in our laboratory, even credited as the world's largest, it is ovbious that more materials and informations are necessary to contribute to the solution of various complicated and difficult problems of human congenital anomalies such as analysis of the relationship of maternal factors associated with a specific type of anomalies or effective monitoring of congenital malformations. For clarifying the pathogenesis more early and late specimens are needed to disclose the whole course of abnormal processes which is finally to be linked to the definite form of malformations found in the newborns or postnatally.

The problems and the weak points of our studies will be discussed from the following three points.

1. LIMITATION OF MATERIALS

First of all, it should be again ascertained if our materials can be regarded as a non-selected sample of the total embryonic population. Analysis of the forms furnished by obstetricians shows some characteristics of the materials [14, 181]. The parents live mostly in urban districts in the central areas of Japan, and the socioeconomic rank of the parent judged by the occupation is estimated neither especially high nor low. The frequency of declared consanguineous marriage is 2.31 per cent and lower than the reported figures in the general population. The average maternal age (30.1) is 2 1/2 years higher and the average parity (1.7) is higher by one than the corresponding figures for total deliveries. Further careful comparison should be made between the population whose pregnancies are terminated by induced abortion and that of deliveries, and at the same time, between the induced abortion group as a whole in Japan and our group from which relatively undamaged embryonic specimens are obtained. For instance, as for parity, it may be explained that majority of the pregnant women consider induced abortion after they get a baby and that undamaged embryonic specimens from nullipara are generally more difficult to obtain than those from multipara. However, it may be concluded that our materials generally represent the total early intrauterine population.

Our collection shows clearly that a certain stage (Carnegie stages 14–16) of human embryonic specimens is relatively easy to get but those at other stages, especially the earlier ones, are extremely difficult to obtain. It is just because the women at such early phase of gestation may not consult obstetrician for abortion suspecting the possibility of pregnancy. The exceptional cases may be obtained at hysterectomy. It should be stressed again here that the acquisition of embryonic materials depend mainly by chance by the method of dilatation and curettage. Even by most skillful obstetricians the embryos are somewhat damaged in majority of the cases. It is especially true in cases of the older embryos and early fetuses which are difficult to pass the minimumly dilated cervical canal. Even if a patient is suspected for having a malformed embryo and carefully operated, the chance to get a good specimen suitable for morphological study is extremely low. Therefore, case study is difficult. Epidemiological study may not be affected if the chance of damage is equal.

Changes of trends for contraception or fertility control in Japan should be considered for continuation of the study. The cases of induced abortion, especially in the fetal stage, are sharply decreasing. As for methods for interruption of pregnancy at the second and third months, the vacuume suction method is becoming more popular in Japan as in other countries. This simple method unfortunately damages the embryos completely. Intraamniotic injection of saline may be revived in Japan but it generally results in the macerated fetuses unsuitable for morphological study.

2. LIMITATION ON EXAMINATION

First of all, it is to be noted that most of our materials are fixed with Bouin's fluid. It is an extremely good fixative for morphological studies of small embryonic specimens. Moreover, we found that by transferring the specimens into 10% formalin after 24 hours' fixation with Bouin, they can be preserved for several months at obstetricians' clinics and still good for the usual H.E. stained histology. This is a very good advantage for us because the cooperative obstetricians are located in various parts of Japan and we cannot so often visit them to receive the specimens. However, the specimens fixed with Bouin are not suitable for many special and histochemical staining and especially difficult for sex chromatin identification as many small chromatin particles appear. Recently we have preliminarily tried to use Lillie's acetic alcohol fixative, which is satisfactory for sex chromatin study.

Next, it is to be mentioned that differentiation of artifacts in such small specimens is not easy. The mechanical and pathophysiological damages *in utero* during the operation, mechanical injuries after the operation and physical traumas during the fixation, all cause the troublesome problems. Even histological examination may not give the final clue in some cases. Examples were already described such as nuchal blebs and crater-like rupture of the brain. It should be recognized that even a specimen from hysterectomy has an artifact or damage during the course of operation. Post-mortem changes furnish more difficulties in identifying the specific type of malformations in localized regions. The best way may leave such cases as dead *in utero,* unsuitable for local examination, as the experimental teratologists usually prefer. Thorough examination of internal organs is also practically the problem. Quick screening under stereomicroscope and slow and patient stereographic examination of histological specimens have both advantages and disadvantages in some way or other. Skillful associates in our group have been engaged in microdissection to detect internal anomalies in specimens later than at stage 18.

We have concentrated our efforts in the morphological studies using the relatively undamaged specimens. However, there are varieties of types of congenital anomalies in humans and one of the most important categories is cytogenetic anomalies. Several epidemiological studies in induced or spontaneous abortuses have been reported not describing the morphological states in most cases. The large scaled studies to connect morphology with cytogenetics in the embryonic studies are obviously requested.

3. LIMITATION OF HISTORY TAKING

It is naturally very difficult to get the data on mother's history with uniform preciseness and details from several hundred collaborative obstetricians. Moreover, most of them are at their private clinics. This has some advantage because they can keep the trust in patients resulting in good record in special cases. However, they are usually busy. Therefore, the history taking on genetic items is unsuitable and unreliable for overall screening (not for case study), and we have abandoned the attempt to get many items on genetic history. It is also difficult in Japan to get the good reliable criteria on socioeconimical status by just asking the parents. Obtaining the coital date may also be a troublesome items for obstetricians. However, gradually we are getting specimens arising from a single fruitful coitus and it is expected to enable us to evaluate rhythm method with respect to efficacy and safety of the progeny as its unsuccessful outcome.

For the purpose of monitoring on the potential teratogenic agents, the use of newborns and spontaneous abortuses have been tried by some investigators. Prenatal monitoring

Table 15 Congenital anomalies monitoring.*

		Induced abortus	Spontaneous abortus	Newborn
Population		overall intrauterine legally restricted demand for abortion	a part of intrauterine habitual	hospital or birth certificate
Material	*collection*	difficult	relatively easy for sac but not embryo	easy
	damage	often	most easily damaged	undamaged
Examination	*region*	external and internal	often external	mostly external, if alive
	difficulty	less easy for smallness	least easy for smallness and postmortem change	easy for largeness
Anomalies	*criteria*	fairly easy (development in progress)	difficult (sometimes no embryo found)	easy for external
	frequency	highter	highest	low
	type	limited	very limited	various including functional
History	*taking*	relatively difficult less detailed	fairly easy detailed	easy, biased by anomailes, fairly detailed
	memory	less biased	less biased	easily biased
Cooperation	*doctor*	not easy (confidentiality)	easy	moderate
	patient	less easy	easiest	easy
Monitoring	*speed*	earlier entry	earlier entry	late entry
	completeness	moderate	low	high
Related reporting system		a few	almost none	many (birth record, certificate)

* From TANIMURA, T.: The use of induced abortuses for monitoring. In: Shepard, T. H. et al. (eds.) Methods for Detection of Environmental Agents that Produce Congenital Defects. pp. 197–201, North-Holland, Amsterdam, 1975.

with fetal wastage was discussed by SHEPARD et al. [182], NELSON et al. [183] and MILLER and POLAND [184]. Advantages and disadvantages of induced abortus monitoring are summarized in Table 15. It may be concluded at present that all three methods should be attempted in order to compensate deficiencies each other.

For further scopes of the systematic studies with early prenatal human specimens, special efforts should be done for obtaining the very early human embryos, better history taking and use of partially damaged embryos. As for the last items, they can be utilized for studies of special types of malformation such as limb defects if such regions exist. They may facilitate the monitoring on such defects.

Due to the advance in technology, use of fresh (unfixed) and frozen specimens has been extensively widened. Some biochemical parameters such as enzymes patterns may be utilized for monitoring for not only teratogens but also mutagens. Electromicroscopic studies are also to be greatly encouraged.

Since the specimens of human early prenatal stage are still precious materials, and many laboratories of embryology may have kept some cases, the author would like to propose international registry of undamaged specimens which can furnish the mutual comparison of stored specimens on the same criteria and be utilized by every scientist in the world who concerns normal and abnormal development. Special attention should be made to abnormal embryos and early embryos before stage 10. Description of stage, crown-rump length, condition in preservation, state of abnormalities and history should be included and photographs, gross and histological, should be provided. When the author examined the Carnegie Collection now transferred into Davis Campus, University of California, U.S.A., it is the author's regret that color of many histological slides is fading despite the careful efforts for preservation. It is also hoped that monkey embryonic specimens should be included. The value of non-human primates has been discussed as a test animal for detection of human teratogenic agents, and it is essential to have the good comparative knowledge on developmental progress in both man and monkey to evaluate and extrapolate the monkey experiments.

Recently, the legistrative threat to research on human congenital defects by restricting the studies on live human embryonic and fetal materials was called for attention in the United States [185]. On the other hand, many countries including many States in U.S.A. have liberated the induced abortion. Most of the aborted materials are lost without contribution to the individual and the society. It is of course self-evident that any research using the human materials even at the earliest phase of life should be performed under the strictest ethical consideration. The ethical review of the present studies is summarized in the following : First, there is no physical risk to the patients directly related to the project, because only dead embryonic and fetal specimens obtained from the patients after routine treatments which are performed by the collaborative obstetricians independently from the research project. The project does not alter the clinical descision or operative procedures of the collaborative obstetrician. Secondly, the investigators obtain through the collaborative obstetrician the parent's consent of the subjects for its dissection and preservation as a specimens for scientific purposes. Thirdly, the investigators believe that the potential benefits of this activity outweigh any probable psychological risks to the patients. Usually the offering the dead embryonic and fetal specimens for the important medical purpose is considered to satisfy the philanthropic thought of the parents, since otherwise the specimens are cremated. Moreover, the investigators will inform the related obstetricians the result of the dissection of the specimens when abnormal findings are found, and also provide the mothers with the useful data on genetic counseling. From the foregoing data and discussions, it is the author's sincere hope that the epidemiological studies of abnormal development in the early prenatal stage may give more beneficial information on individuals and public in the present and the future through better cooperation of obstetricians and patients as well as understanding of health science authorities.

SUMMARY

Collection of human embryos and early fetuses in Department of Anatomy, Kyoto University has become the world's largest through the fifteen year efforts and by the collaboration of many obstetricians. Characteristics of the present specimens were described and some standards on normal development were established.

The early prenatal population showed remarkably high prevalences of most types of malformations as compared with those found in the perinatal period. Some maternal factors associated with malformations were evaluated. Pathogenesis of a certain types of malformations were also presented.

Finally, advantages and disadvantages of monitoring human teratogens in the early prenatal population were discussed.

ACKNOWLEDGEMENTS

The author expresses his sincere gratitude to Professor emeritus HIDEO NISHIMURA, M.D., former Head of the Third Division, Department of Anatomy, Faculty of Medicine, Kyoto University for the encouragement and guidance of the studies as well as permisssion to cite the works done in the Department. He is also indebted to Drs. M. Yasuda, O. Tanaka, Y. Yasuda, R. Semba, K. Shiota, K. Yamanaka, K. Ezaki, S. Lee and other colleagues of the Department of Anatomy, Kyoto University for their cooperative studies in various areas: Miss C. Uwabe and Miss H. Fukushima for their laboratory help; and Miss R. Chiba, Miss Y. Teraoka and Miss M. Uemura for their help in analysis.

Special thanks to more than 1,000 collaborative obstetricians, present and past, are expressed for their cooperation in supplying the specimens.

This study was in part supported by the Award of Lalor Foundation (to Dr. Tanimura). The major part of the research was supported by Association of Crippled Children, U.S.A., National Institutes of Health (HD 01401), U.S.A., World Health Organization, Population Council, Japanese Ministry of Health, Japanese Ministry of Education, and the Fujiwara Memorial Foundation, Kyoto, Japan (to Dr. Nishimura).

REFERENCES

1. His, W.: Anatomie Menschlicher Embryonen, I-III. Verlag von F.C.W. Vogel, Leipzig, 1880–1885.

2. Keibel, F.: Normentafeln zur Entwicklungsgeschichte der Virbertiere. Verlag von Gustav Fischer, Jena, 1908.

3. Mall, F.P.: On stages in the development of human embryos from 2 to 25 mm long. Anat. Anz. 46; 78, 1914.

4. Streeter, G.L.: Developmental horizons in human embryos. Description of age group XI, 13 to 20 somites, and age group XII, 21 to 29 somites. Carnegie Contr. Embryol. 30; 213, 1942.

5. Streeter, G.L.: Developmental horizons in human embryos. Description of age group XIII, embryos about 4 or 5 millimeters long and age group XIV, period of indentation of the lens vesicle. Carnegie Contr. Embryol. 31; 29, 1945.

6. Streeter, G.L.: Developmental horizons in human embryos. Description of age groups XV, XVI, XVII and XVIII, being the third issue of a survey of the Carnegie collection. Carnegie Contr. Embryol. 32; 133, 1948.

7. Streeter, G.L.: Developmental horizons in human embryos. Description of age groups XIX, XX, XXI, XXII and XXIII, being the fifth issue of a survey of the Carnegie collection. Carnegie Contr. Embryol. 34; 165, 1951.

8. Heuser, C.H. and Corner, G.W.: Developmental horizons in human embryos. Description of age group X, 4 to 12 somites. Carnegie Contr. Embryol. 244; 31, 1957.

9. Hertig, A.T., Rock, J. and Adams, E.C.: A description of 34 human ova within the first 17 days of development. Amer. J. Anat. 98; 435, 1956.

10. O'Rahilly, R.: Developmental Stages in Human Embryos. Part A: Embryos of the First Three Weeks (Stages 1 to 9). Carnegie Institution of Washington, Washington, D.C., 1973.

11. Nishimura, H., Takano, K., Tanimura, T., Yasuda, M. and Uchida, T.: High incidence of several malformations in the early human embryos as compared with infants. Biol. Neonat. 10; 93, 1966.

12. Stratford, B.F.: Abnormalities of early human development. Amer. J. Obstet. Gynec. 107; 1223, 1970.

13. Pearson, A.A., Nishimura, H., Tanimura, T. and Sauter, R.W.: Observations on the development of the external form of the Japanese embryo. Anat. Rec. 160; 489, 1968.

14. Nishimura, H., Takano, K., Tanimura, T. and Yasuda, M.: Normal and abnormal development of human embryos: First report of the analysis of 1,213 intact embryos. Teratology 1; 281, 1968.

15. Nishimura, H., Tanimura, T., Semba, R. and Uwabe, C.: Normal development of early human embryos: Observation of 90 specimens at Carnegie stages 7 to 13. Teratology 10; 1, 1974.

16. Kobyletzki, D. von and Gellen, J.: Zur Vorhersage des embryonalen Entwicklungszustandes beim Menschen. Arch. Gynäk. 209; 293, 1970.

17. Oliver, G. and Pineau, H.: Horizons de Streeter et age embryonnaire. Bulletin de l'Association des Anatomistes 47; 573, 1961.

18. IFFY, L., SHEPARD, T.H., JAKOBOVITS, A., LEMIRE, R.J. and KERNER, P.: The rate of growth in young human embryos of Streeter's horizons XIII to XXIII. Acta Anat. **66**; 178, 1967.

19. JIRÁSEK, J.E.: Development of the Genital System and Male Pseudohermaphroditism. Johns Hopkins Press, Baltimore and London, 1971.

20. AREY, L.B.: Developmental Anatomy, 7th ed. Saunders, Philadelphia and London, 1965.

21. PATTEN, B.M.: Human Embryology, 2nd ed. McGraw-Hill, New York, 1953.

22. WITSCHI, E.: Development of Vertebrates. Saunders, Philadelphia, 1956.

23. TANIMURA, T., KOYAMA, T. and NISHIMURA, H.: Individual variations with respect to organogenesis in early human embryos. Proc. Cong. Anom. Res. Assoc. Jap. **5**; 46, 1965.

24. TANIMURA, T., NELSON, T., HOLLINGSWORTH, R.R. and SHEPARD, T.H.: Weight standards for organs from early human fetuses. Anat. Rec. **171**; 227, 1971.

25. HILL, A.H.: Fetal age assessment by centers of ossification. Amer. J. Phys. Anthropol. **24**; 251, 1939.

26. FLECKER, H.: Time of appearance and fusion of ossification centers as observed by roentgenographic methods. Amer. J. Roentgenol. & Rad. Therapy **47**; 97, 1942.

27. NOBACK, C.R.: Developmental anatomy of human osseous skeleton during embryonic, fetal and circumnatal periods. Anat. Rec. **88**; 91, 1944.

28. NOBACK, C.R. and ROBERTSON, G.G.: Sequences of appearance of ossification centers in human skeleton during the first 5 prenatal months. Amer. J. Anat. **89**; 1, 1951.

29. O'RAHILLY, R. and MEYER, D.B.: Roentgenographic investigation of the human skeleton during early fetal life. Amer. J. Roentgenol. & Rad. Therapy **76**; 455, 1956.

30. NOZAKI, K.: Roentgenographic studies on the appearance of ossification centers of epiphyses of bones in extremities and carpal and tarsal bones in Japanese fetuses and newborns. Igaku Kenkyu **1**; 11, 1927. (in Japanese)

31. SHIMIZU, Y.: Roentgenographic studies on the ossification of fetal skeleton in Japanese. Nippon Fujinkagakkai Zasshi **34**; 1351, 1939. (in Japanese)

32. TANAKA, O. and NISHIMURA, H.: Individual differences in the stage of appearance of several ossification centers in Japanese fetuses. Teratology **6**; 121, 1972.

33. TANIMURA, T. and TANIOKA, Y.: Comparison of embryonic and fetal developments between man and rhesus monkey. In: The Breeding of Simians and their Uses in Developmental Biology. Perkins, F.T. (ed.) International Association of Biological Standardisation, London, 205, 1975.

34. MORIYAMA, Y.: Statistical study on congenital malformations. Sanfujinka no Sekai **16**; 139, 1964. (in Japanese)

35. TSUKAMOTO, S.: Round table discussion on congenital malformations. Sanfujinka no Sekai **8**; 843, 1956. (in Japanese)

36. MITANI, S. and KITAMURA, Y.: Malformations and their classification. Sanfujinka-Chiryo **17**; 265, 1968. (in Japanese)

37. BABA, K., TAKEYA, H., OKADA, T., NAKAMURA, J. and OTSUKA, S.: Twenty-years review of congenital abnormalities born in a hospital in Tokyo. Nichidai Igaku Zasshi **26**; 420, 1967. (in Japanese)

38. NEEL, J.V.: A study of major congenital defects in Japanese infants. Amer. J. Hum. Genet. **10**; 398, 1958.

39. MORIYAMA, Y. and MINAGAWA, S.: Statistical studies on congenital malformations in Japan. Cong. Anom. **14**; 201, 1974. (in Japanese)

40. KNÖRR, K.: Missbildungen und Entwicklungsstörungen nach Blutungen in der Frühschwangerschaft. Geburtsh. u. Frauenheilk. **18**; 414, 1958.

41. SAKAKURA, Y.: Relationship between anomalies and various factors during pregnancy. Proc. Cong. Anom. Res. Assoc. Jap. **6**; 4, 1966.

42. JUNG, H.F. and KLÖCK, K.: Zur Prognose und Therapie der drohenden Frühgeburt und die Ergebnisse nach behandelter Schwangerschaft. Geburtsch. u. Frauenheilk. **27**; 461, 1967.

43. KRAUS, A. and SABBAGH, A.K.: Blutungen in der Frühschwangerschaft. Zbl. Gynäk. **93**; 969, 1971.

44. WALLNER, H., BREITNER, J. and SCHMIDT, M.: Analyse von 480 Geburten nach Blutungen in der Schwangerschaft. Münch. med. Wschr. **113**; 690, 1971.

45. RUMEAU-ROUQUETTE, C., GOUJARD, J. and ETIENNE, C.: Relation entre les métrorrhagies du début de la grossesse et les malformations congénitales. Résultats d'une enquête prospective portant sur 9,525 grossesses. Gynecol. Obstet. **70**; 557, 1971.

46. WALLNER, H.J., WAIDL, E. and WELSCH, H.: Abortus imminens—Therapie und Missbildung-squote. Arch. Gynäk. **214;** 83, 1973.

47. MAU, G. and NETTER, P.: Blutungen in der Frühschwangerschaft: Ein Hinweis auf kindliche Missbildungen? Z. Kinderheilk. **117;** 79, 1974.

48. NAKAJIMA, S., SEKIGUCHI, M. and HIROSAWA, K.: Relationship between ectopic pregnancy and induced abortion. Sanfukinka no Jissai **4;** 413, 1955.

49. WHO Scientific Group: Spontaneous and Induced Abortion. Wld Hlth Org. Techn. Rep. Ser. No. 461, 1970.

50. YASUDA, M. and NISHIMURA, H.: Substandard intrauterine development shown in some of the malformed human embryos. Teratology **7;** A-30, 1973.

51. POLAND, B.J.: Study of developmental anomalies in the spontaneous aborted fetus. Amer. J. Obstet. Gynec. **100;** 501, 1968.

52. ROUX, M.C.: Etude morphologique des embryons humains atteints de trisomie D. C.R. Acad. Sci. Paris **269;** 417, 1969.

53. MIKAMO, K.: Anatomic and chromosomal anomalies in spontaneous abortion. Amer.J. Obstet. Gynec. **106;** 243, 1970.

54. IKEUCHI, T., SASAKI, M., KOHNO, S., HAYATA, I. and FUJIMOTO, S.: Chromosome studies on spontaneous and threatened abortions. Jap. J. Human Genet. **16;** 191, 1972.

55. GEISLER, M., KLINEBRECHT, J. and DEGENHARDT, K.H.: Histologische Analyse von Triploiden Spontaneaborten. Humangenetik **16;** 283, 1973.

56. PAWLOWITZKI, I.H., CENANI, A. and FRISCHBIER, H.J.: Autosomal monosomy (45, XX, C-) in a human embryo with total amelia and further malformations. Clin. Genet. **4;** 193, 1973.

57. HAMERSMA, K.: Anencephalie en Spina Bifida. Drukkerji Romijn, Apeldoorn, 1966.

58. PADGET, D.H.: Neuroschisis and human embryonic maldevelopment: New evidence on anencephaly, spina bifida and diverse mammalian defects. J. Neuropath. Exp. Neurol. **29;** 192, 1970.

59. GARDNER, W.J.: The Dysraphic States from Syringomyelia to Anencephaly. Excerpta Medica, Amsterdam, 1973.

60. PATTEN, B.M.: Embryological stages in the establishing of myeloschisis with spina bifida. Amer. J. Anat. **93;** 365, 1953.

61. LEMIRE, R.J., SHEPARD, T.H. and ALVORD, E.C., Jr.: Caudal myeloschisis (lumbo-sacral spina bifida cystica) in a five millimeter (horizon XIV) human embryo. Anat. Rec. **152;** 9, 1965.

62. DEKABAN, A.S. and BARTELMEZ, G.W.: Complete dysraphism in 14 somite human embryo. A contribution to normal and abnormal morphogenesis. Amer. J. Anat. **115;** 27, 1964.

63. TANIMURA, T.: Complete dysraphism in human embryos. Teratology **8;** 107, 1973.

64. DeMYER, W., ZEMAN, W. and PALMER, C. G.: The face predicts the brain: Diagnostic signi-ficance of median facial anomalies for holoprosencephaly (arhinencephaly). Pediatrics **34;** 256, 1964.

65. LESER: Ein Fall von Cyklopie. Zbl. Prakt. Augenheilk. **35;** 366, 1911.

66. MALL, F. P.: Cyclopia in the human embryo. Carnegie Contr. Embryol. **6;** 5, 1917.

67. POLITZER, G.: Arhinencephalie bei einem menschlichen Embryo von 7 mm gr. L. Z. Anat. Entw. **93;** 188, 1930.

68. MITANI, S. and HASHIZUME, H.: Three cases of cyclopia and a case of cebocephaly. Nihon Ika Daigaku Zasshi **12;** 331, 1941. (in Japanese)

69. LLORCA-RODRIGO, J. P.: El ojo de un embrion ciclope humano de veintidos milimetros (emb. mom.). Arch. Soc. Oftalmol. Hispano-Americana **12;** 184, 1952.

70. ORTS LLORCA, F.: Le cerveau et l'oeil de deux embryons humains cyclopes de 37 et 45 jours. Acta Anat. **23;** 379, 1955.

71. SUZUMURA, M., MINE, M. and KASAMATSU, T.: A case of abortion of cyclopia at the fourth month of pregnancy. Sanfujinka no Sekai **10;** 296, 1958. (in Japanese)

72. ASAMI, I.: Cyclopie in einem 10.4 mm. menschlichen Embryo, mit besonderer Rücksicht auf seine Gesichtsgestaltung. Acta Anat. Nippon. **41;** 176, 1966. (in Japanese)

73. TANIMURA, T. and UWABE, C.: Eighty-one cases of holoprosencephaly in Japanese embryos. Proc. Cong. Anom. Res. Assoc. Jap. **11;** 37, 1971.

74. ROGERS, K. T.: Experimental production of perfect cylopia in the chick by means of LiCl, with a survey of the literature on cyclopia produced experimentally by various means. Dev. Biol. **8;** 129, 1963.

75. Warkany, J.: Congenital Malformation. Notes and Comments. Year Book, Chicago, 1971.

76. Kraus, B. S., Kitamura, H. and Ooe, T.: Malformations associated with cleft lip and palate in human embryos and fetuses. Amer. J. Obstet. Gynec. **86**; 321, 1963.

77. Maurer, H.: Die Entstehung der Lippen-Kieferspalte bei einem Keimling von 22 mm. Z. Anat. Entw. **105**; 359, 1936.

78. Veau, V.: Hasenscharten menschlicher Keimlinge auf der Stufe 21–23 mm. S. St. L. Z. Anat. Entwicklungsgesch. **108**; 459, 1938.

79. Ströer, W. F. H.: Über die Hasenscharte eines menschlichen Embryos von 18 mm. Z. Anat. Entwicklungsgesch. **109**; 339, 1939.

80. Kitasato, Y.: Zur Genese der Missbildungen der menschlichen Embryonen. III. Über die eigentümliche Gesichtsmissbildung (Aprosopie) im Anfangsstadium ihrer Entstehung. Nagasaki Igakukai Zasshi **17**; 1571, 1939. (in Japanese)

81. Töndury, G.: Zum Problem der Gesichtsentwicklung und der Genese der Hasenscharten. Acta Anat. **11**; 303, 1950.

82. Politzer, G.: Zur normalen und abnormen Entwicklung des menschlichen Gesichts. Z. Anat. Entw. **116**; 332, 1952.

83. Kitamura, H. and Kraus, B. S.: Visceral variations and defects associated with cleft lip and palate in human fetuses: A macroscopic description. Cleft Palate J. 99, 1964.

84. Kawarada, M. and Handa, S.: A case of human embryo with cleft lip. Kyushu Journal of Medical Science **15**; 105, 1964.

85. Matsuda, M., Koyama, T. and Tanimura, T.: Harelips found in Japanese early embryos. Jap. J. Human Genet. **11**; 94, 1965. (in Japanese)

86. Iizuka, T.: High incidence of cleft lip and cleft palate in the human embryos and early fetuses. Okajimas Fol. Anat. Jap. **50**; 259, 1973.

87. Kobayashi, Y.: A genetic study on harelip and cleft palate. Jap. J. Human Genet. **3**; 73, 1958. (in Japanese)

88. Tanaka, T.: A clinical, genetic and epidemiologic study on cleft lip and/or cleft palate. Jap. J. Human Genet. **16**; 278, 1972. (in Japanese)

89. Akasaka, Y.: Statistical and cytogenetic study on the cleft lip, alveolus and/or palate. Jap. J. Human Genet. **15**; 35, 1970. (in Japanese)

90. Fogh-Andersen, P.: Inheritance of Harelip and Cleft Palate. Nordisk Forlog. Arnold Busch., Copenhagen, 1942.

91. Fraser, C.R. and Calnan, J.S.: Cleft lip and palate: Seasonal incidence, birth weight, birth rank, sex, site, associated malformations and parental age. A statistical survey. Arch. Dis. Child. **36**; 420, 1961.

92. Iizuka, T.: Stage of the formation of the human upper lip. Okajimas Fol. Anat. Jap. **50**; 307, 1973.

93. Iizuka, T.: Stage of the closure of the human palate. Okajimas Fol. Anat. Jap. **50**; 249, 1973.

94. Fulton, J.T.: Closure of the human palate in embryo. Amer. J. Obstet. Gynec. **74**; 179, 1957.

95. Wood, P.J. and Kraus, B.S.: Prenatal development of the human palate. Some histological observations. Arch. Oral Biol. **7**; 137, 1962.

96. Kitamura, H.: Epithelial remnants and pearls in the secondary palate in the human abortus: A contribution to study of the mechanism of cleft palate formation. Cleft Palate J. **3**; 240, 1966.

97. Kraus, B.S., Kitamura, H. and Latham, R.A.: Atlas of Developmental Anatomy of the Face. Hoeber, New York, 1966.

98. Burdi, A.R. and Faist, K.: Morphogenesis of the palate in normal human embryos with special emphasis on the mechanism involved. Amer. J. Anat. **120**; 149, 1967.

99. Burdi, A.R.: Distribution of midpalatine cysts: a reevaluation of human palatal closure mechanisms. J. Oral Surg. **26**; 41, 1968.

100. Burdi, A.R. and Silvey, R.G.: Sexual differences in closure of the human palatal shelves. Cleft Palate J. **6**; 1, 1969.

101. Hikita, Y.: Incidence of harelip and cleft palate in Nagasaki city. Nagasaki Igakukai Zasshi **28**; 1371, 1953. (in Japanese)

102. Sanui, Y.: Clinical statistics and genetics on the cleft-lip and the cleft-palate. Jap. J. Human Genet. **7**; 194, 1962. (in Japanese)

103. Frederiks, E.: Vascular patterns in normal and cleft primary and secondary palate in human embryos. Brit. J. Plast. Surg. **25**; 207, 1972.

104. YASUDA, M.: Early morphogenesis of preaxial polydactyly in human embryos. Acta Anat. Nippon. **45**; 32, 1970. (in Japanese)

105. YASUDA, M.: Pathogenesis of preaxial polydactyly in human embryos. J. Embryol. Exp. Morph. **33**; 745, 1975.

106. O'RAHILLY, R., GARDNER, E. and GRAY, D.J.: The ectodermal thickening and ridge in the limbs of staged human embryos. J. Embryol. Exp. Morph. **4**; 254, 1956.

107. SWINYARD, C.A. and PINNER, B.: Some morphological considerations of normal and abnormal human limb development. In: Limb Development and Deformity: Problems of Evaluation and Rehabilitation. Swinyard, C.A. (ed.) Charles C Thomas, Springfield, Ill., 1969.

108. YASUDA, Y.: Differentiation of human limb buds in vitro. Anat. Rec. **175**; 561, 1973.

109. YASUDA, M.: Early morphogenesis of cleft hand in human embryos. Acta Anat. Nippon. **46**; 19, 1971. (in Japanese)

110. YASUDA, M.: Early morphogenesis of postaxial polydactyly in human embryos. Proc. Cong. Anom. Res. Assoc. Jap. **11**; 36, 1971.

111. YASUDA, M. and NAKAMURA, H.: Early pathogenesis of polydactyly: Pre- or postaxial tubercle on the hand plate of human embryos at the stage of digital ray formation. Teratology **6**; 125, 1972.

112. ASAMI, I.: Beitrag zur Entwicklung des Kammerseptums im menschlichen Herzen mit besonderer Berücksichtigung der sogenannten Bulbusdrehung. Z. Anat. Entwicklungsgesch. **128**; 1, 1969.

113. KRAMER, T.C.: The partitioning of the truncus and conus and the formation of the membranous portion of the interventricular septum in the human heart. Amer. J. Anat. **71**; 343, 1942.

114. VERNALL, D.G.: The human embryonic heart in the seventh week. Amer. J. Anat. **111**; 17, 1962.

115. O'RAHILLY, R.: The timing and sequence of events in human cardiogenesis. Acta Anat. **79**; 70, 1971.

116. MALL, F.: On the development of the human heart. Amer. J. Anat. **13**; 249, 1912.

117. TAKANO, K., NAKAO, Y., SAKAKIBARA, T., KUROTANI, Y. and NISHIMURA, H.: Incidence of cardiovascular malformations in human embryos. Proc. Cong. Anom. Res. Assoc. Jap. **7**; 38, 1967.

118. SEMBA, R., NAKAO, Y., NISHIWAKI, Y. and NISHIMURA, H.: High prevalence of cardiac malformations in human embryos arising from ectopic pregnancy. Proc. Cong. Anom. Res. Assoc. Jap. **11**; 36, 1971.

119. CHUAQUI, B. J. and BERSCH, W.: The periods of determination of cardiac malformations. Virchows Arch. Abt. A. Path. Anat. **356**; 95, 1972.

120. LEE, S. and TANIMURA, T.: Urogenital anomalies found in Japanese embryos. Proc. Cong. Anom. Res. Assoc. Jap. **7**; 44, 1967.

121. ZONDEK, T.: Notes on the topography of the foetal horseshoe kidney. Brit. J. Urol. **24**; 201, 1952.

122. JOLY, J. S.: Fusion of the kidneys. Proc. Roy. Soc. Med. **33**; 697, 1940.

123. CAMPBELL, M. F.: Urology, 3 volumes. Saunders, Philadelphia, 1963.

124. LEE, S. and TANIMURA, T.: A case of crossed ectopic kidney with fusion in a human embryo. Teratology **6**; 112, 1972.

125. LEE, S.: High incidence of true hermaphroditism in the early human embryos. Biol. Neonate **18**; 418, 1971.

126. WILSON, K. W.: Origin and development of the rete ovaries and the rete testis in the human embryo. Carnegie Contrib. Embryol. **17**; 69, 1926.

127. GILLMAN, J.: The development of the gonads in man, with a consideration of the role of the fetal endocrines and the histogenesis of ovarian tumors. Carnegie Contrib. Embryol. **32**; 133, 1948.

128. OVERZIER, C.: True hermaphroditism. In: Overzier Intersexuality. Academic Press, New York and London, 1963.

129. MERRILL, J. A. and RAMSEY, J. E.: True hermaphroditism. A report of a case and review of the literature. Obstet. Gynec. **22**; 505, 1963.

130. JONES, H. W. and SCOTT, W. W.: Hermaphroditism. Genital Anomalies and Related Endocrine Disorders. Williams & Wilkins, Baltimore, 1958.

131. LEE, S. and TAKANO, K.: Sex ratio in human embryos obtained from induced abortion: Histological examination of the gonad in 1,452 cases. Amer. J. Obstet. Gynec. **108**, 1294, 1970.

132. Sasaki, M., Makino, S., Muramoto, J. I., Ikeuchi, T. and Shimba, H.: A chromosome survey of induced abortuses in a Japanese population. Chromosoma **20**; 267, 1967.

133. Schultze, K. W.: Geschlechtsbestimmungen bei Abortus verschiedener Genese. Zbl. Gynäk. **83**; 56, 1961.

134. Tanimura, T.: Internal anomalies combined with external malformations in human embryos. Teratology **6**; 121, 1972.

135. Shiota, K., Uwabe, C., Tanimura, T. and Nishimura, H.: Nuchal blebs occasionally found in human seven week-embryos. Teratology **8**; 105, 1973.

136. Töndury, G., Schenk, R. and Morger, R.: Menschliche Keimlinge mit Nackenblasen. Biol. Neonate **1**; 68, 1959.

137. Ullrich, O.: Embryo-fetale Hautshwellungen als phänogenetische Gestaltungsfaktoren. Mschr. Kinderheilk. **98**; 416, 1950.

138. Singh, R. P. and Carr, D. H.: The anatomy and histology of XO human embryos and fetuses. Anat. Rec. **155**; 369, 1966.

139. Kitasato, Y.: Zur Genese der Missbildungen der menschlichen Embryonen. II. Supravitales Experiment über den Entstehungsmechanismus der Exencephalie bei menschlichen Embryonen. Nagasaki Igakukai Zasshi **17**; 664, 1939. (in Japanese)

140. Steiner, K.: Über Hautbezirke mit starker Zellvermehrung bei menschlichen Embryonen. Arch. Dermatol. Syphilis **162**; 576, 1931.

141. Knapp, K.,Lenz, W. and Nowack, E.: Multiple congenital abnormalities. Lancet **2**; 725, 1962.

142. Kita, M. and Lenz, W.: Die Thalidomidembryopathie in Japan. Arch. Kinderhilk. **177**; 244, 1968.

143. Warkany, J., Beaudry, P.H. and Hornstein, S.: Attempted abortion with amniopterin (4-amino-pteroylglutamic acid). Amer. J. Dis. Child. **97**; 274, 1959.

144. Emerson, D.J.: Congenital malformation due to attempted abortion with aminopterin. Amer. J. Obstet. Gynec. **84**; 356, 1962.

145. Milunsky, A., Graef, J.W. and Gaynor, M.F.: Methortrexate-induced congenital malformations. J. Pediat. **72**; 790, 1968.

146. Tanimura, T.: Supernumerary nipples in human embryos. Acta Anat. Nippon. **49**; 73, 1974. (in Japanese)

147. Iwai, T.: Relation of polymastia to multiparous birth. Lancet **2**; 818, 1907.

148. Hirasawa, M.: Über akzessorische Brüste. Zbl. Gynäk. **56**; 585, 1932.

149. Sawazaki, S.: Statistical studies on accessory breasts. Tokyo Iji Shinshi No. **2970**; 583, 1936. (in Japanese)

150. Kamei, E.: Genetic studies on human accessory breasts. Nihon Ika Daigaku Zasshi **26**; 151, 1959. (in Japanese)

151. Sakamoto, U.: Axial breast and its development. Tokyo Iji Shinshi No. **2425**; 1362, 1925. (in Japanese)

152. Araumi, K., Murata, T. and Nishimura, N.: Statistical and clinical studies on accessory breasts in Japanese women. Osaka Iji Shinshi **6**; 1551, 1935. (in Japanese)

153. Mori, T.: Studies on accessory breasts in the elementary school boys and girls. Nippon Iji Shinpo No. **409**; 1482, 1930. (in Japanese)

154. Schmidt, Hugo: Über normale Hyperthelie menschlicher Embryonen. Anat. Anz. **11**; 702, 1896.

155. Schmidt, Hugo: Über normale Hyperthelie menschlicher Embryonen und über die erste Anlage der menschlichen Milchdrüsen überhaupt. Morph. Arb. **7**; 157, 1897.

156. Schmidt, Heinrich: Über die Entwicklung der Milchdrüse und die Hyperthelie menschlicher Embryonen. Morph. Arb. **8**; 236, 1898.

157. Berk, F.: Beitrag zur Kenntnis der ersten Anlage der menschlichen Brustdrüse. Julius Abel, Greifswald, 1913.

158. Lustig, H.: Zur Entwicklungsgeschichte der menschlichen Brustdrüse. Arch. f. mikr. Anat. **87**; 38, 1915.

159. Dawson, A.B.: The origin and occurrence of the single umbilical artery in normal and abnormal human fetuses. Anat. Rec. **24**; 321, 1922.

160. Benirschke, K. and Brown, W.H.: A vascular anomaly of the umbilical cord. Obstet. Gynec. **6**; 399, 1955.

161. Tanimura, T.: Effects on macaque embryos of drugs reported or suspected to be teratogenic to humans. Acta Endocrinol. **166** (Suppl.); 293, 1972.

162. LITTLE, W.A.: Umbilical artery aplasia. Obstet. Gynec. **17**; 696, 1961.
163. BENIRSCHKE, K. SULLIVAN, M.M. and MARINPADILLA, M.: Size and number of umbilical vessels. Obstet. Gynec. **24**; 819, 1964.
164. MONIE, I.W.: Genesis of single umbilical artery. Amer. J. Obstet. Gynec. **108**; 400, 1970.
165. TANIMURA, T. and EZAKI, K.: Single umbilical artery found in Japanese embryos. Proc. Cong. Anom. Res. Assoc. Jap. **8**; 27, 1968.
166. EZAKI, K., TANIMURA, T. and FUJIKURA, T.: Genesis of single umbilical artery. Teratology **5**; 105, 1972.
167. SOMA, H., YOSHIDA, K. TATSUOKA, O., NAKAI, S. and OKAMOTO, M.: Relationship between abnormal umbilical vessels and congenital anomalies. Nippon Sanka-Fujinka Gakkai Zasshi **15**; 1050, 1963. (in Japanese)
168. NISHIMURA, K., IWATSUBO, T., HISATOMI, F. and ISHII, A.: Clinical significance of babies with single umbilical artery. Shonika **10**; 1178, 1969. (in Japanese)
169. KIMURA, Y.: A single umbilical artery. Sanka to Fujinka **41**; 211, 1974. (in Japanese)
170. WILLIS, R.A.: The Borderland of Embryology and Pathology. Butterworth, London, 1958.
171. TANIMURA, T. and UWABE, C.: Regression of the tail and variation of the caudal end of the spinal cord in human embryos. Teratology **10**; 100, 1974.
172. KUNITOMO, K.: The development and reduction of the tail and of the caudal end of the spinal cord. Carnegie Contr. Embryol. **8**; 161, 1918.
173. IKEDA, Y.: Beiträge zur normalen und abnormalen Entwicklungsgeschichte des caudalen Abschnittes des Rückenmarks bei menschlichen Embryonen. Z. Anat. Entw. **92**; 380, 1930.
174. POLITZER, G.: Die Ursachen der abwegigen Entwicklung des Schwanzmarkes beim Menschen. Roux' Arch. Entw. -mechan. **145**; 293, 1951.
175. SCHUMACHER, S.: Über die sogenannte Vervielfachung des Medullarrohres (bzw. des Canalis centralis) bei Embryonen. Z. mikrosk.-anat. Forschg. **10**; 35, 1927.
176. TOURNEUX, F. and HERMANN, G.: Sur la persistance de vestiges médullaries coccygiens pendant toute la période foetale chez l'homme et sur le rôle de ces vestiges dans la production des tumeurs sacrococcygiennes congénitales. J. Anat. Physiol. **23**; 498, 1887.
177. LEMIRE, R.J.: Variations in development of the caudal neural tube in human embryos (horizons XIV-XXI). Teratology **2**; 361, 1969.
178. STREETER, G.L.: Factors involved in the formation of the filum terminale. Amer. J. Anat. **25**; 1, 1919.
179. KERNOHAN, J.W.: The ventriculus terminalis: its growth and development. J. Comp. Neurol. **38**; 107, 1924.
180. NAKAGAWA, H.: Über den Schwanz und den Steisshöcker in Japanischen Embryonen. Mit. Med. Gesels. Osaka **42**; 297, 1943. (in Japanese)
181. NISHIMURA, H.: Incidence of malformations in abortions. In: Congenital Malformations. Fraser, F.C. (ed.) Excerpta Medica, Amsterdam, 1970.
182. SHEPARD, T.H., NELSON, T., OAKLEY, G.P. Jr. and LEMIRE, R.J.: Collection of human embryos and fetuses: A centralized laboratory for collection of human embryos and fetuses: Seven years experience: I. Methods. In: Monitoring, Birth Defects and Environment. Hook, E.B., Janerich, D.T. and Porter, I.H. (eds.) Academic Press, New York and London, p. 29, 1971.
183. NELSON, T., OAKLEY, G.P., Jr. and SHEPARD, T.H.: Collection of human embryos and fetuses: A centralized laboratory for collection of human embryos and fetuses: Seven years experience: II. Classification and tabulation of conceptual wastage with observations on type of malformations, sex ratio and chromosome studies. In: Monitoring, Birth Defects and Environment. Hook, E.B., Janerich, D.T. and Porter, I.H. (eds.) Academic Press, New York and London, p. 45, 1971.
184. MILLER, J. R. and POLAND, B. J.: Monitoring of human embryonic and fetal wastage. In: Monitoring, Birth Defects and Environment. Hook, E. B., Janerich, D. T. and Porter, I. H. (eds.) Academic Press, New and London, p. 65, 1971.
185. SHEPARD, T. H., HAUSCHKA, S. and BLANDAU, R.: Legislative threat to research on human congenital defects. Teratology **8**; 243, 1973.

Author index

Subject index